Immunity

This book explores the essence of immunity. After an initial review of hypotheses, models, and theories proposed to explain immune phenomena in humans and mice, it summarizes the results from synchronic organism-level analyses and diachronic analyses tracing phylogeny. These results suggest that immunity is coextensive with life and is equipped with functions similar to the nervous system. Philosophical reflection with reference to Spinoza and Canguilhem suggests immunity is part of the essence of life—and the essence of immunity embraces mental elements with normativity. Approaching the essence of any phenomenon in this way is called "metaphysicalization of science." This book demonstrates the potential of this approach and contributes to a richer understanding of nature.

Key Features

- Reviews the history of immunological theories
- Discusses and integrates science and philosophy
- Provides a biological framework for cognition and self vs. nonself
- Inspired by Auguste Comte's "The Law of Three Stages"

Immunity
From Science to Philosophy

Hidetaka Yakura

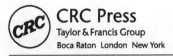

CRC Press
Taylor & Francis Group
Boca Raton London New York

CRC Press is an imprint of the
Taylor & Francis Group, an **Informa** business

Designed cover image: Shutterstock contributor Corona Borealis Studio

First edition published 2025
by CRC Press
2385 NW Executive Center Drive, Suite 320, Boca Raton FL 33431

and by CRC Press
4 Park Square, Milton Park, Abingdon, Oxon, OX14 4RN

CRC Press is an imprint of Taylor & Francis Group, LLC

© 2025 Hidetaka Yakura

ISBN: 978-1-032-77659-0 (hbk)
ISBN: 978-1-032-78214-0 (pbk)
ISBN: 978-1-003-48680-0 (ebk)

DOI: 10.1201/9781003486800

Typeset in Times
by codeMantra

A philosophy of life comprises the philosophy of the organism and the philosophy of mind.[1]

Hans Jonas

I have distinguished two methods of unveiling the secrets of nature: one I called Promethean and one I called Orphic.[2]

Pierre Hadot

I think originality is what one looks for when one looks for books to read. You don't look or at least I don't look for clever solutions to old problems. You look for people who sweep the old problems off the board and set up the pieces in a new way.[3]

Richard Rorty

---

[1] Jonas, H. (2001). *The Phenomenon of Life: Toward a Philosophical Biology.* Northwestern University Press. (Originally published 1966). 1.

[2] Hadot, P. (2006). *The Veil of Isis: An Essay on the History of the Idea of Nature* (M. Chase, Trans.). Harvard University of Press. (Originally published 2004). 155.

[3] McReynolds, P. (2015). *The American Philosopher: Interviews on the Meaning of Life and Truth.* Lexington Books. 34.

Contents

Acknowledgments

This book is a slightly modified version of my book, *From Immunity to Science as Philosophy* (*Men-eki kara Tetugaku toshiteno Kagaku he*), published in Japanese by Misuzu Shobo in March 2023. I have benefited from many people in the process of producing this book. Because this discussion begins with the results in immunology, I imagine that the influence of many researchers with whom I interacted during my research in that field is reflected in invisible ways. After entering the field of philosophy, I have been indebted to the following people: Dr. Marc Daëron (Pasteur Institute), who introduced me to the field of philosophy of medicine; the late Dr. Jean Gayon (Paris 1 Panthéon-Sorbonne University), who accepted me as a Master's student; Dr. Alain Leplège (Paris Cité University) for his generous guidance as my doctoral supervisor; Drs. Geoffrey Butcher (Babraham Institute), Anne Fagot-Largeault (Collège de France), Anne-Marie Moulin (Paris Cité University), and Thomas Pradeu (University of Bordeaux) for their valuable comments on my thesis; Dr. Maël Lemoine (University of Bordeaux) for inviting me as a visiting researcher at the University of Tours; and Drs. Wiep van Bunge (Erasmus University Rotterdam), Henri Atlan (Institute of Advanced Scientific Studies), and Pascale Gillot (University of Tours) for valuable opportunities to exchange views on Spinoza's philosophy. Finally, I thank Dr. Chuck Crumly and Ms. Kara Roberts of CRC Press/Taylor & Francis Group for their thoughtful editorial decision and cooperation.

Author

Hidetaka Yakura, M.D., Ph.D. (Pathology), Ph.D. (Epistemology, History of Science and Technology), is the director of the Institute for Science and Human Existence. He started his career with 7 years of research in immunology at the Dana–Farber Cancer Institute in Boston and the Memorial Sloan Kettering Cancer Center in New York City. After serving as the director of the Department of Immunology and Signal Transduction at the Tokyo Metropolitan Institute for Medical Research, he embarked on philosophical investigations of immunity in Paris in 2007, receiving his Ph.D. from Sorbonne University Paris Cité (presently, Paris Cité University) in 2016. He is currently exploring new perspectives on nature, life, and human existence.

Introduction

Is there anything more daring, anything newer than to announce [...] to biologists that life will only be understood through thought?[1]

Henri Bergson

As my research career as a scientist in the field of immunology came to an end, I felt a great sense of inadequacy. I realized that while I had worked in the field for many years, the essence of immunity and, more importantly, the nature of science itself had eluded me. I concluded that to overcome this sense of inadequacy, I would need time and inner space to think freely, unencumbered by deadlines or other concerns, and I chose to live in France. During what I call my "holistic life," which began in the fall of 2007, I have deepened my thoughts through nine years of graduate studies and autodidactic pursuits in history and philosophy of science in Paris. It is said that science questions nature to find consensual answers. In contrast, philosophy is a paradoxical activity in that while it seeks truth, it does not always guarantee an answer leading to consensus. In other words, while science progresses by reaching a consensus on each research question, philosophy is an eternally open search. During my years as a scientist and throughout my contemplative life in France, my thoughts on the phenomenon of immunity gradually matured, and this book analyzes and reconstructs them in a way that has never been done before.

Specifically, it is based on a process of the "metaphysicalization of science" (MOS), which looks beyond the facts revealed by science about the phenomenon of immunity to arrive at a new level of knowledge (Yakura, 2013, 2020, 2022, 2023). This approach is inspired by the Law of Three Stages proposed by Auguste Comte (1798–1857), the founder of sociology and advocate of positivism. The Law of Three Stages, which Comte identified by reviewing the history of humankind, refers to the three stages of the human spirit's development. The first is the theological stage, a spiritual world in which all natural phenomena are explained by imagination and supernatural activity. Next is the metaphysical stage, in which abstract concepts of human thought replace supernatural elements in explaining natural and social phenomena. Last is the empirical and scientific stage, considered the highest state the human mind can reach. There, metaphysical knowledge obtained through reflection and intuition is rejected, and laws are identified through observation and experimentation (Comte, 1893). When I first learned of Comte's Law in 2008, soon after having moved from science to philosophy, I felt that the denial of metaphysics and theology had robbed our thinking of its richness and depth, for a new world could be opened up by reexamining nature from theological or metaphysical perspectives. This recognition became the initial experience that led to the conception of the "theologico-metaphysicalization of science" (TMOS), or MOS for short.

Later, through observing society and politics, I came to believe that the MOS, which I had conceived only for science, could be valid for many specialties beyond science. I theorized the process of metaphysicalization in three steps. The first step, called "scientific abstraction," is to gather as many scientific results as possible on the subject of one's research and then extract the essential elements common to them. In the second step, called "philosophical reflection," a wide range of knowledge is mobilized from philosophy, history, and theology, among other disciplines. Guided by logic and reason, one then reflects, searching for concepts corresponding to the extracted content and thereby attempting to approach its essence. This process presumes that the content includes aspects that cannot be discovered through science alone and whose discovery will enrich our understanding of nature. I believe that examining both the surface and the depth produces a more profound understanding, not only in the realm of science but also of everyday events. Therefore, in the third "dissemination" step, the importance of such attempts and the specific results revealed from them will be communicated not only to scientists but also to the public at large, for example, by holding talk sessions and conferences or publishing books such as this one.

Modern science seems to distance itself from philosophy. In contrast, there is a pronounced effort in philosophy to avoid the errors of the past by adopting a more scientific approach. Since many past errors arose from a priori methods, much of philosophy seems to be now oriented toward science's a posteriori thought. Some scholars conceive of a philosophy directly related to science and even useful to it. The trend of subordinating philosophy to science seems uninteresting, however, especially to those such as myself who entered philosophy from science and do not want to see philosophy's scope narrowed. That trend not only diminishes philosophy's value but also seems to erase aspects of its approach that address what science cannot know. In terms of Comte's Law, the MOS could be described as the fourth stage in the development of the human spirit. This idea is based on the recognition that as long as we remain in Comte's third stage (i.e., scientific thinking to the exclusion of philosophical thoughts), we will likely create many social problems and impoverish our inner world. I believe that by entering a new fourth stage, we will be able to advance to a deeper level of awareness by mobilizing philosophical thinking in addition to scientific thinking.

This book is the first serious attempt to utilize this recognition to metaphysicalize science. It is not an attempt to settle the question, "What is immunity?" Instead, it presents a dynamic viewpoint that must continually evolve, thereby shaking up our perception of immunity and hopefully providing an opportunity for contemplation about the field of science. Here, I briefly introduce the book's contents.

In Chapter 1, I present a comprehensive and integrated overview of how immunity has been viewed throughout human history. Specifically, I review the theories and hypotheses proposed between the end of the 19th century, when modern immunology was born, and the present, reinterpreting the entire explanatory efforts. In this process, I uncover the interaction between science and philosophy and clues to immunity's essence.

In Chapter 2, I consider an unavoidable part of immunology: the distinction between self and nonself and the concomitant danger of the immune system attacking the self. That danger was recognized at the beginning of the 20th century when the first theory of immunity was proposed, and it was seen as something to be eliminated. Subsequent research has revealed that through a mechanism governed by chance, the immune system prepares itself for reactivity to all elements in the external world and even to all substances in the universe. Consequently, the immune system may attack some of its own components. In cases of severe autoreactivity, a condition known as autoimmune disease arises. Once reactivity to the self was found under physiological conditions, however, it was proposed that autoimmunity is essential to the regulation of biological functions. It has also been shown that while nonself is eliminated in other cases, paternal genes do not cause fetuses to be rejected by their mothers, and microorganisms, including bacteria, coexist in many living organisms. Such phenomena are not necessarily consistent with the theory of immunity, which is based on identifying and eliminating nonself components. Is symbiosis a phenomenon that deviates from the immune mechanism, or can it be explained within the immune mechanism? Microbial symbiosis is so widely observed in nature that it is the rule rather than the exception. This phenomenon raises both biological and philosophical questions about how to define organisms. How to think about symbiosis is a question that also forces us to examine our view of nature. Throughout this part of the book, I deepen my thoughts on these issues.

In Chapter 3, I present a synchronic analysis of immunity at the organism level. In the history of immunology, the significance of immunity has been elucidated mainly by analyzing the immune system of mammals such as humans and mice at the organism level. The result has been to blur boundaries, both between the immune system's subsystems and between the immune system and the nervous, endocrine, and metabolic systems (among others). Until recently, immunity was understood to comprise two distinct arms: acquired immunity, which was characterized by specificity and memory, and innate immunity, which was thought to lack both of those characteristics. However, various discoveries have cast doubt on this classical classification, and the boundary between the two is becoming fuzzy. Furthermore, it is now clear that innate immunity is essential to the operation of acquired immunity, and the two are deeply intertwined. Additionally, the immune system is more closely interconnected with the nervous, endocrine, and metabolic systems than previously thought, and distinguishing them is becoming increasingly difficult. In other words, when the immune system is viewed at the organism level, its contours become blurred, and immunity reappears in a new guise, as a function carried out by the entire organism.

In Chapter 4, I expand this view to the entire living world and examine the mechanism of immunity from a diachronic perspective that traces the phylogenetic tree. Results have shown that despite significant differences in their structural formation, nearly all organisms have an immunity function, and by comparing the immune systems of different species, it is possible to determine the minimum functional components that are common to them all. Four common components have already been identified in the bacterial immune system: recognition, information processing, appropriate responses to the external and internal worlds, and a memory of these experiences. In addition to being recognized as parts of the immune system, these components closely resemble the basic functional elements of the nervous system. In this book, I use the term "cognition" to denote the set of these four components. However, it is important to note that the structures responsible for cognitive function in these two systems are naturally very different. Along with the classical view of immunity as a defense system, I move away from it and rethink immunity from the perspective of a cognitive apparatus responsible for recognition and memory.

In Chapter 5, I reflect on the meaning and possibilities inherent in the function of immunity as revealed by scientific analysis. For this, I use the MOS method (Yakura, 2013, 2020, 2022, 2023). Immunity, which is exclusive to living organisms and helps preserve life by confronting the internal and external environments, reminds me of Spinoza's concept of *conatus*: the effort toward self-preservation exercised by all beings. An examination of the relationship between the concept of *conatus* in Spinoza's philosophy and the context of immunity reveals that immunity corresponds to "appetite" (*appetitus*), a subconcept of *conatus*, the basic activity related to the body and mind of organisms. Furthermore, it becomes apparent that the polarity between good and bad in Spinoza's *conatus* resembles the biological polarity between normality and pathology that is regulated by the immune system. Therefore, I reflect further on immunity with reference to the philosophy of Georges Canguilhem (1904–1995), who examined the normativity of life, and approach immunity's essence.

This book concludes with Chapter 6, where I review the analysis and articulate the new philosophy of life we should aim for in the future.

NOTE

1 Bergson, H. (2007). *The Creative Mind: An Introduction to Metaphysics.* (M. L. Andison, Trans.). Dover Publications. (Originally published 1934). 216.

REFERENCES

Comte, A. (1893). *The Positive Philosophy of Auguste Comte. Vol. 1.* (H. Martineau, Trans.). Kegan Paul, Trench, Trübner. (Originally published 1830). 1–4.

Yakura, H. (2013). Science in the 21st century, or a new "ethics of knowledge." *Igaku no Ayumi (Journal of Clinical and Experimental Medicine), 244,* 572–576.

Yakura, H. (2020). Immunity in light of Spinoza and Canguilhem. *Philosophies, 5,* 38. doi: 10.3390/philosophies5040038.

Yakura, H. (2022). *Meditative Life of an Immunologist in Paris.* Ishiyaku Publishers. 241–287.

Yakura, H. (2023). *From Immunity to Science as Philosophy.* Misuzu Shobo. 246–252.

1 What Has Immunology Tried to Explain?

> Knowledge continues. [...] but if philosophy is not knowledge, philosophy probably cannot continue. Philosophy always begins. [...] All philosophers said, I begin. [...] (At the beginning) there is a new interpretation of the past tout ensemble.[1]
>
> **Alain Badiou**

In a world filled with living organisms, each organism lives in relationship to many others in an invisible network that extends throughout the natural world. Humans are also members of this network, and we must coexist with bacteria, fungi, and viruses (whose status as living organisms remains undetermined). Some of these may be pathogens that threaten our survival. However, recent studies have shown that while only a few microorganisms pose a threat, many others are integral to other organisms and essential to their survival. The physiology and pathology of many organisms, including humans, are determined by the delicate balance between them and their surrounding environments, and the defense system called immunity is of the utmost importance. This book seeks immunity's essence.

Originally guided by the philosophy of René Descartes (1596–1655), modern scientific endeavors have turned toward analyzing objects by dividing them into simpler parts to make them easier to solve. Descartes also advocated a return from the simple to the complex whole, but the search for the whole currently lacks an effective methodology and fails to yield concrete results. If truths in science are always partial and tentative, a historico-philosophical approach emerges to elucidating truths that are as universal as possible. Albert Einstein (1879–1955) stresses the importance of historical analyses of scientific theories for a deeper understanding of a particular theme. He said the following:

> There is always a certain charm in tracing the evolution of theories in the original papers; often such study offers deeper insights into the subject matter than the systematic presentation of the final result, polished by the words of many contemporaries.
>
> **Einstein (2005)**

I want to begin by reflecting on how immunology addresses some basic questions about immune phenomena—for instance, how the immune system processes diverse microorganisms and how immune responses are initiated and regulated for that purpose—including the hypotheses and theories it has proposed. This reflection should reveal what immunology has and has not understood. It should also uncover many historical facts that lie hidden in the background, inaccessible to those who focus solely on established knowledge. Moreover, by introducing new interpretations of the history of immunology, I hope that new images and questions about immunity will emerge.

1.1 ON THE TERM "IMMUNITY" OR METAPHOR

Before going into the main topic, I briefly review the word "immunity." The word has a very long history and is said to derive from *immunitas*, which in ancient Rome indicated exemption from political obligations or burdens (*munus*). It referred to the exemption of certain persons or groups from responsibilities, tax payments, military service, execution of sentences, and so on, prescribed

DOI: 10.1201/9781003486800-1

by law for all Roman citizens. In other words, it was not initially a biological term but a political and legal term referring to exceptions to the responsibilities and obligations that applied only to certain persons in a community. This meant that legal exemption would be a privilege. Immunity represented a kind of anomalous condition rather than a rule (Cohen, 2009). This status is problematic from the perspective of the law, which, by its very nature, must be applied fairly. Roberto Esposito noted that the word "immunity" focuses more on a difference from the condition of others than on the notion of exemption per se and that the true antonym of *immunitas* is not *munus* but the *communitas* of those who support it. It is noncommunal because those subject to it do not fulfill their obligations as a member of the community. A person who does not fulfill their duties as a member of the community becomes noncommunal, and the exempt person is considered an impediment to social customs and placed outside of society. If we trace the original meaning of the word "immunity," we can see there are inherent issues of rule and exception, and the whole and the part (Esposito, 2011).

It took a long time before *immunitas* came to be used in the sense of immunity in medicine. According to the French medical historian Anne-Marie Moulin, there are records of antecedents in the 17th and 18th centuries (Moulin, 1983b). In 1616, the German alchemist Michael Maier (1568–1622), a counselor to the Holy Roman Emperor Rudolf II (1552–1612), recommended gold, symbolizing eternity, as a remedy, claiming that it could bring about "freedom from corruption" (*a corruptione immunitas*). In this case, however, it is used rather ambiguously, as if the cure with gold could bring eternal freedom from disease or a new kind of life force. In 1775, Gerard van Swieten (1700–1772), a Dutch physician working in Austria, commenting on the writings of his teacher Herman Boerhaave (1668–1738), wrote that it would be necessary to find a method "to obtain in a healthy body the same effect as in those who have once contracted a disease or who, by virtue of their constitution, are not subject to contagion, in a word to obtain immunity to disease" (Moulin, 1983a). This word appears to reflect an ancient Greek episode, which will be described in Section 1.2 of this chapter, and is close to the modern understanding of immunity. However, it would take another century for the medical meaning of immunity to be clearly stated and for it to become widely accepted. In the late 19th century, Émile Littré (1801–1881) added the medical meaning of "exempt from disease" to the word "immunité" in his *Dictionary of the French Language*, which he compiled between 1863 and 1872.

This meaning would be metaphorical since the word "immunity," derived from political and legal terms, is used in the field of medicine. Etymologically, the word "metaphor" comes from the Greek *metaphorá* (*meta*; on, over + *pherein*; to carry), which includes the meaning to carry something beyond to another place. Metaphor functions as a medium for understanding certain things, linking the unknown with the known to make the unfamiliar familiar. Because they are sometimes ambiguous, they can carry expansive poetic meanings and even be associated with creativity, which is important when observing and thinking about this world. Applying the political definition of exemption from duty used in ancient Rome to the field of medicine, we can see that getting sick is a rule (one might even say an inevitability), and immunity is a privileged mechanism to be exempt from it.

Historically, however, metaphors were seen as something to be avoided in strict discussion. For example, Aristotle (384–322 BC) recognized metaphor as a kind of decoration and a powerful tool for effective communication but believed that words should be used as they mean in rigorous argument (Aristotle, 1909). John Locke (1632–1704) also held that rhetorical language should be avoided since it would allow false ideas to enter the mind, influence emotions, and ultimately lead to incorrect judgments (Locke, 1825). Metaphors appear to have been avoided in the realm of science. However, a closer look at biomedical domains, for example, reveals that not only are they used abundantly, but some of them have become technical terms. Thomas Kuhn (1922–1996) saw metaphors as playing an important role in linking the abstract language of science with the everyday world (Kuhn, 1993). We will see that metaphors are also helpful in understanding and explaining the immune phenomena we will be examining. If we fully understand the rich functions of metaphors, we may be able to express the hidden meaning of immunity through the power of metaphors.

Taking the form "A is B" could lead to defining A. It is sometimes said that poetry is close to philosophy. To come up with such a form requires a penetrating philosophical perspective that approaches the essence of A. If a B is discovered that no one has thought of before, it could open up a new world that would change our perception of A. We may have to invent metaphors to reach the essence, even against the criticism that it is poetic (i.e., not scientific). Because if we can do this in the field of immunology, we may be able to get to the essence of immunity.

1.2 WHAT HAD BEEN REVEALED BEFORE MODERN IMMUNOLOGY WAS ESTABLISHED

Phenomena related to immunity were already observed at least as far back as the ancient Greeks. It is the phenomenon of being able to protect oneself from infectious diseases by becoming infected. In Chapter 7 of Book II of his *History of the Peloponnesian War* (Thucydides, 1914b), Thucydides (c. 460–400 BC) records in detail the condition of plague during the Peloponnesian War (431–404 BC). This war broke out between the Delian League, led by Athens, and the Peloponnesian League, led by Sparta, resulting in many casualties. Thucydides, who was present and infected himself, wrote that he wanted to try to describe the symptoms, leaving the search for the cause to others. The first casualties occurred after the Peloponnesian League took Attica, when an Athenian soldier died. The symptoms were like nothing doctors had ever seen before, and not only were they unable to help him, but because they had many patients to care for, they also fell victim to it. This situation overlaps with what we experienced especially in the early days of the pandemic of novel coronavirus disease (COVID-19) caused by severe acute respiratory syndrome coronavirus 2 (SARS-CoV-2). It was initially suspected that the Peloponnesian League had poisoned the wells. However, this suspicion could not explain why the town was flooded with victims. In addition, while it was expected that all would suffer and then die, Thucydides describes it this way:

> Yet it was with those who had recovered from the disease that the sick and the dying found most compassion. These knew what it was from experience, and had now no fear for themselves; for the same man was never attacked twice—never at least fatally. And such persons not only received the congratulations of others, but themselves also, in the elation of the moment, half entertained the vain hope that they were for the future safe from any disease whatsoever.

Thucydides (1914a)

This testimony indicates that our bodies remember previous encounters with pathogens and that some people erroneously believed that this experience was effective against all pathogens. In other words, the history of immunity began with a statement suggesting that immunity has a phenomenon of memory and specificity to pathogens. In this regard, the record by Thucydides some 2,500 years ago is extremely important. In humans and other highly evolved animals, immunological memory was considered a characteristic function of acquired immunity performed by B and T cells. However, it has recently become apparent that it is also found in innate immunity, for which other immune cells are responsible. Furthermore, mounting evidence indicates that an immunological memory exists in almost all organisms, including animals, plants, and bacteria that do not have B or T cells, although its structure and mechanisms differ greatly (Rimer et al., 2014; Gourbal et al., 2018; Lau and Sun, 2018). This issue will be discussed in detail in Chapters 3 and 4. These facts mean that any theory or hypothesis explaining immunity must be able to account for immunological memory and specificity.

At the turn of the 18th century, the English physician and scientist Edward Jenner (1749–1823) reasoned, based on his observation that milkmaids often did not contract smallpox, that this might be due to their contact with the pus of cowpox, a cow disease similar to smallpox. To test the validity of his hypothesis, based on his outstanding observations and reasoning, he inoculated the gardener's eight-year-old son, James Phipps, with the pus of a milkmaid, Sarah Nelms, who had been diagnosed with cowpox on May 14, 1796. However, no serious symptoms developed, so he inoculated James with smallpox 6 weeks later to test the preventive effect of an initial inoculation and found no infectious symptoms. This is believed to be the first case of vaccination. Jenner first sent his paper to the Royal Society of London. However, they refused to publish it in their journal, *Philosophical Transactions*. So, 2 years later, he published Phipps and other cases in a book entitled *An Inquiry into the Causes and Effects of the Variolae Vaccinae* (Jenner, 1798). The success of Jenner's smallpox vaccination may have influenced Émile Littré to add the biological meaning of "exempt from disease" to the word "immunité" in the late 19th century.

Some view this event as the birth of immunology and Jenner as the "father of immunology." However, similar prophylactic methods had been used before Jenner, and others attempted to popularize them. Mary Wortley Montagu (1689–1762) stayed in Constantinople, where her husband, a diplomat, was posted, for 18 months from 1717. During her stay in the Ottoman Empire, she became aware of the inoculation against smallpox practiced there, in which pus from a mildly infected smallpox patient was inoculated into the skin of a non-infected person by scarring it. She called this process "engrafting." She then introduced this method in England and worked to spread its use upon her return. It is said that she lost her beauty and her brother to smallpox before leaving for Turkey. So it is not hard to imagine that this experience may have contributed to her interest in this disease. Not only did she apply this method to her son in Turkey, but she also gave smallpox to her daughter when smallpox struck London in 1721.

Louis Pasteur (1822–1895) came on the scene almost a century after Jenner. He proposed the mechanism of fermentation and the germ theory of disease. Furthermore, he developed a method of sterilization by heating to 100 degrees Celsius or less, named "pasteurization," and a method of prevention against chicken cholera, anthrax, and rabies using attenuated pathogens. Pasteur gave this prophylaxis the name "vaccination" (from the Latin *vacca*, meaning cow) as a sign of his respect for the immense service rendered by Jenner, "one of England's greatest men" (Vallery-Radot, 1919). In light of these accomplishments, Niels Jerne (1911–1994; Nobel Prize in Physiology or Medicine 1984) named Pasteur the "father of immunology" (Jerne, 1974). However, at this point, the mechanisms of immunization and vaccination in the modern sense had not been clearly explained. Therefore, immunology as a discipline that studies and explains the mechanisms of biological phenomena was still in its infancy. It was not until the 1880s that discussions on the actual mechanisms began. If we consider this period as the beginning of modern immunology, we can see that it is a relatively new discipline that developed rapidly over only a hundred or so years after its overwhelmingly long prehistory. In the rest of Chapter 1, I will focus on the most recent century and trace the progress toward understanding immune phenomena.

1.3 BIRTH OF MODERN IMMUNOLOGY

What exactly happened at the end of the 19th century? The history of immunology provides several examples of multiple theories and models being proposed for important issues. Many people are interested in these issues and immediately turn to examine them. Consequently, one theory may be correct and the other incorrect. It is also possible that each of the opposing claims is partially correct. The first theoretical conflict in immunology resulted in the latter. The point of contention was what constitutes immunity and how it protects the organism from pathogen attack.

1.3.1 CONFLICT BETWEEN THE CELLULAR AND HUMORAL THEORIES

Two schools of thought arose regarding the actors responsible for immunity. One, called the cellular theory, was advocated by Élie Metchnikoff (1845–1916; Nobel Prize in Physiology or Medicine 1908), a French scientist from Russia (present-day Ukraine, near Kharkiv) who worked at the Pasteur Institute in Paris. He identified the main players in the immune system as phagocytes, derived from the Greek word *phagein*, meaning to eat. The other was the humoral theory, which states that factors named "antibodies" in the blood are responsible for infection defense, proposed by German scientists Paul Ehrlich (1854–1915; Nobel Prize in Physiology or Medicine 1908 with Metchnikoff) and Emil von Behring (1854–1917; First Nobel Prize in Physiology or Medicine 1901). Von Behring's research was supported by Shibasaburō Kitasato (1853–1931), who would have won the Nobel Prize jointly in modern times. It is probably only in the last 40 or so years that the Nobel Prize has come to recognize the contributions of junior collaborators. In the field of immunology, the joint award went to César Milstein (1927–2002; Nobel Prize in Physiology or Medicine 1984) and Georges Köhler (1946–1995; Nobel Prize in Physiology or Medicine 1984), who invented a method for the production of monoclonal antibodies in Milstein's laboratory. In addition, Linda Buck (1947–), who moved from immunology to neuroscience to conduct pioneering research on the olfactory system with Richard Axel (1946–), shared the 2004 Nobel Prize in Physiology or Medicine with Axel. Incidentally, Metchnikoff and Ehrlich were jointly awarded the Nobel Prize in 1908, and it was recognized that both the cellular and humoral theories explained part of the immune phenomena. This conflict between the cellular and humoral theories lasted about 20 years from the end of the 19th century, and some believe that the Franco-Prussian War (1870–1871) was behind it (Silverstein, 1989b). Despite the intense hostility between French and German scientists, scientific discussions and exchanges were fruitful, laying the foundation for immunology.

Let us look a little closer at the research conducted in the two camps. At the end of the 19th century, Metchnikoff conducted an experiment in Messina, Italy, that would change his life. There is a famous episode (Metchnikoff, 1921). According to his wife Olga, one day when the whole family had gone to see the circus, he stayed home alone, observing the life in the mobile cells of a transparent starfish larva under a microscope. When a new thought suddenly flashed across his brain that similar cells might serve in the defense of the organism against intruders, he was so excited. If this hypothesis was correct, then rose thorns introduced into a starfish larva should be surrounded by mobile cells. It is a remarkable imagination. He quickly experimented and the next morning found that his hypothesis was correct. From there, he laid the foundation for his phagocytosis theory, which states that cells with phagocytic activity are also responsible for defense against pathogens (Metchnikoff, 1883). However, he was not the first to observe phagocytosis or to show that mobile cells destroy invading bacteria. His theory was that under certain conditions, phagocytes defend the body by swallowing and destroying harmful invaders through phagocytosis. In other words, the inflammatory process was not a passive, host-damaging phenomenon, as previously thought, but an active, beneficial process that protected the host from microbial invasion. This theory is considered the first example of an explanation of the immune phenomenon of defense against microorganisms based on a scientific theory comprising phagocytes and phagocytosis (Chernyak and Tauber, 1988).

It should be noted that Metchnikoff saw the role of phagocytes not only in pathological phenomena but also in the physiological process of development through which the organism's shape forms. Starting out as a developmental biologist, he believed that competition occurs between cells in an organism during development and that the organism changes its shape through "physiological inflammation" caused by phagocytes recognizing other cells as "foreign," so to speak. In other words, he believed that the developmental process is not a passive phenomenon but a process in which phagocytes are actively involved, thereby maintaining the organism's identity. Since physiology precedes pathology, the original role of phagocytes, which he considered responsible for the function of immunity, was to maintain identity during the developmental process, and their role in defending the organism against microorganisms after birth was to maintain integrity. Inevitably, he imagined that the biological defense involved in maintaining the organism's integrity was merely subordinate to the function of maintaining identity (Tauber, 1992).

In 1890, Emil von Behring and Shibasaburō Kitasato discovered that a substance exists in the blood of animals immunized with diphtheria or tetanus bacteria that can specifically protect other individuals from infection (von Behring and Kitasato, 1890). This observation was the discovery of antibodies. Since this discovery, a controversy arose about whether phagocytes or antibodies were more important for immunity. However, the cellular theory was confronted with serious problems

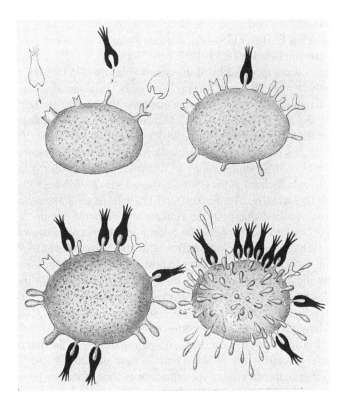

FIGURE 1.1 Ehrlich's side-chain theory. Cells express many types of receptors called "side chains" on the surface (top left). When an antigen binds to one type of corresponding receptor (upper right–lower left), it causes the cell to produce and secrete the same type of receptor (lower right). (From Ehrlich, P. (1900). Croonian lecture. On immunity with special reference to cell life. *Proceedings of the Royal Society of London*, 66: Plate 6.)

such as the nonspecific activity of phagocytes, the difficulty of experiments using cells, and the lack of a quantitative explanation. In contrast, as will be discussed below, research on antibodies occupied a central position in immunological research in the first half of the 20th century, thanks to the convincing picture presented by Ehrlich in 1900 to explain his theory (Figure 1.1), the success of serum therapy by von Behring, and the explanation of immunological phenomena by rigorous chemistry (Tauber, 1992). This research included applying these fundamental discoveries to treat disease and exploring the questions constituting the basis of immunology: how immunological specificity in the antigen–antibody reaction is determined and how antibodies are produced.

1.3.2 Conflict between the Selection and Instruction Theories

1.3.2.1 Early Selection Theories

In the 1900 Croonian Lecture in London, Paul Ehrlich, with remarkable foresight, proposed the first serious theory of antibody production, called the side-chain theory (Ehrlich, 1900). It introduced chemical and quantitative elements into the analysis of biological phenomena. At the same time, he stressed the importance of in vivo dynamics of substances such as toxins. This line of research might be called pharmacodynamics in today's terminology. He did not look at the cell from a morphological perspective but considered its constituents from a purely chemical perspective. He finally concluded that the "protoplasm" in the parlance of the time (including the plasma membrane, cytoplasm, and nucleus) was equipped with atomic groups that could fix certain nutrients vital for cellular life. He named the atomic group expressed on the cell surface a "side chain," and applied this hypothesis to the relationship between toxins and cells. This side chain would be the first conceptualization of the molecule now called the "receptor."

In experiments where tetanus toxin was mixed with homogenates of guinea pig brain material, Ehrlich showed that brain cells could remove the toxin's ability to cause lethal disease. His results suggested that structures must exist in normal brain cells that act as antitoxins and have an affinity for tetanus toxin. He further speculated what happens in the normal immune process as follows. It was that there are side chains (receptors) with diverse specificities on a single cell in the body, and that when an antigen enters the body, it binds to the corresponding side chain and induces the production of the same side chain, releasing part of it into the blood or tissue fluid when its amount becomes excessive (Figure 1.1). This hypothesis, born of his extraordinary imagination, was strongly persuasive partly because of the vividness of the figure he used to illustrate it. Of particular importance here is that Ehrlich postulated that the body's cells normally possess a repertoire of antigen-specific side chains before their exposure to the antigens and made the presence of antibody-like molecules in the blood a prerequisite for his hypothesis. Furthermore, he proposed that the production of antitoxins should be considered analogous to normal metabolic processes. If interpreted as the antigen selecting its corresponding side chain, this theory would be the first selection theory in immunity.

This perspective would be raised and modified half a century later by Niels Jerne in his natural selection theory of antibody formation (Jerne, 1955), which will be discussed in Section 1.4.1, Chapter 1. A little later, the Australian virologist Frank Macfarlane Burnet (1899–1985; Nobel Prize in Physiology or Medicine 1960) adopted this basic framework of Ehrlich's theory to propose the clonal selection theory (Burnet, 1957), which became the paradigm in modern immunology (Section 1.4.2, Chapter 1). The overall structure of the side-chain theory, which emerged from Ehrlich's unparalleled creative speculation, is remarkably accurate in light of current knowledge and has not faded after more than a century.

However, Ehrlich's selection theory was destined to be abandoned and neglected for about half a century. The reason for this was that the number of antibodies detected increased very early after he proposed the side-chain theory, and the corresponding side chains could not be physically accommodated in a single cell. As a result, this cast doubt on the validity of the side-chain theory, and the results of experiments using haptens and carriers by Austrian chemist Karl Landsteiner (1868–1943; Nobel Prize in Physiology or Medicine 1930) dealt a fatal blow to Ehrlich's theory. Haptens are small molecules that cannot induce antibody production alone (they are not immunogenic). However, they can when combined with large immunogenic proteins called carriers. Therefore, the hapten-carrier system is a very powerful experimental system for analyzing the specificity of immune responses. Landsteiner showed that specific antibodies were not only produced against a number of natural proteins but could be induced by combining synthetic haptens, such as picryl chloride and 2,4-dinitrochlorobenzene, with carriers (Landsteiner, 1936). These observations indicated that the immune system could produce antibodies to an almost unlimited number of antigens, not only those present but also those that could be present. Therefore, Ehrlich's theory, which postulated multiple side chains on a single cell, was rendered physically untenable.

1.3.2.2 Rise and Fall of the Instructive Theory

After the side-chain theory collapsed, various theories and models were proposed for the mechanism of antibody production against an almost infinite number of antigens. The most influential of these was the instructive or template theory. In Ehrlich's side-chain theory, the antigen was not directly involved in the side chain or antibody production process, but merely selects and binds to the corresponding side chain physicochemically. In contrast, the basic premise of the instructive theory is that the antigen actively participates in the antibody production process. Several arguments in the vein of the instructive theory had already been recognized since the 1910s, the first reliable one being the direct template theory proposed by Friedrich Breinl (1888–1936) and Felix Haurowitz (1896–1987) (Breinl and Haurowitz, 1930). They examined the amino acid composition of proteins present in serum before and after the immunization of individuals with hemoglobin and found no difference between them. While their analysis may not have been exact, they deduced from their results that the differences between the antibodies produced after immunization and the normal proteins were due to differences in amino acid sequence or three-dimensional structure. According to the theory of Breinl and Haurowitz, the antigen enters the cell and acts as a template at the site of antibody production, directly instructing the amino acid residues to constitute the configuration complementary to the antigen's reaction site. Jerome Alexander and Stuart Mudd, independently proposed a similar theory (Alexander, 1932; Mudd, 1932).

Such an instructive theory was further refined by Linus Pauling (1901–1994; Nobel Prize in Chemistry 1954 and Nobel Peace Prize 1962). He did not take the inductive approach of integrating the extensive and complex published experimental data to explore the antibody production mechanism. Instead, Pauling chose the deductive path of theory building, searching for the simplest conditions for antibody structure based on information about intermolecular and intramolecular forces (Pauling, 1940). He was unconvinced by the direct template theory of Breinl and Haurowitz (Breinl and Haurowitz, 1930), which advocated that the antigen directly modifies the amino acid sequence of the antibody. Instead, he believed there was no difference in the composition of the polypeptide chains of both antibody molecules and normal globulins and that the difference lay in their three-dimensional structure. In other words, he believed that the function of the antigen was to direct the antibody's antigen-binding site to form a complementary three-dimensional structure to it (Figure 1.2). This theory was widely accepted partly due to Pauling's fame as a star in the scientific world but also due to the convincing picture he prepared to explain his theory, like in the case of Ehrlich's side-chain theory (Figure 1.1).

Surprisingly, even in the 1960s, when most immunologists abandoned the instructive theory, there were still those who faithfully supported it. For example, according to Melvin Cohn (1922–2018), a theoretical immunologist who was also involved in the founding of the Salk Institute, the French immunologist Alain Bussard (1917–2010) waited until the end of his life for solid evidence to support the instructive theory to appear (Cohn et al., 2007). Bussard's episode illustrates the extent of the influence of the instructive theory.

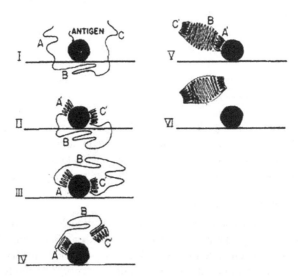

FIGURE 1.2 Pauling's instructive theory. The six stages of antibody production in reaction with antigen (●) are shown. The ends (A and C) (I) of the normal globulin molecule (hand-drawn curve) take stable forms (A' and C') complementary to the antigen (II–IV) and finally constitute the antibody molecule (V–VI). (From Pauling, L. (1940). A theory of the structure and process of formation of antibodies. *Journal of American Chemical Society*, 62: 2645.)

The direct template theory requires the presence of an antigen during the entire period of antibody production, but there was no evidence for this. The enhanced secondary response also cannot be explained by this theory. With this in mind, Macfarlane Burnet proposed the adaptive enzyme theory (Burnet, 1941). According to this theory, when an antigen enters the cell and comes into contact with an enzyme involved in the elimination of waste products, the enzyme adapts similarly to its normal substrates, synthesizing an antibody specific for the initial antigen. Furthermore, Burnet and Frank Fenner (1914–2010), also a virologist, presented a refined indirect template theory (Burnet and Fenner, 1949). The theory postulated that a new self-replicating system regulated by gene is present in the cell which can be caused to multiply by the appropriate stimulus, guaranteeing antibody production in the absence of antigen.

However, these theories failed to explain several crucial immunological phenomena. First, natural antibodies existing before encountering the antigen cannot be explained by theories that assume the antigen is involved in the antibody production process, whether directly or indirectly. Second, they cannot explain immunological memory, where the second and subsequent antigenic stimuli induce a faster and stronger response than the first. Third, they cannot explain the phenomenon of antibody affinity maturation, in which antibodies produced late in the immune response bind to the antigen more effectively than the antibody initially produced. Fourth, it was later shown that each cell produces only one type of antibody in principle, and a theory implying that a single cell produces an unlimited variety of antibodies is simply untenable. The instructive theory, which could not solve these problems, was discarded, and the selection theory prevailed in the 1960s.

In the conflict between the cellular and humoral theories, it was clear that both contained some truth in their claims, but in the controversy between the selection and instructive theories, the latter was utterly wrong. It has been suggested that one reason why Pauling and others who advocated the instructive theory were unable to draw the correct conclusions was that they, despite their biological interests, had a very hierarchical view of science and saw physics and chemistry above biology (Silverstein, 1989c; Moulin, 1991b). This reductionist view of science dictates that all sciences or knowledge can eventually be reduced to physics and chemistry. In this mental framework, the problems specific to other disciplines including biology are often overlooked or neglected. For Pauling, searching for the theory of antibody formation was like an intellectual application of his physicochemical view of proteins to a biological phenomenon, but the problem itself may not necessarily have attracted his genuine interest. In addition, Pauling's attitude was that of a theorist with a deductive mind who tried to interpret biological phenomena in mechanical and simplified terms (Moulin, 1991b).

1.4 THE EMERGENCE OF NEW SELECTION THEORIES

Arthur Silverstein, an American historian of medicine, saw a shift in the perspective of analysis from the physicochemical to the biological during the 1940s and 1950s (Silverstein, 1989a). At that time, there were two competing theories: the direct template theory proposed by Breinl and Haurowitz (1930) and by Pauling (1940) and the indirect template theory by Burnet and Fenner (Burnet, 1941; Burnet and Fenner, 1949). However, the more biologically oriented scientists such as Niels Jerne, David Talmage (1919–2014), Macfarlane Burnet, and Joshua Lederberg (1925–2008; Nobel Prize in Physiology or Medicine 1958) had begun to conceive of a new theory in which the specificity repertoire of antibodies (the totality of antigen specificity possessed by an individual) is prepared in an antigen-independent manner beforehand and the antigen simply selects the corresponding antibody (Jerne, 1955; Burnet, 1957; Talmage, 1957; Burnet, 1959; Lederberg, 1959; Talmage, 1959).

1.4.1 NIELS JERNE'S NATURAL SELECTION THEORY

In 1955, Niels Jerne advocated the theory of natural selection of antibody production in opposition to the instructive theory (Jerne, 1955). His theory was that there are small amounts of antibody molecules, which he called "natural antibodies," in animal blood that react to all antigens to which the animal might react. The premise of this theory is the existence of a mechanism for the a priori production of globulin molecules with numerous specificities. Jerne considered the role of antigens as follows: The role of the antigen is not to serve as a template, as proponents of the instructive theory claim (Breinl and Haurowitz, 1930; Alexander, 1932; Mudd, 1932; Pauling, 1940), or to induce modified enzymes, as Burnet and Fenner suggest (Burnet, 1941; Burnet and Fenner, 1949), but to select and bind to an already existing antibody that has an affinity for it. He assumed that once the antigen–antibody complex is internalized into the cell, the antibody dissociates from the complex and becomes a signal that induces the synthesis of an antibody with the same specificity.

The natural selection theory explained phenomena that the instructive theory could not explain. For example, the presence of antibodies in the absence of antigen was incorporated as a premise of this theory. In addition, immunological memory, where the second and subsequent reactions are faster and stronger than the first, could be explained by the antigen encountering a higher antibody concentration in the second and subsequent reactions. Moreover, the affinity maturation or the change in the properties of antibodies during the immune reaction could be explained if antibodies with high affinity are naturally selected. Furthermore, the absence of autoantibodies could be explained by assuming that autoantibodies are eliminated by binding to the body's own components. Therefore, the natural selection theory appealed to researchers who sought answers to the biological problem of antibody production. However, Jerne's theory conflicts with scientific data in two respects. According to Jerne, it is not the antigen but the antibody that induces antibody production. If this were the case, antibody production would increase when antibodies were administered, but the opposite is observed instead. Additionally, the very idea that proteins function as replication units was beginning to lose credibility as it became clear that it is not the protein but the genetic material that is inducing the replication of the protein (Watson and Crick, 1953).

Furthermore, Jerne received several allegations from different camps after the publication of this theory. One was that his theory merely reaffirmed Ehrlich's side-chain theory, and it was unfair not to mention Ehrlich's name in the paper. According to one of his biographies, *Science as Autobiography: The Troubled Life of Niels Jerne* (Söderqvist, 2003a), written by a Swedish medical historian who is said to have had access to all the documents, while Jerne denied intentionally neglecting to mention Ehrlich's contribution, Ehrlich's name was clearly written in the draft of his 1955 paper. This fact may indicate that Jerne was well aware of the similarities between the two theories: that antibodies with many specificities had already been prepared and that the involvement of the antigen in the antibody production process was limited or none. However, as will be discussed in the next section, there were differences between the two theories. In Jerne's theory, selection by antigen occurs at the level of humoral antibodies, whereas in Ehrlich's theory, selection occurs at the level of receptors on the cell surface. As we will see below, Ehrlich's foresight was superior in this regard.

1.4.2 MACFARLANE BURNET'S CLONAL SELECTION THEORY–PARADIGM IN IMMUNOLOGY

David Talmage, who was studying allergy in the United States, became interested in antibody production and specificity, believing that if an allergy was due to antibodies, then the problem of allergic sensitization could largely be reduced to that of antibody production. He was one of the first to recognize Ehrlich's ideas in Jerne's natural selection theory, but he also recognized that the two theories differed in mechanism (Talmage, 1957). In the case of Ehrlich's theory, selection occurs through interactions between the antigen and the side chains (receptors) on the cell surface. In contrast, Jerne's theory postulates that the antigen selects natural antibodies already present in the circulatory system to form a complex, which is then taken up into the cell, where the antibodies induce further large-scale antibody production. In other words, while they both agree on placing antibodies at the center of their selection theories, Jerne's selection and replication unit was at the level of extracellular natural antibodies, whereas Ehrlich's basic unit was the receptor on the cell surface. Based on experimental data, Talmage supported the idea that the replication unit is the cell (cellular selection theory) for several reasons. First, the antibody's shape was thought to be determined by the information contained in the cell's genetic material. Second, the time required for an immune response to occur in vivo was longer than the time required for the intracellular components to increase. Third, it had been suggested that cell division was still occurring after the antigen disappeared. Based on this reasoning, Talmage concluded that the replication unit of the antibody reaction was not the antibody but the cell that produces it (Talmage, 1957, 1959). The confusion that had persisted for more than half a century since Ehrlich first proposed his theory was finally settled by the reversion of the replication unit from the free antibody back to the cell with the antibody on its surface.

In 1957, Burnet published a paper entitled "A modification of Jerne's theory of antibody production using the concept of clonal selection" (Burnet, 1957). The concept described in this paper explains the occurrence of antibody diversity without the active involvement of antigens and was called the clonal selection hypothesis. In this case, a clone is a cellular clone, meaning all cells that arise from a cell with one specificity. At the beginning of this landmark paper, he discusses his approval or disapproval of three theories circulating at that time: two versions of the instructive theory—the direct template theory (Breinl and Haurowitz, 1930; Pauling, 1940) and the indirect template theory (Burnet and Fenner, 1949)—and the natural selection theory (Jerne, 1955). To briefly summarize them once again, the direct template theory holds that the antigen functions as a specific template for the antibody produced, whereas the indirect template theory postulates a secondary template incorporated in the genetic process of the antibody-producing cell. In contrast, the natural selection theory proposes that the antigen is not directly involved in the antibody production process but selects the one with the corresponding specificity from among the natural antibodies.

By the time Burnet's paper was published, many had come to believe that the direct template theory could not satisfactorily explain immune phenomena. Burnet was struggling with explaining immunological tolerance (the lack of reactivity to one's own components) and antibody production that persists after antigen disappearance. He evaluated Jerne's natural selection theory mainly for two reasons. One was that antibodies with a wide range of specificities existed in the body beforehand as natural antibodies, and the other was the explanation that the lack of autoreactivity was due to the adsorption of autoantibodies on the body's own antigens. However, Burnet saw in Jerne's theory the problem that there was no precedent for explaining how partially denatured antibodies stimulate the production of the same molecules in the cell and that no mechanism had been proposed for this process. Burnet also recognized Talmage's contribution in proposing the theory of natural selection at the cellular level because he thought Talmage's theory of cellular selection could potentially remove the shortcomings of Jerne's theory and rescue it as a theory. Burnet combined Talmage's cellular selection theory with Jerne's natural selection theory, so to speak, to explain the generation of antibody diversity and immune tolerance.

The clonal selection theory was proposed to examine the immune system from a clonal perspective. In modern terms, his arguments can be summarized as the following four postulates:

1. The entire repertoire of immune specificity is generated by some unknown mechanisms and predates encounter with antigens.
2. Each cell has a single type of receptor with a single specificity.
3. The response to an antigen involves the proliferation of cells with the corresponding receptors, the descendants of which include antibody-producing plasma cells and lymphocytes that perform the same function (memory cells).
4. Lymphocytes with receptors for "self" will be removed early in embryonic development (central tolerance).

Burnet's view of the immune system assumes that there is a vast number of cells, each with one type of receptor on the surface, before exposure to an antigen (postulates 1 and 2), a kind of axiom of his theory. Postulate 3 concerns the proliferation and differentiation of clonal cells and immune memory, and postulate 4 concerns immune tolerance. These postulates made it possible to logically explain many immune phenomena, such as generating diverse specificity, immunological memory, and tolerance to self-components. Burnet's theory is reminiscent of Darwin's (1809–1882) theory of evolution by mutation and natural selection (Darwin, 1859). In the modern synthesis of evolution (neo-Darwinism), genetic variation is thought to preexist in a population and individuals with mutations suitable for reproduction and survival are selected for in a changing environment. If genetic variation corresponds to different receptors on the cell surface in Burnet's theory, and environmental factors correspond to antigens that select for receptors, then the clonal selection theory overlaps with neo-Darwinism. This overlap would indicate that Burnet was strongly influenced by evolutionary theory. In addition, while there are differences in the types of receptors on a single cell, as Talmage noted (Talmage, 1957), Burnet's theory was also a rediscovery of Ehrlich's side-chain theory from half a century earlier (Ehrlich, 1900).

There are several conjectures about Burnet's decision to publish his paper in an Australian journal that was not so highly regarded internationally. For example, some European researchers only publish their research results in European journals. In Burnet's case, however, it is believed that he had no such nationalistic or regionalistic view. Instead, he may have felt an urgency to publish his hypothesis as soon as possible because Talmage's paper had already reached him. Moreover, some have speculated that Burnet thought that if his theory was incorrect, it would not stand out (Nossal, 1995). This event recalls what happened when Darwin and Alfred Russel Wallace (1823–1913) attempted to publish their respective theories of evolution (Darwin and Wallace, 1858). In this case, however, both men had the opportunity to speak at a conference that may have been held under pressure on Darwin's part. Immunologist Donald Forsdyke (1938–) believed that Burnet developed his clonal selection theory independent of Talmage, although Forsdyke admits that, unlike in Darwin's case, no formal records survive (Forsdyke, 1995). Another study stated that there is a record of the theory in the archives of the University of Melbourne, written by Burnet himself 6 or 7 weeks before the publication of his paper, but that it is unknown whether this was before he received the Talmage paper (Hodgkin et al., 2007). In any case, the clonal selection theory gradually gained acceptance and became the paradigm of immunology. It signified the triumph of the biological over the physicochemical view of the phenomenon of immunity. However, this theory did not immediately resolve the mechanisms through which a vast repertoire of antibody specificities is created. It took some time until a clear consensus about the clonal selection theory was reached among scientists.

In response to this problem, Joshua Lederberg attempted to construct his own selection theory based on the principles of genetics developed in the field of microbiology. In 1959, 2 years after Burnet's clonal selection theory was published, Lederberg published nine axioms he had written while visiting Burnet at the Walter Eliza Hall Medical Research Institute in Melbourne (Lederberg, 1959). The paper was titled "Genes and antibodies" and subtitled "Do antigens bear instructions for antibody specificity or do they select cell lines that arise by mutation?" It is apparent that Burnet's clonal selection theory was not widely accepted immediately after its publication. Lederberg's nine propositions are listed below:

1. The stereospecific segment of each antibody globulin is determined by a unique sequence of amino acids.
2. The cell making a given antibody has a correspondingly unique sequence of nucleotides in a segment of its chromosomal DNA: its "gene for globulin synthesis."
3. The genic diversity of the precursors of antibody-forming cells arises from a high rate of spontaneous mutation during their lifelong proliferation.
4. This hypermutability consists of the random assembly of the DNA of the globulin gene during certain stages of cellular proliferation.
5. Each cell, as it begins to mature, spontaneously produces small amounts of the antibody corresponding to its own genotype.

6. The immature antibody-forming cell is hypersensitive to an antigen–antibody combination: it will be suppressed if it encounters the homologous antigen at this time.
7. The mature antibody-forming cell is reactive to an antigen–antibody combination: it will be stimulated if it first encounters the homologous antigen at this time. The stimulation comprises the acceleration of protein synthesis and the cytological maturation which mark a "plasma cell."
8. Mature cells proliferate extensively under antigenic stimulation but are genetically stable and therefore generate large clones genotypically preadapted to produce the homologous antibody.
9. These clones tend to persist after the disappearance of the antigen, retaining their capacity to react promptly to its later reintroduction.

Given the paucity of information on the gene-level mechanisms of antibody production and the cellular components involved in antibody production at that time, it is impressive to witness such rigorous and meticulous logic and prescience. According to Lederberg, proposition 5 is central to the selective theory. The first four propositions are special postulates that can be modified, and the last four concern cellular characteristics of antibody formation and may apply to selective and instructive theories. It is important to note that proposition 6 represents a decisive modification to Burnet's original theory. As shown in his fourth postulate, Burnet believed that the lack of reactivity to self (immune tolerance) is induced during the embryonic stage of an organism through the interaction of autoreactive cells with self-antigens in the internal environment and their subsequent inactivation. However, when it soon became evident that lymphocytes are generated during embryonic development and throughout an organism's life, Burnet's tolerance theory became challenging to reconcile. Lederberg proposed changing the immune tolerance timing from the organism's developmental stage to a cell's maturational stage. It is now generally accepted that the differentiation stage of lymphocytes determines their fate after interacting with an antigen: activation vs. inactivation or immunity vs. tolerance.

The instructive and selection theories are opposing ways of explaining the diversity of the antibody repertoire. The instructive theory considers the antigen involved in producing diverse antibodies as a template. In this sense, the form of the antigen is the most important factor in generating antibody diversity. In addition, the distinction between self and nonself is not an issue in the instructive theory. In contrast, in the selection theory, the antibody repertoire is prepared in advance before reacting with the external world, and the antigen has no role in this process. The structure of the antigen only becomes important when it reacts with the antibody to modulate the immune system. It could also be argued that the diversity of antibodies in our bodies is designed to receive everything from the external world, in the sense that the immune system can recognize all possible substances in the universe in a complementary manner. As will be discussed in Section 1.7.1, this view was further developed in Jerne's idiotypic network theory to the point that our immune system has a complete "internal image"—positive but not complementary—of the external world. However, this theory was never proven.

Another thing to add about the instructive and selection theories is that their controversy reminds us of the difference between empiricism and innatism (Moulin, 1991a). According to the instructive theory, antibodies are produced only after encountering the antigen that directs antibody production. This argument is consistent with empiricism, which holds that the human mind is an innate unwritten board (*tabula rasa*) and that knowledge is established through experience. In contrast, innatism asserts that knowledge exists before contact with the external world. This view is long inscribed in human history and can be traced back to Plato (427–347 BC) (Plato, 2009). However, since innatism claims that "part" of the knowledge exists a priori, it does not fully correspond to the theory of selection, which holds that the "whole" of antibody specificity is prepared before contact with antigens.

Therefore, whether the antibodies are free or bound to the cell, the selection theory assumes that there is an a priori mechanism for generating diversity. Burnet believed that this mechanism should be gene-mediated. He emphasized that genetic variation is involved because, given the enormous diversity, our genetic information cannot generate all the diversity as it is. As we have already seen, Lederberg also considered the importance of genetic variation, and immunologists were also discussing the genetic mechanisms that generate antibody diversity. There were two main camps. One was the germline theory and the other was the somatic mutation theory. The former argued that a germline gene encodes each antibody and that the genome contains an almost infinite repertoire of antibody genes that can be used against an almost infinite number of antigens. In contrast, the somatic mutation theory proposed that the genome does not contain enough antibody or immunoglobulin (Ig) genes for every antigen potentially encountered and that mutations in the sequence of antibody variable regions give rise to their enormous specificity.

In 1976, almost 20 years after the clonal selection theory was published, Susumu Tonegawa (1939–; Nobel Prize in Physiology or Medicine 1987) proposed the framework of the genetic mechanism of antibody diversity generation (Hozumi and Tonegawa, 1976). This experiment examined the genetic composition of antibody light chains in cells of early embryos that had not yet differentiated into antibody-producing cells and in cells that had already differentiated into antibody-producing cells. Their results showed that the genes encoding an antibody's variable region (involved in antigen recognition) and constant region were located far apart on the chromosome in early embryos but contiguous in antibody-producing cells. This finding suggested that antibody diversity may be generated by both the number of genes in germ cells and the combination of gene fragments, called "gene rearrangement." The research that began there has revealed the following overall picture.

The antibody specificity that characterizes each clone results from gene rearrangement during the maturation process of the cells destined to produce the antibody (B cells). The variable region of an antibody is encoded by the V (variable), D (diversity), and J (joining) gene fragments in heavy chains and the V and J gene fragments in light chains. In germ and non-lymphoid cells, the gene fragments encoding the variable region are located at distant positions on the chromosome. However, in mature B cells, gene rearrangement places them as contiguous genes, VDJ for the heavy chain gene and VJ for the light chain gene. Therefore, antibody diversity increases markedly after gene rearrangement. For example, if the human heavy chain variable region contains $100 V$ genes, $30 D$ genes, and $6 J$ genes, their rearrangement will create 16,200 different specificities. Since a similar genetic mechanism operates on the V and J genes in the light chain, the diversity increases dramatically with the combination of heavy and light chains. Furthermore, the addition or deletion of nucleotides at the junctions between gene segments of the variable region significantly increases the diversity of antibodies. Therefore, in addition to diversity created through the rearrangement of gene segments, mutations generating junctional diversity also contribute to generating antibody diversity. However, this mechanism is based on the wasteful creation of gene sequences that do not result in protein synthesis due to mutations. Two-thirds of gene rearrangements do not result in the production of antibody proteins, and many B cells created in the bone marrow die.

The generation of diversity is of paramount importance to life. In addition to the genetic mechanism described above, there is a mechanism called "somatic hypermutation." This is a spectacularly creative process in the periphery in which somatic cells (B cells) generate additional diversity and more effective antigen recognition by introducing point mutations, mainly in the variable regions of heavy and light chains. This level of creativity could only exist in immune cells. I am reminded of "bricolage," a metaphor used by François Jacob (1920–2013; Nobel Prize in Physiology or Medicine 1965) to explain evolution. It refers to weaving together what already exists in a given situation, not creation from nothing (*creatio ex nihilo*), and is not goal-directed (Jacob, 1977). What is created is left to chance since no one knows what will be produced. The genetic mechanism of generating diversity in the immune system is full of the creative power of life.

When the process of generating diversity in the immune system is examined from an economic perspective, it is easy to see that many costs are involved since most antibodies in the immune system's repertoire may never be used in the organism's lifetime. This recognition provokes questions such as why our bodies produce antibodies that are never used or whether they may have unknown physiological roles if one dares to consider them from a teleological perspective, which seems to be avoided in modern science. If we consider the diversity of antibodies as an abundant reserve to respond to any invader or unexpected event, this mechanism would be a hallmark of the immune system's flexibility. Therefore, diversity in response to a nearly infinite number of molecules would inevitably also encompass reactivity to self. Even Burnet realized that autoimmunity was an inevitable consequence of the process of clonal propagation of genetic mutations (Burnet, 1957). The immune system had to weigh the cost of autoimmunity against inadequate protection against pathogens. Indeed, would an organism have chosen a perfect defense strategy even at the risk of autoimmunity during evolution?

A review of the history of immunological theory shows that Ehrlich's theory of selection (Ehrlich, 1900) went through the instructive theories of Breinl and Haurowitz (1930) and Pauling (1940) and then back to the selection theories of Jerne (1955) and Burnet (1957). Furthermore, the site of reaction between the antigen and antibody was the cell surface in the side-chain theory (Ehrlich, 1900), the free antibody in Jerne's natural selection theory (Jerne, 1955), and then the cell surface again in the clonal selection theory (Burnet, 1957; Talmage, 1957). The first theory is resurrected in a more refined form in both transitions. The path to the current theory is a repetition of the paradigm shift seen several times in the history of immunology. Burnet's clonal selection theory was initially received with skepticism, but at the Cold Spring Harbor Symposium held 10 years later, it was accepted as the paradigm of immunology (Burnet, 1967) because it better explained the fundamental problems that immunology faced. The fundamental questions were, for example, how antibodies with a wide variety of specificities are produced, how B cell activation leads to antibody production and memory formation, and by what mechanism autoimmunity does not occur in most cases. Subsequent studies have shown that similar principles hold true for T cells, further solidifying the foundations of this theory.

The issues that Burnet considered important included self-recognition and immune tolerance (Burnet, 1961, 1969), and immunology came to be described as the "science of self–nonself discrimination" (Klein, 1982). However, as research results accumulated, it became clear that Burnet's clonal selection theory did not explain all immunological phenomena. These were autoimmunity that should not occur and symbiosis with fetuses and microorganisms that would normally have to be rejected because they carry nonself genes. These issues will be discussed in Sections 2.2 and 2.3, Chapter 2.

1.5 HOW WERE THE KEY COMPONENTS RESPONSIBLE FOR IMMUNITY DISCOVERED?

We have charted the development of immunological theory through the lens of the mechanism of antibody diversity generation because immunology has regarded this issue as one of the most important. However, the specific cells involved in the immune response were initially unknown. Moreover, it was unclear that the cells responsible for antibody production were B cells and that there were other cells (T cells) responsible for cellular immunity, which does not depend on antibodies. Here, I review how B cells, central to antibody-based humoral immunity, were discovered and how T cells and their receptors, which recognize antigens by a different mechanism from B cells, were identified. I also touch on how the products of the major histocompatibility complex (MHC; the human leukocyte antigen [HLA] system in humans and histocompatibility 2 [H-2] system in mice), another important molecule responsible for acquired immunity that characterizes an individual and is a barrier to transplantation, were discovered and how their intrinsic functions were revealed. This knowledge will be indispensable for understanding the framework of the immune response that will be discussed.

1.5.1 B Cells and T–B Cell Interactions in Antibody Production

As we have already seen, from the end of the 19th century to the first half of the 20th century, the critical question was whether it was antibodies or cells that were responsible for immunity. In their studies of immunity against diphtheria and tetanus, Emil von Behring and Shibasaburō Kitasato demonstrated the importance of antitoxins (antibodies) in the blood. Paul Ehrlich hypothesized that a single cell possesses many different side chains (receptors), each of which can bind the corresponding molecule, and that the binding of the molecule induces the cell to produce and eventually secrete large amounts of identical side chains, although the mechanism was unknown. Consequently, research on antibodies became dominant. However, studies started in the 1930s by Merrill Chase (1905–2004) and Karl Landsteiner at the Rockefeller Institute of Medicine (now Rockefeller University) in Manhattan revealed that an immune response dependent on cells rather than antibodies (cellular immunity) does indeed exist (Landsteiner and Chase, 1942; Chase, 1945). In a paper published in 1942, using the hapten-carrier system, Landsteiner and Chase studied contact hypersensitivity to haptens and delayed hypersensitivity to tuberculin in guinea pigs, demonstrating that these responses were not due to serum components but could be established by adoptive transfer of cellular components from the abdominal cavity to normal guinea pigs.

In the mid-20th century, crucial discoveries were also made in the area related to the B cells responsible for antibody production. In 1952, Ogden Bruton (1908–2003) reported a unique immunodeficiency (Bruton, 1952). The patient, an 8-year-old boy with recurrent sepsis who lacked only gamma globulin among his serum proteins, could not produce antibodies to the typhoid vaccine. However, his symptoms improved with the administration of gamma globulin. He had a primary immunodeficiency disease that would later be named "X-linked agammaglobulinemia." While its pathogenic mechanism could not be determined at the time, it was elucidated 40 years later. Its cause was an abnormality in an enzyme-encoding gene on the X chromosome that inhibited B cell differentiation in the bone marrow, resulting in the absence of mature B cells in the periphery. The enzyme responsible is called Bruton tyrosine kinase (BTK) (Tsukada et al., 1993; Vetrie et al., 1993), whose name is a tribute to the discoverer of the syndrome. The notable aspects of Bruton's discovery were that it suggested that cellular and humoral immunity may divide roles in the immune system, and it was the first report of an "experiment of nature" showing that defective or dysfunctional immune system components could lead to disease development. Indeed, since then, there has been a series of discoveries of primary immunodeficiency diseases caused by defective or dysfunctional molecules that constitute the immune system; as of 2020, 431 had been found (Notarangelo et al., 2020).

Furthermore, in 1956, Bruce Glick and his colleagues discovered the organ in which the B cells responsible for antibody production develop in birds (Glick et al., 1956): the bursa of Fabricius, which is a blind sac-like dorsal diverticulum in the wall of the cloaca. This organ was discovered and published in 1621 by Hieronymus Fabricius (also known as Girolamo Fabrizio; 1533–1619), who taught anatomy at the University of Padua in Italy. Among his students was William Harvey (1578–1657), who published his theory of blood circulation in 1628. More than three centuries had passed since Fabricius' discovery without its function being determined. Indeed, Glick's discovery was the result of sheer chance. Glick, then a graduate student at Ohio State University, was experimenting with removing the bursa of Fabricius to clarify their function. However, he was unable to obtain a clear answer. One day, a fellow graduate student asked him to donate chickens for an experiment he was doing on antibody production against *Salmonella* for undergraduate students. The results showed that chickens without bursae did not produce antibodies, while those with bursae had high antibody titers. After further comparison between the control group and the group whose bursae had been removed at 2 weeks of age, it became evident that the bursa of Fabricius plays a vital role in antibody production (Glick et al., 1956). This finding would not have been possible without a chance request from a colleague. The paper was sent to the journal *Science* but was rejected because the mechanism was not shown. It was published in the more specialized journal *Poultry Science* (Ribatti et al., 2006; Taylor and McCorkle, 2009). Subsequently, homologous organs were searched for in mammals, but none have been identified to date. The mammalian organ involved in B cell production is thought to be the bone marrow. The "B" in B cell is derived from the first letter of the bursa of Fabricius or bone marrow. While these findings suggest a division of roles between humoral and cellular immunity in the immune system, it remained unresolved whether they belong to the same lineage and perform different functions at different stages of differentiation or whether the cells responsible for each function differentiated independently.

The answer to this question became clear in 1965. Max Cooper (1933–) and Robert Good (1922–2003) showed that the cells responsible for humoral and cellular immunity belonged to different lineages (Cooper et al., 1965). Using chickens as a model, they prepared the following groups: one in which the bursa of Fabricius, essential for the antibody response, was removed immediately after birth; one in which the thymus, which was shown to be essential for cellular immunity 4 years earlier (Miller, 1961), was removed; one in which both the bursa and the thymus were removed; and a group in which both organs were left intact. Lymphoid organ histology, antibody production capacity and serum gamma globulin levels as indicators of humoral immunity, and allogeneic skin grafts and delayed hypersensitivity as indicators of cellular immunity were examined in these groups. Their results showed that in the bursectomized (bursa-removed) group, the thymus was normal, the transplanted skin grafts were rejected, and delayed-type hypersensitivity was observed. However, there were no plasma cells (antibody-producing cells) in lymphoid tissues, and no Igs or specific antibodies were produced in the peripheral blood. This manifestation is very similar to that of X-linked agammaglobulinemia. In contrast, the thymectomized (thymus-removed) group had normal plasma cell and Ig levels, but their skin graft and delayed hypersensitivity responses were altered to varying degrees. Interestingly, specific antibody production was suppressed relative to the control group, suggesting that the thymus is involved in antibody production.

Over the next few years, it would be established that T cell–B cell interactions are essential for antibody production (Claman et al., 1966; Miller and Mitchell, 1968; Mitchell and Miller, 1968a; Nossal et al., 1968). Overlooking their results, Cooper and colleagues concluded that there are two immunity axes. One involves the central organs, such as the bursa of Fabricius and the thymus, and peripheral organs, such as the spleen and lymph nodes. The other involves cells controlled by the bursa of Fabricius (B cells) and the thymus (T cells). This categorization has remained unwavering to the present day, and this paper was the starting point for delineating the functional distinction between T cells and B cells 8 years after Macfarlane Burnet published his clonal selection theory.

In 1959, the structure of antibodies was elucidated by Gerald Edelman (1929–2001; Nobel Prize in Physiology or Medicine 1972) of Rockefeller University in New York City and Rodney Porter (1917–1985; Nobel Prize in Physiology or Medicine 1972) of the National Institute of Medical Research at Mill Hill, a suburb of London. By cleaving the antibody with a chemical that reduces the disulfide bond between two sulfur atoms, Edelman showed that the antibody is composed of two polypeptides, the heavy and light chains as we know them today, and that there are two heavy chains and two light chains based on the molecular weight of the antibody (Edelman, 1959; Edelman and Poulik, 1961). Porter's analysis of three nearly identical-sized fragments obtained by treating rabbit antibodies with the enzyme papain revealed that the antibody has a structure with two antigen-binding sites (Fab region) and a constant region (Fc region) that is obtained as a crystal. Furthermore, when antibodies with different specificities were treated, the fragments that formed crystals were constant, whereas the antigen-binding fragments were different (Porter, 1959, 1963). These studies had a major impact on the direction of research because they elucidated immune phenomena at the molecular level, which had been lacking in earlier understanding.

1.5.2 THE T CELL, ITS RECOGNITION MECHANISM, AND THE ROLE OF MHC

In the previous section, I indicated that antibody production depends on both B and T cells (i.e., the interaction between them is necessary). In 1961, Australian Jacques Miller (1931–) showed that T cells were derived from the thymus (Miller, 1961). While previous thymectomies of mature mice had not affected antibody production, Miller performed thymectomy immediately after birth. Consequently, in the thymectomized group, he found decreased blood lymphocytes, germinal centers—the sites of B cell responses in peripheral lymphoid organs (e.g., the spleen and lymph nodes)—and plasma cells, and no rejection of allogeneic skin grafts. Miller proposed several hypotheses based on these findings. One was the possibility that the thymus regulates the production of immune cells (in this case, T cells), serving as the primary site producing such cells and stimulating the production of immune cells in other lymphoid organs by releasing humoral factors. Another was that the thymus produces lymphoid progenitor cells during embryonic life and that immunologically mature cells migrate elsewhere after birth. This paper, published when Miller was 30 years old, clarified the previously unknown function of the thymus and was a landmark discovery that complemented Cooper and Good's findings in that it uncovered the existence of an axis of immune function that was distinct from antibody production, forming the backbone of modern immunology.

In 1968, echoing Bruton's case in B cells, Angelo DiGeorge (1921–2009), a pediatrician at Temple University in Philadelphia, reported a human case of thymus deficiency (DiGeorge, 1968). In the symptoms of this disease, which would later be called "DiGeorge's syndrome," plasma cells and antibody production are unaffected, but cellular immunity is absent. It was found to be caused by a microdeletion on the long arm of chromosome 22 (22q11.2) (de la Chapelle et al., 1981; Kelley et al., 1982).

The question then arose about what molecules (receptors) were responsible for antigen recognition by T cells. Early papers suggested that, by analogy with B cells, antibody or antibody-like molecules may exist on the surface of T cells and that their receptors may be secreted, but this was never confirmed. The situation was changed by Rolf Zinkernagel (1933–; Nobel Prize in Physiology or Medicine 1996) and Peter Doherty (1940–; Nobel Prize in Physiology or Medicine 1996). They began their research at the John Curtin School of Medicine in Canberra, Australia, and reported that the recognition mechanism of T cells was very different from that of B cells.

In 1973, they began working on immune responses to lymphocytic choriomeningitis virus (LCMV). The initial impetus was a paper by Michael Oldstone, Hugh McDevitt (1930–2022), and others that came out earlier that year in which the susceptibility of mice to LCMV varied with the MHC (H-2 in mice) (Oldstone et al., 1973). Zinkernagel and Doherty began their experiments with the hypothesis that the activity of cytotoxic T cells (CTLs) against this virus determined disease severity, which might be related to H-2. They found that CTL activity was involved in LCMV infection (Zinkernagel and Doherty, 1973) and that CTL sensitized by LCMV could not destroy target cells unless at least one H-2 allele was identical to the LCMV-infected target cells (Zinkernagel and Doherty, 1974b). This phenomenon is known as "MHC restriction." For example, if the infected target cells were derived from $H-2^k$ mice, the CTLs were only active if they were derived from mice with one allele identical to the target, such as $H-2^k$ or $H-2^{k/b}$. CTLs from $H-2^b$ or $H-2^{b/d}$ did not kill the target.

At that time, papers had been published on the involvement of H-2 in the CTL response to leukemia viruses (Leclerc et al., 1972) and how T and B cells with different H-2 types did not interact and produce antibodies (Kindred and Schreffler, 1972; Katz et al., 1973), but they had not gone as far as to approach the recognition mechanism by T cells. Of course, neither the structure of the T cell receptor nor the MHC had yet been clarified. Zinkernagel and Doherty prepared and verified two models of CTL recognition (Zinkernagel and Doherty, 1974a). One is a two-receptor model in which different receptors on CTLs recognize viral antigens and the MHC, respectively. In other words, in addition to antigen recognition by the receptor, the MHC present on CTLs and target cells may bind to each other through a self-recognition mechanism. The other model involved a single receptor recognizing an "altered self." The altered self was assumed to be the MHC of the target cell altered by the virus or the MHC bound to the virus. After further investigation, it became clear that a model in which a single CTL receptor recognizes the altered self could explain the experimental results without contradiction (Zinkernagel and Doherty, 1974a).

Since then, controversy has arisen as to the structure of the T cell receptor and the relationship between the MHC and the antigen. I began my research just as these issues were being raised, and I witnessed the process of establishing important scientific facts by submitting and verifying various hypotheses. In 1984, the human and mouse T cell receptor genes were identified (Hedrick et al., 1984; Yanagi et al., 1984), and in 1987, the three-dimensional structure of the human MHC class I antigen was determined (Bjorkman et al., 1987). These results visualized the altered self, with antigen peptides always embedded in grooved pockets in the MHC structure. At the same time, the MHC restriction mechanism by which T cell receptors recognize their own MHC and antigen peptides was also visually illustrated. Zinkernagel and Doherty, who provided the basis for this work, were honored with the Nobel Prize in Physiology or Medicine in 1996 for their discoveries regarding the specificity of cellular immunity.

The MHC has thus been shown to play an important role in the immune recognition process, but let us now look back at the early research history of this molecule. The MHC was discovered between 1936 and 1937 by Peter Gorer (1907–1961), a 29-year-old pathologist at the Lister Institute of Preventive Medicine in London (Gorer, 1936, 1937). He discovered the mouse MHC, now known as H-2. By then, it was known that tumors grew when they were transplanted into genetically identical mice but stopped growing when they were transplanted into genetically different mice, for which two explanations were offered. One was that it was due to differences in tumor malignancy, and the other was that such a mechanism functioned not only in tumors but also in normal tissues.

Since the beginning of the 20th century, when Landsteiner and others reported the biochemical properties of the erythrocyte membrane as represented by the ABO blood type in humans, there had been a series of discoveries of blood types in many animals, including rabbits, dogs, goats, pigs, and sheep. John Burdon Sanderson Haldane (1892–1964), the head of the laboratory that Gorer would join, began to wonder if there might be a link between the success or failure of transplants and the nature of red blood cells. During a trip to the U.S. laboratories in 1933, Haldane realized that genetically uniform inbred mice would be needed to determine whether the success or failure of transplantation was determined by the tumor or by the host response, and he brought back to England three breeding pairs of inbred mice (A, CBA, and C57BL). He then advised Gorer to work in this direction (Klein, 1986).

Unlike humans, mouse sera do not contain antibodies to blood types. Because immunizing mice with whole blood from mice of other strains did not yield antibodies, Gorer immunized rabbits with mouse blood to obtain three antisera. However, since the normal rabbit serum contained antibodies that reacted with all strains of mice, he performed absorption experiments with red blood cells of each strain to determine antibody specificity. Consequently, it was found that the anti-CBA serum contained antibodies that reacted more strongly to CBA and A than to C57BL and was named antibody I. He also deduced that the anti-A serum contained at least two antibodies, antibody I and one that reacted strongly with A, weakly with CBA, and not with C57BL, which he named antibody II (Gorer, 1936). The following year, further transplantation experiments using mammary sarcoma that spontaneously developed in the A strain revealed that the antigen detected by antibody II determined the success or failure of transplantation (Gorer, 1937). Therefore, it was suggested that the antigen II detected by antibody II, which confers resistance to tumor transplantation, is also expressed in normal tissue other than red blood cells. This study led to the discovery of the MHC (H-2) as the molecule that characterizes the self as a barrier to transplantation.

However, few people initially realized the importance of this discovery, and it was forgotten for a while. Later, George Snell (1903–1996; Nobel Prize in Physiology or Medicine 1980), who collaborated with Gorer, developed congenic mice that differed only at specific genetic loci and inbred mice at the Jackson Laboratory in Maine, USA. These mice became indispensable in analyzing the function of genes in certain phenomena to exclude the involvement of other genes and contributed greatly to the development of research in this area. Snell was awarded the Nobel Prize in Physiology or Medicine in 1980, along with Jean Dausset (1916–2009), who discovered HLA, the human MHC, and Baruch Benacerraf (1920–2001), who clarified the function of the MHC.

Unfortunately, Gorer died of lung cancer in 1961 at 54. Many wonder if he might have received the prize if he had lived. While Gorer was the originator of such important research, his research style was very modest. Edward Boyse (1923–2007), a student of Gorer and my mentor, wrote that Gorer was not the type to systematically develop his research, that he was indifferent to many practicalities and did not seek influence in academic circles, and that he led an otherworldly life (Boyse, 1986).

Subsequently, an inquiry began into the mystery of what the MHC is there for because it is difficult to believe that nature has selected the MHC for transplantation, which is an artificial manipulation. The work of Zinkernagel and Doherty mentioned earlier and the analysis of the crystal structure of MHC provided the answer to this question.

1.6 HOW WAS THE INITIATION OF THE IMMUNE RESPONSE EXPLAINED?

As Burnet's clonal selection theory on the antibody diversity generation and the framework of the immune response gained acceptance in the immunologist community, researchers' interest shifted to the question of how the immune response is initiated (i.e., how immune cells are activated). In this section, I look back at how immunologists have explained the initiation of the immune response.

1.6.1 Burnet and Lederberg's B Cell Activation Model

I will begin by discussing the model advocated by Burnet. According to his model, antigen recognition induces B cell activation, proliferation, and differentiation. To ensure that the immune response is directed only to the nonself component, self-reactive cells must be inactivated or eliminated from the immune system. Burnet initially thought self-reactive cells are eliminated at an immature developmental stage by reacting with the body's own components. However, hematopoietic cells are produced throughout an organism's life, not just during the embryonic stage. Burnet adopted Lederberg's theory (Lederberg, 1959) and modified his explanation that it is at the immature stage of differentiation of cells, rather than at the immature developmental stage of the organism that elimination of self-reactive cells occurs.

In this model, the recognition of the antigen by the B cell (i.e., the binding of the antigen to its receptor) is the key factor in determining the cell's fate. In other words, while immature autoreactive cells are destined to die when they encounter self-antigens, mature cells become activated and differentiate into antibody-producing cells when they interact with the antigen. A version of this model was presented at the Cold Spring Harbor Symposium in 1967 (Burnet, 1967) and came to be considered the central theory of immunology.

1.6.2 Bretscher and Cohn's Two-Signal Model

The situation, however, was not so simple. As experimental data accumulated, it became clear that mature cells could also be rendered unresponsive to antigens, and other explanations were required. Peter Bretscher and Melvin Cohn thought that even if there were a mechanism by which autoreactivity could be eliminated a priori from the genome, it would not be beneficial from an evolutionary perspective since the mere introduction of a mutation in a gene could result in autoimmunity or autoimmune diseases. Indeed, there is no such mechanism for self–nonself discrimination at the genetic level. Instead, B cells are dividing cells and should constantly mutate and produce autoreactive cells, but in most cases nothing happens. From this, they deduced that a mechanism at the somatic cell level must control the response of mature B cells to self-antigens.

In 1968, they proposed a "two-signal model" to explain this seemingly paradoxical situation (Bretscher and Cohn, 1968). The premise of this model is that antigen receptors on the B cell surface can transmit two qualitatively different signals. As we have already seen, Landsteiner analyzed the specificity of the immune response in the early 20th century using the hapten-carrier system (Landsteiner, 1936). Haptens are small molecules that cannot induce antibody production by themselves, whereas carriers are large immunogenic proteins. Landsteiner's experiments revealed that immunization with haptens bound to carriers not only induced antibody production against the carriers but also the haptens with remarkable accuracy. Integrating the results obtained from the hapten-carrier system, Bretscher and Cohn proposed a hypothesis for the conditions leading to activation and inactivation ("paralysis" in their terminology) of B cells based on the following logical sequence.

First, they supposed that an antigen has multiple regions (determinants) that are recognized and bound by antibodies (receptors) on the B cell surface. If only one antigenic determinant binds to the receptor, it generates a signal that leads to inactivation of the B cell. However, if two or more antigenic determinants bind to the receptor simultaneously, the receptor's three-dimensional structure changes to a "stretched" state, which, for some reason, generates a signal that leads to the activation of the B cell. Furthermore, they envisioned a molecule that could bind to the antigen, ensuring that multiple antigenic determinants bind to a single receptor, which they called a "carrier antibody." This mechanism is in marked contrast to Lederberg's model, which assumes that the stage of cell maturation determines the cell's fate, with immature B cells being inactivated and mature B cells being activated (Lederberg, 1959). This difference is because Bretscher and Cohn argued that the same cell could have two different fates depending on how it is stimulated.

In 1970, Bretscher and Cohn published a more sophisticated version of the "two-signal model" (Bretscher and Cohn, 1970). The important point was that the carrier antibody envisioned in the previous paper could transmit an activation signal called "signal 2" that is independent of "signal 1," which is generated by an antigenic determinant binding to an antigen receptor, but they could interact, meaning the two signals are not mutually exclusive and the cell integrates these signals to determine its fate. According to the data accumulated up to that point (see Section 1.5, Chapter 1), antibody production occurs due to the proper interaction of two cell types—that is, B cells derived from the bone marrow and T cells "educated" in the thymus (Claman et al., 1966; Mitchell and Miller, 1968b). These results led Bretscher and Cohn to consider T cells as generating "signal 2." These cells would later be called helper T (Th) cells since they assist in activating B cells and other cells.

As mentioned above, the danger of antigen receptor gene mutation exists even in mature cells, giving rise to autoreactive cells. Unless the immune system has a mechanism to suppress autoreactivity, we will suffer from autoimmune diseases induced by increased reactivity to our own components. Bretscher and Cohn thought such pathology could be avoided by postulating a two-step mechanism in which an immune response cannot be initiated unless two cells that recognize different antigenic determinants in a single antigen are activated. The process is that antigen recognition (signal 1) alone leads to the inactivation or death of the B cell. However, the receipt of an appropriate auxiliary signal (signal 2) from the Th cell induces the B cell to differentiate into an antibody-producing cell. Th cells are activated in response to antigen peptides presented with MHC proteins on the B cell surface and secrete humoral factors such as interleukin (IL)-2, IL-4, IL-5, and IL-6 as signal 2, or express the CD40 ligand or CD40L (CD154), which reacts with the CD40 protein on the B cell surface, contributing to B cell activation. A ligand is a substance that binds specifically to a particular receptor. Furthermore, similar mechanisms were found to regulate T cell activation and inactivation, affirming the validity of the basic framework of the two-signal model.

In the 1970s, it became clear that leukocyte surface molecules, which came to be called "differentiation antigens," were useful in identifying differentiation stages and subpopulations of various cell types. From the late 1970s, the question of their functions in cell activation and inactivation became a major theme, and the analysis of these functions began. When I began my research in this domain in the United States, it was at its dawn. Since each laboratory had its own name for these differentiation antigens, it was challenging to distinguish their differences. To resolve this issue, researchers began systematizing the differentiation antigens by assigning CD (Cluster of Differentiation) numbers to them through regular international workshops starting in 1982.

The cytotoxic T-lymphocyte-associated protein 4 (CTLA4, also called CD152) was the subject of the Nobel Prize in Physiology or Medicine awarded to James Allison (1948–) in 2018. This molecule suppresses T cell activity by binding to its ligands (CD80 and CD86) on an antigen-presenting cell (APC). APCs include dendritic cells, macrophages, and B cells that bind antigen peptides to their MHC and present them to T cells. While CD28 is known to bind to the same ligands and send an activation signal, CTLA4 has a higher affinity for them. Therefore, it was thought that by suppressing CTLA4 activity by administering antibodies that bind to it, which act as a brake on T cell function, it would be possible to unleash the inherent functions of the immune system. Based on this hypothesis, Allison has shown that it is possible to treat certain types of cancer (Leach et al., 1996), a method known as "immune checkpoint therapy." If we apply the two-signal model to these molecules, we can see that positive and negative regulators exist within signal 2. Initially, it was thought that the CTLA4 antibody's mechanism was to enhance CTL activity. However, since CTLA4 is also expressed in cells called regulatory T (Treg) cells, or Tregs (see Section 2.1.4, Chapter 2) that suppress immune responses, it is now believed that the CTLA4 antibody enhances immunity by releasing the suppressive function of Treg cells (Wing et al., 2008). Few expected that a molecule so familiar to immunologists could contribute to treating cancer, which had loomed before humankind as an intractable problem. Tasuku Honjo (1942–), a co-winner of the Nobel Prize in 2018, has clearly shown that programmed cell death 1 (PD-1, also known as CD279) and its ligand, programmed cell death-ligand 1 (PD-L1, also known as CD274), are effective target molecules for cancer therapy, which is also a checkpoint therapy by releasing the function of molecules that suppress immune function (Iwai et al., 2002). These developments teach us that the seeds of discoveries that will contribute significantly to humanity are potentially hidden in researchers' daily lives and that it is essential to pursue them relentlessly.

There is another example of Bretscher and Cohn's insight. They foresaw the existence of an intracellular molecule, what they called an "interaction sensing unit," that senses conformational changes in antibody molecules upon binding to antigens and generates some signal in the cell (Bretscher and Cohn, 1970). What corresponds to this unit seems to be the B cell signaling molecules discovered 20 years later, CD79A (also called Ig-α) and CD79B (Ig-β) (Hombach et al., 1990). These transmembrane proteins form a complex with the B cell antigen receptor and transmit signals generated by antigen binding to the receptor into the cell. A similar mechanism operates in T cells, where CD3 and zeta chains (CD247), which form a complex with the T cell receptor, are involved in the transduction of signals resulting from the reaction of the antigen with the T cell receptor (Brenner et al., 1985; Samelson et al., 1985). In any case, the deductive thinking and principle-oriented philosophy of Bretscher and Cohn can be seen behind these developments. This is worthy of special mention in the context of biological research, which tends to neglect principle-oriented thinking in favor of mechanism analysis.

1.6.3 T Cell Activation Depends on Antigen-Presenting Cells

While T and B cells have been the main actors in the model up to this point, a new actor has emerged from the study of T cell activation: graft versus host reaction (GVHR). The GVHR is a cytotoxic reaction in which immunologically active cells (T cells) introduced into a host of the same species with a different MHC are activated and destroy the host's tissues and organs. It acts in the opposite direction to the graft rejection reaction. Curiously, the GVHR was observed to be stronger in allogeneic (between different individuals of the same species) than in xenogeneic (between different species) transplants (Lafferty and Jones, 1969). For example, chicken cells injected into genetically distinct chicken eggs induced a much stronger reaction than when pigeon cells were introduced into chicken eggs. When lymphocytes from sheep or mice were introduced into chicken eggs, there was no GVHR. These results seem to be slightly absurd to our commonsensical perception. However, the authors concluded that the difference in histocompatibility antigen per se is not a determining factor in inducing a strong GVHR. In other words, a greater genetic difference in the histocompatibility antigen, for example, xenogeneic over allogeneic combinations, does not necessarily guarantee stronger reactions.

From this, it was hypothesized that something other than the antigen is necessary to induce a stronger reaction and that introduced cells must interact with genetically different host cells, which then produce a stimulatory factor(s). This theory meant that a T cell must recognize not only an antigen but also receive another factor, which they called an "allogeneic stimulus." This stimulus was thought to determine the strength of the reaction. This model was later revised and generalized to apply to cellular responses to antigens in general (Lafferty and Cunningham, 1975). According to this model, signal 1 (antigen recognition) of the Bretscher–Cohn model (Bretscher and Cohn, 1970) is insufficient to activate Th cells, and another signal is required, what would later be called "co-stimulation," a species-specific factor secreted by APC (Lafferty et al., 1978).

While this model did not initially attract much attention, almost 10 years later, it became clear that in the T cell proliferative response system, chemical treatment of APCs does not cause a proliferative response (i.e., the APCs must be alive to provide a signal 2 for T cell activation) (Jenkins and Schwartz, 1987). As noted by Bretscher and Cohn in B cells (Bretscher and Cohn, 1970), T cells also become unresponsive (anergy) in the absence of co-stimulation with an antigen (Nossal and Pike, 1980). These results strongly suggest that co-stimulation of T cells by APCs is essential for initiating an immune response. The fact that co-stimulation with APCs is essential to activate T cells that are inactive in the steady state raises questions about the specificity of the immune response because APCs cannot discriminate between self and nonself. If they are responsible for initiating the immune response, the question arises as to how specificity is ensured. In other words, the question is how the response to self is controlled and by what mechanism the integrity of the organism is maintained.

1.6.4 Charles Janeway's Discrimination Between "Infectious Nonself" and "Noninfectious Self"

To explain this seemingly contradictory situation, Yale immunologist Charles Janeway (1943–2003), with extraordinary intuition, proposed a hypothesis that would change our perception of the immune system. It answered the question of how nonspecific stimulation of APCs could be integrated into the specific identification of self and nonself, and at the same time had the effect of making visible the thread that links innate and acquired immunity (Janeway, 1989, 1992; Janeway and Medzhitov, 2002). How did he approach this question? The first clue was the use of "adjuvants," which immunologists have used to enhance the immune response to antigens of low immunogenicity (the ability to induce antibody production). The word "adjuvant" comes from the Latin verb *adjuvare*, meaning "to help," and typically contains dead bacteria such as *Mycobacterium tuberculosis* or *Bordetella pertussis*. It has been used routinely in laboratories worldwide for almost a century but without serious thought about its significance in immunity. Janeway called adjuvants the "immunologist's dirty little secret," and he believes that the microorganisms in adjuvants stimulate APCs to produce costimulatory molecules, which are responsible for the effective initiation of immune responses (Janeway, 1989).

Janeway proposed a new theory in the introduction to the Cold Spring Harbor Symposium in 1989: that the immune system evolved not only to allow B and T cells to discriminate between self and nonself in an antigen-specific manner but also to identify molecules that are not present in self but in microorganisms, including pathogens. He described it as a mechanism that discriminates between "noninfectious self" and "infectious nonself" (Janeway, 1989). He further predicted that this discrimination is made by innate immunity, which was thought to be non-specific, and that receptors to recognize specific molecular patterns conserved in microbes are expressed on cells, such as APCs (Janeway, 1992; Janeway and Medzhitov, 2002). He named these receptors "pattern recognition receptors" (PRRs). The specific molecular patterns of microorganisms are called pathogen-associated molecular patterns, or microbe-associated molecular patterns (MAMPs), because non-pathogenic microorganisms also express the molecular patterns of microorganisms. Since these molecular patterns are characteristic of the microorganism and not present in the host, they do not induce a self-targeted immune response. In addition, given that these molecules are important components of microbial physiological processes, their structures are not easily altered, making them perfect recognition sites for the immune system. The binding of MAMPs to the corresponding PRRs activates APCs, which in turn express costimulatory molecules to contribute to T cell activation. Therefore, this mechanism provides an excellent means of communication between the innate immune system of APCs and the acquired immune system of B and T cells.

Notably, APCs are not activated until after the PRRs of APCs encoded by germline genes recognize MAMPs, meaning that APCs, like B and T cells, are not activated in the steady state and must receive an activation signal. Therefore, an immune response cannot be initiated unless APCs recognize a pattern characteristic of the microbe before B and T cells are activated. Furthermore, while the APCs' recognition is nonspecific, the PRRs recognize MAMPs characteristic of the microorganism that is not present in the host, meaning that they respond to nonself while avoiding attacking the self. In other words, discrimination between self and nonself is performed at two levels: innate and acquired immunity.

1.6.5 DISCOVERY OF TOLL-LIKE RECEPTORS

This prediction by Janeway was to be proven by subsequent experiments, from which further unexpected connections emerged. In 1996, the Strasbourg group led by Jules Hoffmann (1941–; Nobel Prize in Physiology or Medicine 1999) discovered that mutating the *toll* gene of *Drosophila melanogaster* made it susceptible to infection by a fungus (*Aspergillus fumigatus*) (Lemaitre et al., 1996). The *toll* gene was identified in 1985 by Christiane Nüsslein-Volhard's (1942–; Nobel Prize in Physiology or Medicine 1995) group in Tübingen as a gene required for determining the dorsoventral axis during *Drosophila melanogaster* development (Anderson et al., 1985). The name *toll* was given to the mutated gene because when Nüsslein-Volhard saw a strange-looking fly larva with an underdeveloped ventral portion of the body, her first reaction was "Das war ja toll!" meaning "That was amazing!" (Hansson and Edfeldt, 2005). The *toll* gene was cloned in 1988 (Hashimoto et al., 1988), and 8 years later, it was discovered that a transmembrane Toll protein had the immune function described above. This discovery accelerated the investigation of the existence of Toll-like molecules in other species and their physiological functions.

Janeway's group was also searching for human PRRs. It was already known that the transcription factor nuclear factor-kappa B (NF-κB) was an important activator of cells involved in innate immunity and that transmembrane receptors with a Toll/IL-1 receptor (TIR) homology region in the intracytoplasmic region activated the NF-κB-mediated signaling pathway. Ruslan Medzhitov (1966–) and colleagues used the genetic method to search for genes with TIR regions in the database from human library, and a year after the Hoffman group's publication, they reported a human homolog of Toll, which they named the Toll-like receptor (TLR) (Medzhitov et al., 1997). The gene contained a leucine-rich repeat rather than a region associated with an already-known microbial receptor. Since then, more than 10 TLRs have been identified in humans and mice, and their structures are conserved throughout the evolutionary process from sponges to humans (Wiens et al., 2007). Furthermore, plants have transmembrane receptors with structures similar to TLRs (Ausubel, 2005; Boller and Felix, 2009), and bacteria secrete molecules containing TIR regions to inhibit host TLR responses (Cirl et al., 2008). While each TLR recognizes pathogen-specific molecules, the entire repertoire of all TLRs allows for detecting diverse viruses, bacteria, and fungi.

How on earth could Janeway have come up with such an idea? One possibility is that his tendency to look at problems from a broader perspective allowed him to address issues that researchers buried in a narrower field might not be aware of. It is also imagined that he may have used deductive thinking that the cause of a phenomenon must be this way. Janeway's hypothesis was a breath of fresh air to the conventional view of the immune system that centered on discriminating self and nonself by T and B cells, and together with Hoffmann's discovery, it opened up a vast field of research. However, his early death at age 60 made further contributions by Janeway himself impossible.

1.6.6 POLLY MATZINGER'S DANGER THEORY

Janeway's hypothesis was undoubtedly a breakthrough but did not solve everything, as noted by Polly Matzinger (1947–). The criticism was that Janeway's view, which centered on identifying microorganisms, could not answer why, for example, an allogeneic graft without microorganisms would be rejected or what could cause autoimmune disease. In the 1990s, Matzinger proposed the danger theory as a framework for understanding phenomena that could not be explained by previously proposed models without contradiction (Matzinger, 1994). While Burnet's self–nonself discrimination theory assumed that it is something foreign, such as a pathogen, that initiates the immune response, the danger theory considered that everything that could be harmful to the host triggered an immune response. It does not matter whether it is an injury from a pathogen, a change due to stress or some other injury, or an internal disruption such as the necrosis of the host cell itself. These changes became known as danger- or damage-associated molecular patterns (DAMPs). In an interview with The New York Times, she used the example of a community to explain the danger theory in this way (Dreifus, 1998). According to her, in the self–nonself discrimination theory, if a cop meets someone he does not usually see, he kills them, no matter who they are. However, in the danger theory, a cop accepts any person, whether a tourist or an immigrant, and will only move to eliminate them from the community if they are destructive in some way. Indeed, it does not matter if the destructor is an outsider or a member of the community. According to the danger theory, immunity acts like a community police officer, patrolling to seek out those who would do harm, regardless of their place of origin.

Danger theory explains better than Janeway's theory, for example, controversial phenomena such as the lack of reactivity to self-components and graft rejection. According to the danger theory, autoimmunity does not automatically occur even if autoreactive cells react with self-components because they must receive co-stimulation from APCs that sense danger in the environment to be activated. In addition, rejection and other reactions are not necessarily predicted by Janeway's theory. While Janeway's theory states that no reaction occurs without microorganisms, rejection also occurs in grafts without microorganisms. According to Matzinger's theory, it is possible to explain rejection by graft injury that occurs during the transplantation procedure.

Matzinger gives many other interesting examples (Matzinger, 2002). Another example I would like to discuss is symbiosis with microorganisms. This issue will be discussed in detail in Section 2.1, Chapter 2, but almost all organisms have symbiotic relationships with microorganisms, and humans are no exception. A recent study shows that we live in symbiosis with approximately the same number of microorganisms as the cells that make up our bodies (Sender et al., 2016). According to Janeway's theory, our immune system exists to react to microbes, but if so, how does one explain the fact that symbiotic microbes are not eliminated? However, according to Matzinger's theory, the reaction does not occur unless they injure the host. Indeed, these microorganisms do not harm us but instead do something beneficial, becoming an integral part of our physiology, our survival.

In principle, Matzinger accepts not only the Bretscher–Cohn two-signal model (B cell activation by antigens and T cells) but also the view advocated by Janeway that it is the APCs that are responsible for initiating the immune response. The difference with Janeway's theory is how APCs are activated. While Janeway posits that the microorganism activates the APCs, Matzinger posits that it is the injured cell or tissue. Medzhitov and Janeway criticized the danger theory as a tautology. They argue that there is no a priori definition of a danger signal that initiates the immune response, and it cannot be known without the immune response's outcome (Medzhitov and Janeway, 2002). Such criticisms are also reminiscent of Herbert Spencer's (1820–1903) attempts to explain Darwin's theory of evolution based on the idea of "survival of the fittest." This one, too, cannot be defined a priori as the fittest because it must be determined a posteriori whether the individual survived or not. In any case, unlike Matzinger, who believes that necrosis and tissue injury are danger signals that trigger an immune response, Janeway considers that the physiological role of inflammation induced by necrosis is to induce a reparative response to tissue injuries because tissue repair appears to be the most logical answer to tissue injury. As proposed in his discrimination theory of infectious nonself and noninfectious self, the initiation of an immune response is controlled by the innate immune system, which identifies molecular motifs derived from microorganisms (pathogens) that are not present in the host (Medzhitov and Janeway, 2002).

However, data are accumulating on the DAMP's physicochemical properties (Matzinger, 2002, 2007; Chen and Nuñez, 2010). Under physiological conditions, the DAMP is processed intracellularly and is not recognized by the immune system. However, when an injury occurs, the cell membrane is disrupted, leading to necrosis, and the DAMP is released outside the cell, triggering inflammation. In contrast, programmed cell death (apoptosis), in which the cell membrane is not injured, is not considered dangerous. DAMPs that have been identified include proteins associated with nuclear chromatin (high mobility group box 1 [HMGB1]), heat shock proteins, DNA, RNA, ATP, other cell-derived substances, and various proteins released from the extracellular matrix (e.g., proteoglycans), and their physicochemical basis is becoming increasingly certain.

Matzinger proposed that the danger theory and Janeway's argument are not mutually exclusive. Instead, innate immunity has two functions. In other words, innate immunity is activated when a defense response against pathogens is induced and when it is required for physiological responses such as tissue repair and remodeling during injury and development (Seong and Matzinger, 2004). Furthermore, she postulated that the receptors involved in this process have evolved to recognize parts of molecules with a low affinity for water (hydrophobic parts). If life began in water, the hydrophobic part of the molecule would typically not be recognized by the receptor because it is hidden inside the molecule but would be a danger to the cell if exposed. In this connection, she also suggests that to explore the evolution of immunity, we should study the systems involved in tissue injury and repair rather than using molecules homologous to those that recognize heterogeneity, such as MHC, as indicators.

Let us now consider the implications of establishing a unified theory such as that presented by Matzinger. Indeed, having a unified theory that explains as many immunological phenomena as possible may be ideal. However, is it possible to establish a unified theory in biology, which may be possible in physics or chemistry? Above all, does the immune system operate under a single principle? Different manifestations may be found in different locations in an organism as complex in structure as humans, and there is no guarantee that different principles are not at work there. Furthermore, if the immune system has used various strategies throughout its long evolution, it begs the question of whether a single theory or paradigm can explain the diversity of immune phenomena (Vance, 2000). As Russell Vance noted, many arguments by the proponents of the danger theory are based on the two-signal model, downplaying or ignoring signal 1, which is involved in recognizing self and nonself and emphasizing the importance of signal 2, which derives from APCs (Matzinger, 1994, 1998, 2002). While there are exceptions to the self–nonself discrimination model, as in the danger theory, it can explain many important phenomena such as MHC restriction (T cells recognize antigens on APCs with MHC identical to their own), positive selection (leaving T cells in the system that react moderately with their own MHC), negative selection (excluding T cells from the system that react strongly with their own antigens), rejection of allogeneic skin grafts, and acceptance of syngeneic grafts. He argued that while there is certainly some difficulty in defining the self, there is no reason to abandon the self–nonself discrimination model. He also suggested that it is unrealistic to think that the immune response follows a limited set of laws and that instead of seeking a unified theory or relying on a single paradigm, the immune system should be viewed as a set of diverse mechanisms brought together in the course of evolution (Vance, 2000).

This point is important, I think, because it relates to philosophical issues about science in general and is tied to the direction that immunology should take. In other words, the question is how to think about the importance of understanding the whole picture of a particular biological phenomenon and the fundamental principles that supposedly exist in it. Beyond that, the question arises of whether it is possible to understand the fundamental principle. The question of whether we should seek to understand the whole and the root of the matter is normative in nature. However, the possibility should also be subject to scientific consideration. Since the discussion between Vance and Matzinger in 2000, we do not seem to have heard anything on this topic. Have immunologists only analyzed local phenomena in the lungs, skin, bones, and brain? Or have they studied more general phenomena that intersect with other areas, such as aging, cancer, and metabolism? Should immunologists be content to become specialists in increasingly limited areas and discover new diagnostics and therapies? To rephrase this question, is this pragmatic pursuit the only purpose of immunology? Today, the trend toward pragmatism is becoming stronger and more valued. If this trend is accepted uncritically, the viewpoint that seeks to understand the fundamental nature of immunity and its inherent principles will gradually weaken. It will be necessary from now on to promote thinking from a broader and different perspective while emphasizing a viewpoint that moves toward the local.

1.7 NEW THEORETICAL ATTEMPTS TO COUNTER THE CLONAL SELECTION THEORY

Janeway's discrimination theory and Matzinger's danger theory began as a challenge to Burnet's clonal selection theory. Indeed, these theories clarified the understanding of the initial process by which the immune system is activated and the fundamental role of innate immunity. However, they still appear to be within Burnet's framework in that they did not abandon the clonal perspective. Therefore, it would make sense to consider them as important modifications of the clonal selection theory but not its denial. However, there are examples in the history of immunology in which theories have been built on quite different foundations. A notable example is Niels Jerne's idiotypic network theory. This theory attracted many of the best scientists of the time and was studied for almost 15 years, but unfortunately was never scientifically proven. It is now almost completely forgotten, and young researchers may not even know it exists. The developments surrounding this theory provide interesting material when trying to understand how the scientific mind works in scientific activity and what kind of activity science is in the first place. Here, I reflect on this theory's details and what exactly was going on around it.

1.7.1 NIELS JERNE'S IDIOTYPIC NETWORK THEORY—A CREATIVE BUT UNPROVEN HYPOTHESIS

All the theories examined thus far have concerned how the immune system recognizes an almost infinite number of antigens and what initiates the immune response locally. Most theories also saw clonal propagation as initiated by discriminating self and nonself or by identifying what is or is not harmful to self. In this sense, they all fit within Burnet's clonal view of immunity. However, the idiotypic network theory proposed by Niels Jerne differed completely from the previous theories (Jerne, 1974). Jerne sought to understand the immune system as a whole. His theory was the first to attempt to conceptualize the immune system's function without relying on the Burnetian self–nonself discrimination. While this theory was based on scientifically proven facts, it resulted from deductive and metaphysical thinking. Let us begin our discussion with the foundations of this theory.

An antibody molecule has a constant region, whose structure is similar among antibodies, and a variable region, whose structure differs among antibodies, the latter of which is involved in antigen recognition. Therefore, antibodies have the function of recognizing antigens, but at the same time they are recognized by other antibodies. The side that sees the antigen turns to the side that is seen because antibodies have three types of antigenic determinants: isotypes (from the Greek *iso* meaning "equal" and *typos* meaning "form"), allotypes (*allo* meaning "other"), and idiotypes (*idio* meaning "unique"). The isotypes (also called classes) are defined by differences in the amino acid sequence of the antibody's constant region. For example, humans and mice have five isotypes that serve different functions: IgM, IgD, IgG, IgA, and IgE. These isotypes are present in all individuals of one species. Allotypes, like isotypes, are defined by differences in the amino acid sequence of the constant region, which varies from individual to individual in humans and from strain to strain in mice. Therefore, antibodies to an isotype are not produced in the same species and require heterologous immunization, while antibodies to an allotype may be produced by homologous immunization.

The idiotype in question in Jerne's theory was discovered independently by Henry Kunkel (1916–1983) of Rockefeller University (Kunkel et al., 1963) and Jacques Oudin (1908–1985) of the Pasteur Institute (Oudin and Michel, 1963). It is a structure characteristic of each and every antibody molecule and is present in its variable region. Jerne calls the antigen recognition site of an antibody a paratope. Paratopes recognize not only foreign antigens but also idiotypes of other antibody molecules, which are antigenic determinants (epitopes) of antibodies. In other words, idiotypes can also function as antigens that initiate immune responses. Based on these facts, Jerne developed an ingenious theory that paratopes of one antibody bind to idiotypes of other antibodies, forming a network that spans the entire immune system. According to Jerne, the immune system is not open to the external world but a closed, self-sufficient, self-referential system.

While the immune system is believed to have the capacity to produce antibodies to an almost infinite number of specificities, the antibodies actually used during an organism's lifetime are thought only to be a fraction of its repertoire. Proponents of Burnet's clonal selection theory view the immune system as a kind of large reservoir, so the system is flexible to react in any emergent situation. In a sense, antibodies are ready and waiting for the right time, notably during an intrusion of pathogenic microorganisms. In contrast, Jerne, with a touch of teleology, poses the following two questions: For what purpose does the immune system prepare antibodies that are never used? Why do antibodies exist in our bodies in a steady state? These are questions about the raison d'être of antibodies. In reflecting on these questions, Jerne turned his attention to the idiotype enabling antibodies to bind to each other.

Let us consider his theory in more detail. Suppose we have a B cell (let us call it B-1). Its cell surface expresses an antibody (Ab-1) as an antigen receptor with a paratope (P-1) that can bind to the antigen. It also expresses an idiotope (Id-1), a discrete antigenic determinant within the specific idiotype of this antibody. All other B cells (B-2, -3, -4, etc.) likewise have their own paratope and idiotope. For example, the idiotope (Id-1) of Ab-1 is recognized by the paratope (P-2) of B-2 cells, and that recognition activates the B-2 cell. At the same time, P-1 recognizes an idiotope (Id-3) in another cell (e.g., B-3), which activates the B-1 cell. In this way, the antibodies in the body form a network that extends throughout the immune system through the binding of their paratopes and idiotopes, and this network has mechanisms to positively and negatively regulate the immune response (Jerne, 1974).

According to this view, the steady state of the immune system is not dormant but an equilibrium maintained by the dynamic interactions of antibodies with each other. When an antigen enters the system, it disturbs the equilibrium state of the idiotope–paratope network, affecting not only the first reacting paratope but all components connected via the immune system network. This situation may be visualized as a situation in which a stone is thrown into a pond, causing a wave that gradually spreads over its entire surface and extends to its depths but regains its original calm over time. This theory differs from Burnet's theory in the following ways. Jerne's theory views the immune response as a holistic response involving all cells that comprise the idiotypic network. In contrast, Burnet's theory sees the immune response as a localized antigen–antibody response with no apparent relationship to the other immune system components. Jerne's view is somewhat reminiscent of the ancient Greek philosophy of Hippocrates of Kos (c. 460–c. 370 BC), who believed that disease is an overall change caused by a disturbance in the balance of the humoral factors that make up the body and that the whole body can heal itself. According to Jerne's theory, immunological memory is instilled during the signal's propagation through a web of interactions in the system, which is felt deep within the body as a disturbance in the network (Jerne, 1974). The explanation is abstract and literary and lacks molecular and cellular basis.

What is interesting about this theory is that the paratope (P-1) of a single antibody on the surface of B-1 cells is supposed to recognize not only the epitope of the external antigen but also the idiotopes of other antibodies in the system. The immune system envisioned by Jerne would have within the individual a repertoire of all antigenic determinants present in the external world in the form of antibody idiotopes, which he named the "internal image." From this, Jerne deduced that the immune system evolved to recognize the internal image rather than to respond to antigens in the external world. This theory was reminiscent of the "monad" (from the Greek *monas* meaning "unit") advocated by Leibniz (1646–1716) in his *Monadology* (1714). In other words, it is a metaphysics that holds that the things that exist in nature are composed of a monad with no parts that is a living mirror of the world so that its interior reflects the external world. Anne-Marie Moulin noted that the immune system is compatible with Leibniz's philosophy in the sense that it is equipped with a reflection of the antigens present in the world in the form of antigen receptors without relating it to Jerne's theory (Moulin, 1991c). This view is also consistent with Jerne's attempt to reflect nature deep within his soul, and his theory appears to be an attempt to fuse his philosophy and science (Söderqvist, 2003b).

The first version of the idiotypic network theory concerned B cells and antibodies but was later expanded to include T cells and the regulation of molecules secreted by them. The theory's applicability to the entire immune system attracted many brilliant and enthusiastic researchers studying immune regulation. They came to view the idiotypic network theory as the leading clue to a unified understanding of immune phenomena. However, even at its height, it was severely criticized by the likes of Melvin Cohn (Cohn, 1981; Cohn, 1989a). Cohn believed that the discrimination between self and nonself is the fundamental principle in immunity and that this was the reason for the control exercised by the immune system. However, his criticisms were drowned out by the enthusiasm for Jerne's theory. Ultimately, however, the theory was not accepted by the scientific community.

When we reflect on the idiotypic network theory, we see that Jerne's thinking leaped from the experimental fact that the idiotype of one antibody is recognized by the paratope of another antibody to the proposal of a theory that encompasses the entire immune system. Science is not only the accumulation of falsifiable data but also the public discussion of creative minds, and Jerne seems to have regarded the latter function as particularly important. He believed that the leap from experimental data to an original theory was not only right but was the most important step in science. However, as will be discussed in Section 1.7.2, Chapter 1, in the case of Jerne's theory, there seemed to be many problems in the process of deduction to confirm or deny it. Melvin Cohn identified two fundamental failures in Jerne's process of formulating his theory (Cohn, 1989a). The first was his failure to view the immune system from an evolutionary perspective. Second, he did not recognize and actively confront other competing concepts in his analysis of the phenomenon.

Einstein made the following points:

> There is an unbridgeable gap between the concept and the observation. It is a total mistake to think that concepts can be created simply by piecing together observations.
> [...] Every conceptual thing is a construct and cannot be derived from direct experience by logical means. In other words, we are, in principle, completely free to choose even the basic concepts on which we base our descriptions of the world.
>
> **Einstein (1992)**

From this perspective, there is no fault in what Jerne was trying to do. Rather, it would have been desirable. However, there may have been inadequacies in the method of verification that should have been accounted for in arriving at a universal concept or principle. The theory he arrived at was never experimentally proven, even with intensive research from 1975 to 1990 (Eichmann, 2008b; Yakura, 2011). After the downfall of Jerne's theory, immunologists stopped trying to put forward an integrated theory that would explain the entire system and seemed to spend their time analyzing the control mechanisms of its parts without having a holistic conception of the system.

1.7.2   REFLECTIONS BY AN IDIOTYPIC NETWORK RESEARCHER

Why, then, were so many brilliant minds attracted to one fictitious theory for so long and to draw the same erroneous conclusions? Klaus Eichmann (1935–), a German immunologist at the center of Jerne's research circle and former director of the Max Planck Institute for Immunobiology (now the Max Planck Institute for Immunobiology and Epigenetics) in Freiburg, confronted himself starkly with the same question. While searching for the general nature of science, he came across a book, *Genesis and Development of a Scientific Fact* (Fleck, 1935), published in German in 1935 by the Polish physician Ludwik Fleck (1896–1961). Although this book did not receive much attention for a long time, it finally attracted the attention of sociologist Robert Merton (1910–2003), and an English translation was published in 1979 (Fleck, 1979b).

In this book, which examines the development of the Wassermann reaction used to diagnose syphilis, Fleck finds that knowledge acquisition is based on scientific and medical foundations but is also subject to change according to political conditions and the way research is conducted. Scientific knowledge is acquired through human activity and is, therefore, consciously or unconsciously influenced by the social environment. He wrote about this situation as follows: At least three-quarters if not the entire content of science is conditioned by the history of ideas, psychology, and the sociology of ideas and is thus explicable in these terms (Fleck, 1979a).

From this research, Fleck developed important concepts. One was "thought style" (Denkstil), and the other was "thought collective" (Denkkollectiv). A thought style refers to a mode of thinking in which empirical facts are constrained by the subjective fictions of a tradition or group that transcends experience. This thought style is shared by a group of individuals, often forming a closed community in a particular area of study. Fleck called such a group a "thought collective." In his bestseller *The Structure of Scientific Revolutions* (1962), Thomas Kuhn credits Fleck's work as an inspiration for the concept of "paradigm" (Kuhn, 1962). Eichmann was struck by the similarities between the history of idiotypic network theory and that of the Wassermann reaction and used the word "collective" as a tribute to Fleck in the title of his book, *The Network Collective: Rise and Fall of a Scientific Paradigm* (Eichmann, 2008b).

In the chapter entitled "Origins, Rise, and Fall of the Network Paradigm," Eichmann details the scientific saga of the idiotypic network theory by analyzing scientific developments in related fields, such as neuroscience and cybernetics, that influenced the formulation of the idiotypic network theory. This approach is important in light of Fleck's original observation that elements from distinct fields or their thought styles can be incorporated into a new thought style, which becomes a driving force for scientific developments but may also lead to an erroneous paradigm. Because of Jerne's charismatic character, those who belonged to the idiotypic network collective gradually came to think that the idiotypic network theory was not a hypothesis to be tested but must be an already established genuine theory. As a result, negative results were not discussed or interpreted from different perspectives but discarded as meaningless based on technical or other reasons. When testing a hypothesis or theory, results that are unexpected or do not conform to expectations should lead to its revision or reconstruction. However, according to Eichmann, this obvious step was ignored and forgotten in the network collective. It is surprising that a group of supposedly outstanding researchers did not follow this principle. However, while the scientists' motivations may differ, it is worth considering that such things can happen under certain conditions. When the investigations were expanded to the T cell field, experimental materials including polyclonal antibodies (antibodies with many specificities) and congenic mice (strains differing only in certain genetic regions) were problematic, making it difficult to interpret experimental results. Ultimately, the theory was branded fictitious and disappeared from the immunological scene.

In the chapter entitled "Hindsight: Personal Interviews," there is a hint as to why so many talented people were attracted to this project. I could see there a desirable interactive scientific ambiance and some philosophical attitudes against impersonal reductionist approaches that are missing in present-day science. For example, Pierre André Cazenave of the Pasteur Institute made comments in a slightly sentimental way:

Independently of the idiotypic network, I think it was a time of discussion between people, those working on [the] idiotypic network, but also with people outside of the field or even against the network, just think of Mel Cohn. I think these were very interesting interactions among scientists. This is no more the case.

Eichmann (2008a)

He further stated in a strong anti-reductionist manner:

At the present time we see a very reductionist approach. Most people are working on signaling, this is interesting, you have to know the signal chains, but you cannot explain how the immune system works. [...] Signaling is important for cell biology but not for how the immune system works as a system, and a system connected with others, which is one of the most important fields in immunology at the present time. [...] There is nobody now who has a larger view on regulation. This is the case in basic immunology, and even more so if we move to immunophysiopathology.

Eichmann (2008a)

Most of the scientists interviewed in this book agree that at present, there is no comparable paradigm that explains immunological phenomena in an integrative manner. As already discussed in Section 1.6, Chapter 1, the following two questions reappear: Is it necessary to search for a unified theory in immunology, as in physics? Is it feasible to establish one in a field as diverse as immunology? From a practical perspective, developing a therapeutic method without a unified theory is possible. However, the real question is whether scientists are really satisfied with a situation in which we do not have precise ideas about what immunity is or how the immune system functions. Most scientists in the field probably have nothing else to do but continue their work as it is. As Eichmann discussed in the chapter "Science between Fact and Fiction," there is nothing wrong with interpreting data using scientists' imagination because that is the very essence of science. What is important is to remember and be conscious of the fictional nature of scientific concepts, as evidenced by the fact that among at least 15 theories of antibody formation and specificity proposed, Frank Macfarlane Burnet's clonal selection theory is the sole survivor of paradigmatic theory in immunology.

1.7.3 IRUN COHEN'S COGNITIVE PARADIGM

According to clonal selection theory, the immune system's primary function is to discriminate between self and nonself. Self-reactivity or autoimmunity is controlled by exporting only lymphocytes with receptors reactive with nonself from the central lymphoid organs (bone marrow and thymus) to the periphery. Furthermore, since several mechanisms in the periphery check self-reactivity, the distinction between self and nonself is ensured. Therefore, according to this theory, autoimmunity is not expected to be observed under physiological conditions and is due to a random genetic aberration or an accident within the workings of the immune system. If this is the case, the antigens recognized by self-reactive clones would be diverse, and autoimmune diseases would also be diverse. However, their specificity is limited, and autoreactive T and B cells are present even in healthy individuals. These facts have led to the supposition that autoimmunity may be an intrinsic feature of the immune system rather than an abnormality.

The Israeli immunologist Irun Cohen (1937–) accepts the clonal activation of the clonal selection theory but claims that it cannot explain the physiological autoimmunity found in healthy individuals (Cohen, 1992b). He then stated that the immune system exists to enhance adaptation and ensure survival. This role requires the recognition process to effectively discriminate between important signals and noise, selecting when and where to respond and the appropriate type of immune response. While the clonal selection theory is reductionist, mechanical, and clear-cut, Cohen believes it lacks this subtle and holistic view and proposes a "cognitive paradigm" to complement the incomplete clonal selection theory (Cohen and Young, 1991; Cohen, 1992a, 1992b, 2000). As the word "cognitive" implies, he views the immune system as an information-processing system comparable to the central nervous system. A cognitive system extracts information and transforms it into an effective means of coping with the external world using already accumulated information and experience. This cognitive system must know what it is supposed to be looking for and in what context it is supposed to react and must be internally equipped with the information corresponding to the external world in advance. This is reminiscent of Jerne's "internal image" (Jerne, 1974). While we may see intentionality in the cognitive paradigm, it does not imply the involvement of anything like human consciousness, and clearly denies the consciousness of lymphocytes, insects, or plants (Cohen, 1992a). This issue will be discussed in detail in Chapters 4 and 5.

1.7.4 CAROSSELA–PRADEU–VIVIER'S DISCONTINUITY THEORY

Thomas Pradeu (1978–) and Edgardo Carosella (1951–) proposed the hypothesis of continuity (Pradeu and Carosella, 2004, 2006). They criticized the concept of self and nonself and sought new conditions for what triggers the immune response. First, they took examples incompatible with the Burnetian view of discrimination of self and nonself. For example, as will be discussed in detail in Chapter 2, the autoimmunity phenomenon certainly exists. Autoantibodies are present in serum, and autoreactivity is a physiological requirement during T cell maturation. The process of self-tolerance, in which autoimmunity is suppressed, is not without error. Furthermore, nonself components such as the intestinal microbiota are present in an organism, and the mother accepts a fetus with gene products derived from the father that are foreign to her. Based on these discrepant results, Pradeu and Carosella noted the inadequacy of the self–nonself discrimination theory and determined a new condition of immunogenicity, proposing the theory of continuity.

What is important in this theory is the continuity in space and time within the body and the equilibrium state of the immune system. According to this theory, the immune system is activated only when it senses the disruption of this continuity by reacting with the antigenic difference. An important difference from the clonal selection theory is that activation occurs at the level of spatiotemporal continuity rather than at the level of self and nonself. The key factors influencing the initiation of an immune response are (1) the amount of antigen, (2) the degree of molecular difference from the antigens usually encountered, and (3) the speed at which new antigens appear (Pradeu and Carosella, 2006).

Pradeu and Eric Vivier (1964–) refined this theory and renamed it the discontinuity theory, postulating that immune responses are caused by antigen discontinuities (Pradeu et al., 2013). They postulated that an immune response is triggered by the appearance of molecular motifs that differ qualitatively and quantitatively from those the immune system had previously encountered regularly. This idea recalls the theory proposed by Donald Forsdyke in 1968 concerning the determination of self and nonself reactivity (Forsdyke, 1968). According to Forsdyke's theory, antigens of foreign nature are not always present, and their concentration is almost zero most of the time. In contrast, self-antigens are always present at a particular concentration. It is not the physicochemical properties of the antigen itself but the quantitative changes in time and space that trigger the immune system's response. In any case, the discontinuity theory divides reaction types into three categories. First, the sudden appearance of a structurally different motif triggers a strong immune response, and the disappearance of the antigen terminates it. Second, an unusual but persistent motif will first trigger an immune response but will subsequently lead to the termination of an immune response. Third, the slow appearance of a structurally different motif results in a limited response and leads to tolerance. In this model, immunogenicity depends on the antigen's presentation mode to the immune system but not on its physicochemical nature. Thus, whether an immune response will occur cannot be predicted solely by the nature of the antigen. Spatiotemporal and context-dependent factors always determine the initiation of the immune response. This theory is supported by the data on immune checkpoints in viral infections, cancers, and allergies (Pradeu and Vivier, 2016).

1.7.5 Approaches From a Biosemiotics Perspective

In the realm of the immune system, interactions are constantly taking place. Lymphocytes interact not only with antigens and with soluble factors, such as interleukins and chemokines, but also with other cells; T cells interact with B cells and APCs, and so forth. Such interactions often determine the fate of the cells involved. B cells interact with antigens via the B cell receptor, which has complementary structures for the antigen. In the case of the T cell receptor, the target molecule is a complex of an antigenic peptide and the MHC (see Section 1.5, Chapter 1). So-called lock-and-key mechanisms mediate interactions between immunocytes and interleukins or chemokines.

Immunologists frequently use anthropomorphic expressions. For example, lymphocytes "recognize" antigens or T cells are "educated" in the thymus, to name just a few. During those processes, the immune system interprets or deciphers information-bearing molecules. The terms such as "signal" and "information" are used daily in immunology today without being clearly defined. Biosemiotics sees the entity to be recognized as a "sign" and tries to understand biological processes by analyzing signs, meanings, and codes (Prodi, 1988; Kawade, 2006; Barbieri, 2008). The existence of the genetic code inspired the supposition that codes exist in nature, although it may not be a real code but a linguistic metaphor. Furthermore, many related questions can be raised from the perspective of biosemiotics, for example, whether meanings exist in nature. However, would immunology ever benefit from this kind of analysis?

In the early 1980s, Tomio Tada (1934–2010) used the term "immunosemiotics" as a discipline that could unravel the intricacies of communication between lymphocytes. He defined it as the study of the general principles underlying the structure of sign systems perceived by different cells of the immune machinery (Sercarz et al., 1988a). In 1984, the idea of organizing a meeting on this theme arose from a conversation among four immunologists: Eli Sercarz (1934–2009), Franco Celada (1931–), Avrion Mitchison (1928–2022), and Tomio Tada. These immunologists were influenced by Jerne's idiotypic network theory. A meeting on "The Semiotics of Cellular Communication in the Immune System" was held in 1986 at Il Ciocco, Italy (Sercarz et al., 1988b). The meeting aimed to broadly consider the problem of communication among lymphocytes by bringing together people in science and humanities. This meeting's organizers anticipated holding a series of meetings and even aspired to establish a new area of immunosemiotics. However, this anticipation was betrayed because they misunderstood the relation of science to the humanities. As Italian semiotician and novelist Umberto Eco (1932–2016), a participant at this meeting, aptly points out, while semiotics may merit from this type of interaction, it is doubtful that immunology gains from semiotics (Eco, 1988). A similar relationship can be observed between science and philosophy. In any event, the second meeting on this topic was never held.

Indeed, it is very difficult, if not impossible, to integrate the natural sciences with the humanities. The reason for this is that scientific research can be conducted without a background in the humanities, and many scientists avoid bringing philosophical elements into science because it appears that doing so is a condition for being a fine scientist. In such a situation, the natural science side will not accept the humanities unless the humanities offer suggestions that are actually useful to science. It is the scientific side that is narrowing its own field of knowledge. This is in contrast to the situation between different fields of science. Immunogenetics, for example, appeared as a new domain in the early 1970s, combining immunology and genetics. This area remains active even today because this was a combination of different disciplines in science. It is clearly different from a marriage between science and the humanities. However, if the knowledge derived from the natural sciences is always incomplete and reveals only part of the truth of nature, then the humanities, including philosophy, may have a critical role to play. The road to finding this role will be a tough one. However, I believe such integration will become increasingly important for a more complete understanding of nature, as this book demonstrates.

1.7.6 Philippe Kourilsky's Systems Approach

As we have already seen, there were virtually no attempts to understand the immune system as a whole after the collapse of the idiotypic network theory. I imagine this was due to the difficulty of such attempts and the increasing demand to seek what is useful in medicine in the short term. However, some researchers recognize the significance of theorizing to come to the whole, even if it fails. For example, in his recent book *The Game of Chance and Complexity: The New Science of Immunology* (Kourilsky, 2014b), Philippe Kourilsky (1942–), who was Director General of the Pasteur Institute and professor emeritus at the Collège de France, attempted to construct a holistic picture of immunity using existing scientific knowledge as a starting point. The basis of his book is a viewpoint that sees the biological defense system as having three devices for quality control, surveillance, and repair of abnormalities while differentiating "living" and "surviving" functions in the immune system. To survive, we must deal appropriately not only with pathogens and natural physical influences but also with internal enemies—abnormalities in the structure and function of cells, proteins, and genes that cause autoimmune diseases, cancer, neurodegenerative diseases, and so on. Predicting when and where encounters with pathogens and internal abnormalities occur is impossible since they are governed by chance. The biological defense system that fights against external and internal disturbances is complex, and creating such an apparatus is also subject to chance. Mistakes made by seemingly inconvenient coincidences drive evolution, giving rise to creativity in living organisms.

Kourilsky proceeded to analyze the complexity of biological defense systems using the concepts of modularity and robustness, which are used in engineering. Modularity refers to the ability of a system to organize modules, which are reasonable units of the elements (molecules and cells) that comprise an organism. Specifically, he defined about 20 modules, including inflammatory modules (A), modules characteristic of acquired immunity (B), and transversal modules (C), and attempted to gain a fuller picture of the system by identifying the rules between them. The inflammatory module included traumatic inflammation (A1), immediate local inflammation (A2), T cell-assisted inflammation (A3), and immediate hypersensitivity inflammation (A4). The acquired immunity module included natural antibodies (B1), T cell-independent antibody production (B2), T cell activation by APCs (B3), T cell-dependent antibody production (B4), production of specific CTLs (B5), and regulation by Treg cells (B6). The transversal modules included cytokines (C1), chemokines (C2), small inflammatory molecules (C3), neuroendocrine mediators (C4), natural killer (NK) cells or killer lymphocytes in innate immunity (C5), antibody-armed cells (C6), innate memory (C7), and acquired memory (C8) among others. He then attempted to examine which modules each immune response uses. Robustness is the ability to function properly even when disturbed by internal and external events detrimental to the organism and governed by chance. Kourilsky sees the biological defense system, the key to survival, as a manifestation of robustness.

His approach was more an attempt to theoretically explain the details that occur within the framework of the immune system as it has been understood, rather than attempting to force a modification of the framework itself. Kourilsky believes that such an attempt would not reach the level of the whole organism, and he is probably right. Nevertheless, he believes that more attempts should be made at all levels to explain the whole phenomenon of immunity. It could be the whole from a historical, philosophical, or metaphysical perspective, not just a scientific one. All of these, one imagines, would lead to a richer understanding of the phenomenon of immunity.

1.8 THAT WHICH CREATES NEW THEORETICAL FRAMEWORKS

We have seen that various hypotheses have been proposed to understand immunological phenomena. Some did not explain immunity correctly, but were the attempts to propose hypotheses in vain? Of course, it would be better if the hypothesis was correct, but proposing a hypothesis or theory may give ongoing science time to pause and think, which may give life to science. Polly Matzinger, who proposed the danger theory, sees the problem as follows: the value of presenting a hypothesis is not that it will be correct—if it is wrong, someone will correct it—but that it will generate debate, and the phenomenon will be better understood. It is the activity of science, and such scientists contribute to science (Cooper, 1997). Hans Selye (1907–1982), a proponent of stress theory who will appear in Chapter 3, takes a similar position. Peter Galison (1955–), a science historian at Harvard University, believes that rather than placing falsifiability or proof at the center of the debate, the contribution of a hypothesis or theory should be measured by whether or not it has led to a new direction or has shown a connection with other fields. In other words, hypotheses should be evaluated not by their success or failure, but by the magnitude of their impact on the discipline (Galison, 2007). If we take these views, when Jerne's theory was dominating the world, there were frequent exchanges between different disciplines that had been forgotten, and beyond immunology, it influenced neuroscience, linguistics, and philosophy. Some people are still developing speculations based on this theory, even though it has lost its legitimacy in immunology. Given these facts, we must admit that these attempts had a certain significance.

Notably, the scientists who appeared in this Chapter have one thing in common: they were not initiated in immunology. Immunology is a new discipline, and the first professional journal in the United States (the *Journal of Immunology*) was first published in 1916, but the journal of the European Federation of Immunological Societies (the *European Journal of Immunology*) in 1971, and the Japanese Society for Immunology's journal (*International Immunology*) in 1989. When I started my research in Japan in the early 1970s, almost no university departments called themselves immunology, and most research was conducted in laboratories in internal medicine, pediatrics, pathology, biochemistry, bacteriology, and microbiology, among others. Therefore, it was obvious in the case of those before immunology was established but this characteristic can be seen in researchers who emerged after immunology was established. Not only in immunology but also in other fields, researchers usually start their careers in a specific laboratory and develop their research in their own laboratory while inheriting the research done in their initial laboratory. In doing so, they often accept the assumptions made there as given, forgetting that they are tentative and subject to renewal. Humans always think elsewhere. To think about something or to come to the truth, one must physically—or at least mentally—leave the place.

Paul Ehrlich, who advocated the first integrative side-chain theory, began his research with histology and hematology. Karl Landsteiner was well-versed in chemistry. Linus Pauling consciously tried to apply his own specialty, chemistry, to solving the mysteries of immunity. Niels Jerne studied physics at the University of Leiden and then received his medical education at the University of Copenhagen. He became familiar with the philosophy of Søren Kierkegaard (1813–1955), Friedrich Nietzsche (1844–1900), and Henri Bergson (1859–1941), and seems to have loved André Gide (1869–1951) and Marcel Proust (1871–1922) in literature. Macfarlane Burnet's specialty was virology. Peter Bretscher, who proposed the two-signal model, was a graduate student in X-ray crystallography at the Institute of Molecular Biology in Cambridge, England, when he met Sydney Brenner (1927–2009; Nobel Prize in Physiology or Medicine 2002), César Milstein, and Francis Crick (1916–2004; Nobel Prize in Physiology or Medicine 1962). He recalls that he became interested in immunology through contact with these people (Bretscher, 2019). Irun Cohen had done philosophy before entering medicine. Jules Hoffman, who paved the way for innate immunity, went from studying hormones in the development and reproduction of the grasshopper to immunological studies of *Drosophila melanogaster*. Ruslan Medzhitov, born in Tashkent, Uzbekistan, studied science at a local university and earned a degree in biochemistry at Moscow State University before heading to the United States. He studied biochemistry at the University of California, San Diego, before beginning a post-doctoral fellowship at Yale University in Charles Janeway's laboratory. Susumu Tonegawa went from molecular biology and Tasuku Honjo from biochemistry to immunology. James Allison seemed to consider himself an outsider (Dreifus, 2020). Notably, Polly Matzinger was not even a researcher. After working in various jobs, including as a bunny girl at a Playboy Club, professors at the University of California, Davis, discovered her talent as a scientist while waitressing in California (Dreifus, 1998).

They could have looked at immunology from the outside. Being outside would have enabled them not only to see the subject as something unusual and interesting but also to direct their gaze toward the subject as a whole. In some sense, critical and philosophical thinking was likely at work. In his provocative article "How to defend society against science," the philosopher of science Paul Feyerabend (1924–1994) said the following:

> The progress of science, of good science, depends on novel ideas and on intellectual freedom: science has very often been advanced by outsiders (remember that Bohr and Einstein regarded themselves as outsiders).

Feyerabend (1975)

Melvin Cohn, who proposed the two-signal model 30 years ago, made the following harsh criticism of the tendency to emphasize pragmatism and neglect theoretical research:

> The institutional environment does not value, much less reward, such efforts [the search for universal principles]. [...] No wonder that, despite their interdependence, they have come to award prizes for purely technical rather than conceptual achievements. [...] The tragedy is that we no longer revere understanding as the goal of science.

Cohn (1989b)

Behind these trends, an increasingly radical and expansive economic logic is seething, and a situation seems to be unfolding right now that is incomparable to what it was 30 years ago. As Philippe Kourilsky noted, science has developed based on what might be called a figment of the imagination (Kourilsky, 2014a). While unfortunately never confirmed, the idiotypic network theory shows traces of Niels Jerne's extraordinary imagination. Shouldn't we be more tolerant of attempts at holistic explanations that are often viewed coldly by scientists in the field who only want hard data on local events?

NOTE

1 Badiou, A. (2010). *Beyond positivism and nihilism*: Lecture at the European Graduate School. http://www.youtube.com/watch?v=i_kvL1Sg6ms&feature=plcp.

REFERENCES

Alexander, J. (1932). Some intracellular aspects of life and disease. *Protoplasma, 14*, 296–306. doi: 10.1007/BF01604907.

Anderson, K. V., Bokla, L., & Nüsslein-Volhard, C. (1985). Establishment of dorsal-ventral polarity in the drosophila embryo: The induction of polarity by the *Toll* gene product. *Cell, 42*, 791–798. doi: 10.1016/0092-8674(85)90275-2.

Aristotle. (1909). *The Rhetoric of Aristotle*. (R. C. Jebb, Trans.). Cambridge University Press. 149–159.

Ausubel, F. M. (2005). Are innate immune signaling pathways in plants and animals conserved? *Nature Immunology, 6*, 973–979. doi: 10.1038/ni1253.

Barbieri, M. (2008). Biosemiotics: A new understanding of life. *Naturwissenschaften, 95*, 577–599. doi: 10.1007/s00114-008-0368-x.

Bjorkman, P. J., Saper, M. A., Samraoui, B., Bennett, W. S., Strominger, J. L., & Wiley, D. C. (1987). Structure of the human class I histocompatibility antigen, HLA-A2. *Nature, 329*, 506–512. doi: 10.1038/329506a0.

Boller, T., & Felix, G. (2009). A renaissance of elicitors: Perception of microbe-associated molecular patterns and danger signals by pattern-recognition receptors. *Annual Review of Plant Biology, 60*, 379–406. doi: 10.1146/annurev.arplant.57.032905.105346.

Boyse, E. A. (1986). Working with Gorer, 1957-1960. *Immunogenetics, 24*, 350–351. doi: 10.1007/BF00377951.

Breinl, F., & Haurowitz, F. (1930). Chemische untersuchung des präzipitates aus hämoglobin und anti-hämoglobin-serum und bemerkungen über die natur der antikörper (Chemical examination of the precipitates from hemoglobin and anti-hemoglobin serum and observations on the nature of the antibodies). *Zeitschrift für Physiologische Chemie, 192*, 45–47.

Brenner, M. B., Trowbridge, I. S., & Strominger, J. L. (1985). Crosslinking of human T cell receptor proteins: Association between the T cell idiotype beta subunit and the T3 glycoprotein heavy subunit. *Cell, 40*, 183–190. doi: 10.1016/0092-8674(85)90321-6.

Bretscher, P., & Cohn, M. (1970). A theory of self-nonself discrimination. Paralysis and induction involve the recognition of one and two determinants on an antigen, respectively. *Science, 169*, 1042–1049. doi: 10.1126/science.169.3950.1042.

Bretscher, P. A. (2019). The history of the two-signal model of lymphocyte activation: A personal perspective. *Scandinavian Journal of Immunology, 89*, e12762. doi: 10.1111/sji.12762.

Bretscher, P. A., & Cohn, M. (1968). Minimal model for the mechanism of antibody induction and paralysis by antigen. *Nature, 220*, 444–448. doi: 10.1038/220444a0.

Bruton, O. C. (1952). Agammaglobulinemia. *Pediatrics, 9*, 722–728. doi: 10.1542/peds.9.6.722.

Burnet, F. M. (1941). *The Production of Antibodies.* Macmillan.

Burnet, F. M. (1957). A modification of Jerne's theory of antibody production using the concept of clonal selection. *Australian Journal of Science, 20*, 67–69. doi: 10.3322/canjclin.26.2.119.

Burnet, F. M. (1959). *The Clonal Selection Theory of Acquired Immunity.* Cambridge University Press.

Burnet, F. M. (1961). Immunological recognition of self. *Science, 133*, 307–311. doi: 10.1126/science.133.3449.307.

Burnet, F. M. (1967). The impact of ideas on immunology. *Cold Spring Harbor Symposia on Quantitative Biology, 32*, 1–8. doi: 10.1101/SQB.1967.032.01.005.

Burnet, F. M. (1969). *Self and Not-Self.* Cambridge University Press.

Burnet, F. M., & Fenner, F. (1949). *The Production of Antibodies.* (Second Ed.). Macmillan.

Chase, M. W. (1945). The cellular transfer of cutaneous hypersensitivity to tuberculin. *Proceedings of the Society for Experimental Biology and Medicine, 59*, 134–135. doi: 10.3181/00379727-59-15006P.

Chen, G. Y., & Nuñez, G. (2010). Sterile inflammation: Sensing and reacting to damage. *Nature Reviews Immunology, 10*, 826–837. doi: 10.1038/nri2873.

Chernyak, L., & Tauber, A. I. (1988). The birth of immunology: Metchnikoff, the embryologist. *Cellular Immunology, 117*, 218–233. doi: 10.1016/0008-8749(88)90090-1.

Cirl, C., Wieser, A., Yadav, M., Duerr, S., Schubert, S., Fischer, H., Stappert, D., Wantia, N., Rodriguez, N., Wagner, H., Svanborg, C., & Miethke, T. (2008). Subversion of Toll-like receptor signaling by a unique family of bacterial Toll/interleukin-1 receptor domain-containing proteins. *Nature Medicine, 14*, 399–406. doi: 10.1038/nm1734.

Claman, H. N., Chaperon, E. A., & Triplett, R. F. (1966). Thymus-marrow cell combinations. Synergism in antibody production. *Proceedings of the Society for Experimental Biology and Medicine, 122*, 1167–1171. doi: 10.3181/00379727-122-31353.

Cohen, E. (2009). *A Body Worth Defending: Immunity, Biopolitics, and the Apotheosis of the Modern Body.* Duke University Press. 1–7.

Cohen, I. R. (1992a). The cognitive paradigm and the immunological homunculus. *Immunology Today, 13*, 490–494. doi: 10.1016/0167-5699(92)90024-2.

Cohen, I. R. (1992b). The cognitive principal challenges clonal selection. *Immunology Today, 13*, 441–444. doi: 10.1016/0167-5699(92)90071-E.

Cohen, I. R. (2000). *Tending Adam's Garden: Evolving the Cognitive Immune Self.* Academic Press.

Cohen, I. R., & Young, D. B. (1991). Autoimmunity, microbial immunity and the immunological homunculus. *Immunology Today, 12*, 105–110. doi: 10.1016/0167-5699(91)90093-9.

Cohn, M. (1981). Conversations with Niels Kaj Jerne on immune regulation: Associative versus network recognition. *Cellular Immunology, 61*, 425–436. doi: 10.1016/0008-8749(81)90390-7.

Cohn, M. (1989a). Forward: Clippings from one immunologist's journal. (R. E. Langman, Ed.). *The Immune System. Evolutionary Principles Guide Our Understanding of This Complex Biological Defense System.* Academic Press. xxxvii.

Cohn, M. (1989b). Forward: Clippings from one immunologist's journal. (R. E. Langman, Ed.). *The Immune System. Evolutionary Principles Guide Our Understanding of This Complex Biological Defense System.* Academic Press. xlv–xlvi.

Cohn, M., Mitchison, N. A., Paul, W. E., Silverstein, A. M., Talmage, D. W., & Weigert, M. (2007). Reflections on the clonal-selection theory. *Nature Reviews Immunology, 7*, 823–830. doi: 10.1038/nri2177.

Cooper, G. (1997). Clever Bunny. *The Independent.* https://www.independent.co.uk/life-style/clever-bunny-1267594.html.

Cooper, M. D., Peterson, R. D. A., & Good, R. A. (1965). Delineation of the thymic and bursal lymphoid systems in the chicken. *Nature, 205*, 143–146. doi: 10.1038/205143a0.

Darwin, C. (1859). *On the Origin of Species by Means of Natural Selection, or the Preservation of Favoured Races in the Struggle for Life.* John Murray.

Darwin, C., & Wallace, A. (1858). On the tendency of species to form varieties; and on the perpetuation of varieties and species by natural means of selection. *Journal of the Proceedings of the Linnean Society of London. Zoology, 3*, 45–62. doi: 10.1111/j.1096-3642.1858.tb02500.x.

de la Chapelle, A., Herva, R., Koivisto, M., & Aula, P. (1981). A deletion in chromosome 22 can cause DiGeorge syndrome. *Human Genetics, 57*, 253–256. doi: 10.1007/BF00278938.

DiGeorge, A. M. (1968). Congenital absence of the thymus and its immunologic consequences: Concurrence with congenital hypoparathyroidism. *Birth Defects Original Article Series, 4*, 116–121.

Dreifus, C. (1998, June 16). A conversation with Polly Matzinger; Blazing an unconventional trail to a new theory of immunity. *The New York Times.* https://www.nytimes.com/1998/06/16/science/conversation-with-polly-matzinger-blazing-unconventional-trail-new-theory.html.

Dreifus, C. (2020). The contrarian who cures cancers. *Quanta Magazine.* https://www.quantamagazine.org/the-contrarian-who-cures-cancers-20200203/#:~:text=James%20P.,of%20cancer%20survivors%20vindicate%20him.

Eco, U. (1988). On semiotics and immunology. (E. E. Sercarz, F. Celada, N. A. Mitchison, & T. Tada, Eds.). *The Semiotics of Cellular Communication in the Immune System.* Springer-Verlag. 3–15.

Edelman, G. M. (1959). Dissociation of γ-globulin. *Journal of the American Chemical Society, 81*, 3155–3156. doi: 10.1021/ja01521a071.

Edelman, G. M., & Poulik, M. D. (1961). Studies on structural units of the γ-globulins. *Journal of Experimental Medicine, 113*, 861–884. doi: 10.1084/jem.113.5.861.

Ehrlich, P. (1900). Croonian lecture. On immunity with special reference to cell life. *Proceedings of the Royal Society of London, 66*, 424–448. doi: 10.1098/rspl.1899.0121.

Eichmann, K. (2008a). *The Network Collective: Rise and Fall of a Scientific Paradigm.* Birkhäuser Verlag AG. 142.

Eichmann, K. (2008b). *The Network Collective: Rise and Fall of a Scientific Paradigm.* Birkhäuser Verlag AG. 1–274.

Einstein, A. (1992). Create. (T. Kaneko, Ed.). *Einstein Documents: I Want to Solve God's Puzzle.* (J. Tanaka, Trans.). Tetsugaku Shobo. 44–45.

Einstein, A. (2005). *The New Quotable Einstein.* Princeton University Press. 230.

Esposito, R. (2011). *Immunitas: The Protection and Negation of Life.* Polity. 5–6.

Feyerabend, P. (1975). How to defend society against science. *Radical Philosophy, 11*, 8.

Fleck, L. (1935). *Entstehung und Entwicklung einer wissenschaftlichen Tatsache. Einführung in die Lehre vom Denkstil und Denkkollektiv (Origin and Development of a Scientific Fact. Introduction to the Doctrine of Thought Style and Thought Collective).* Schwabe AG.

Fleck, L. (1979a). *Genesis and Development of a Scientific Fact.* (F. Bradley & T. J. Trenn, Trans.). University of Chicago Press. (Originally published 1935). 21.

Fleck, L. (1979b). *Genesis and Development of a Scientific Fact.* (F. Bradley & T. J. Trenn, Trans.). University of Chicago Press. (Originally published 1935). 1–203.

Forsdyke, D. R. (1968). The liquid scintillation counter as an analogy for the distinction between "self" and "non-self" in immunological systems. *Lancet, 291*, 281–283. doi: 10.1016/S0140-6736(68)90126-8.

Forsdyke, D. R. (1995). The origins of the clonal selection theory of immunity. *FASEB Journal, 9*, 164–166. doi: 10.1096/fasebj.9.2.7781918.

Galison, P. (2007). Sur quels critères juger une Théorie? (What are the criteria for judging a theory?) *La Recherche, 411*, 42.

Glick, B., Chang, T. S., & Jaap, G. (1956). The bursa of Fabricius and antibody production. *Poultry Science, 35*, 224–225. doi: 10.3382/ps.0350224.

Gorer, P. A. (1936). The detection of antigenic differences in mouse erythrocytes by the employment of immune sera. *British Journal of Experimental Pathology, 17*, 42–50.

Gorer, P. A. (1937). The genetic and antigenic basis of tumour transplantation. *Journal of Pathology and Bacteriology, 44*, 691–697. doi: 10.1002/path.1700440313.

Gourbal, B., Pinaud, S., Beckers, G. J. M., Van Der Meer, J. W. M., Conrath, U., & Netea, M. G. (2018). Innate immune memory: An evolutionary perspective. *Immunological Reviews, 283*, 21–40. doi: 10.1111/imr.12647.

Hansson, G. K., & Edfeldt, K. (2005). Toll to be paid at the gateway to the vessel wall. *Arteriosclerosis, Thrombosis, and Vascular Biology, 25*, 1085–1087. doi: 10.1161/01.ATV.0000168894.43759.47.

Hashimoto, C., Hudson, K. L., & Anderson, K. V. (1988). The *Toll* gene of Drosophila, required for dorsal-ventral embryonic polarity, appears to encode a transmembrane protein. *Cell, 52*, 269–279. doi: 10.1016/0092-8674(88)90516-8.

Hedrick, S. M., Cohen, D. I., Nielsen, E. A., & Davis, M. M. (1984). Isolation of cDNA clones encoding T cell-specific membrane-associated proteins. *Nature, 308,* 149–153. doi: 10.1038/308149a0.

Hodgkin, P. D., Heath, W. R., & Baxter, A. G. (2007). The clonal selection theory: 50 years since the revolution. *Nature Immunology, 8,* 1019–1026. doi: 10.1038/ni1007-1019.

Hombach, J., Tsubata, T., Leclercq, L., Stappert, H., & Reth, M. (1990). Molecular components of the B-cell antigen receptor complex of the IgM class. *Nature, 343,* 760–762. doi: 10.1038/343760a0.

Hozumi, N., & Tonegawa, S. (1976). Evidence for somatic rearrangement of immunoglobulin genes coding for variable and constant regions. *Proceedings of the National Academy of Sciences of the United States of America, 73,* 3628–3632. doi: 10.1073/pnas.73.10.3628.

Iwai, Y., Ishida, M., Tanaka, Y., Okazaki, T., Honjo, T., & Minato, N. (2002). Involvement of PD-L1 on tumor cells in the escape from host immune system and tumor immunotherapy by PD-L1 blockade. *Proceedings of the National Academy of Sciences of the United States of America, 99,* 12293–12297. doi: 10.1073/pnas.192461099.

Jacob, F. (1977). Evolution and tinkering. *Science, 196,* 1161–1166. doi: 10.1126/science.86013.

Janeway, C. A., Jr. (1989). Approaching the asymptote? Evolution and revolution in immunology. *Cold Spring Harbor Symposia on Quantitative Biology, 54,* 1–13. doi: 10.1101/sqb.1989.054.01.003.

Janeway, C. A., Jr. (1992). The immune system evolved to discriminate infectious nonself from noninfectious self. *Immunology Today, 13,* 11–16. doi: 10.1016/0167-5699(92)90198-G.

Janeway, C. A., Jr., & Medzhitov, R. (2002). Innate immune recognition. *Annual Review of Immunology, 20,* 197–216. doi: 10.1146/annurev.immunol.20.083001.084359.

Jenkins, M. K., & Schwartz, R. H. (1987). Antigen presentation by chemically modified splenocytes induces antigen-specific T cell unresponsiveness in vitro and in vivo. *Journal of Experimental Medicine, 165,* 302–319. doi: 10.1084/jem.165.2.302.

Jenner, E. (1798). *An Inquiry into the Causes and Effects of the Variolae Vaccinae: A Disease Discovered in Some of the Western Counties of England, Particularly Gloucestershire, and Known by the Name of the Cow Pox.* Sampson Law.

Jerne, N. K. (1955). The natural-selection theory of antibody formation. *Proceedings of the National Academy of Sciences of the United States of America, 41,* 849–857. doi: 10.1073/pnas.41.11.849.

Jerne, N. K. (1974). Toward a network theory of the immune system. *Annales d'Immunologie, 125C,* 373–389.

Katz, D. H., Hamaoka, T., & Benacerraf, B. (1973). Cell interactions between histoincompatible T and B lymphocytes. II. Failure of physiologic cooperative interactions between T and B lymphocytes from allogeneic donor strains in humoral response to hapten-protein conjugates. *Journal of Experimental Medicine, 137,* 1405–1418. doi: 10.1084/jem.137.6.1405.

Kawade, Y. (2006). *Biosemiotics: The Biology of Subjectivity.* Kyoto University Press.

Kelley, R. I., Zackai, E. H., Emanuel, B. S., Kistenmacher, M., Greenberg, F., & Punnett, H. H. (1982). The association of the DiGeorge anomalad with partial monosomy of chromosome 22. *Journal of Pediatrics, 101,* 197–200. doi: 10.1016/s0022-3476(82)80116-9.

Kindred, B., & Schreffler, D. C. (1972). H-2 dependence of co-operation between T and B cells in vivo. *Journal of Immunology, 109,* 940–943. doi: 10.4049/jimmunol.109.5.940.

Klein, J. (1982). *Immunology: The Science of Self-Nonself Discrimination.* Wiley.

Klein, J. (1986). Seeds of time: Fifty years ago Peter A. Gorer discovered the H-2 complex. *Immunogenetics, 24,* 331–338. doi: 10.1007/BF00377947.

Kourilsky, P. (2014a). *Le Jeu du hasard et de la complexité: La nouvelle science de l'immunologie (The Game of Chance and Complexity: The New Science of Immunology).* Odile Jacob. 109.

Kourilsky, P. (2014b). *Le Jeu du hasard et de la complexité: La nouvelle science de l'immunologie (The Game of Chance and Complexity: The New Science of Immunology).* Odile Jacob.

Kuhn, T. S. (1962). *The Structure of Scientific Revolutions.* University of Chicago Press. xli.

Kuhn, T. S. (1993). Metaphor in science. (A. Ortony, Ed.) *Metaphor and Thought.* Cambridge University Press. 533–542.

Kunkel, H. G., Mannik, M., & Williams, R. C. (1963). Individual antigenic specificity of isolated antibodies. *Science, 140,* 1218–1219. doi: 10.1126/science.140.3572.1218.

Lafferty, K. J., & Cunningham, A. J. (1975). A new analysis of allogeneic interactions. *Australian Journal of Experimental Biology & Medical Science, 53,* 27–42. doi: 10.1038/icb.1975.3.

Lafferty, K. J., & Jones, M. A. (1969). Reactions of the graft versus host (GVH) type. *Australian Journal of Experimental Biology & Medical Science, 47,* 17–54. doi: 10.1038/icb.1969.3.

Lafferty, K. J., Warren, H. S., Woolnough, J. A., & Talmage, D. W. (1978). Immunological induction of T lymphocytes: Role of antigen and the lymphocyte costimulator. *Blood Cells, 4,* 395–406.

Landsteiner, K. (1936). *The Specificity of Serological Reactions.* Charles C. Thomas.

Landsteiner, K., & Chase, M. W. (1942). Experiments on transfer of cutaneous sensitivity to simple compounds. *Proceedings of the Society for Experimental Biology and Medicine, 49*, 688–690. doi: 10.3181/00379727-49-13670.

Lau, C. M., & Sun, J. C. (2018). The widening spectrum of immunological memory. *Current Opinion in Immunology, 54*, 42–49. doi: 10.1016/j.coi.2018.05.013.

Leach, D. R., Krummel, M. F., & Allison, J. P. (1996). Enhancement of antitumor immunity by CTLA-4 blockade. *Science, 271*, 1734–1736. doi: 10.1126/science.271.5256.1734.

Leclerc, J. C., Gomard, E., & Levy, J. P. (1972). Cell-mediated reaction against tumors induced by oncornaviruses. I. Kinetics and specificity of the immune response in murine sarcoma virus (MSV)-induced tumors and transplanted lymphomas. *International Journal of Cancer, 10*, 589–601. doi: 10.1002/ijc.2910100318.

Lederberg, J. (1959). Genes and antibodies: Do antigens bear instructions for antibody specificity or do they select cell lines that arise by mutation? *Science, 129*, 1649–1653. doi: 10.1126/science.129.3364.1649.

Lemaitre, B., Nicolas, E., Michaut, L., Reichart, J. M., & Hoffmann, J. A. (1996). The dorsoventral regulatory gene cassette *spätzle/Toll/cactus* controls the potent antifungal response in Drosophila adults. *Cell, 86*, 973–983. doi: 10.1016/s0092-8674(00)80172-5.

Locke, J. (1825). *An Essay Concerning Human Understanding*. Thomas Tegg. (Originally published 1689). 372–373.

Matzinger, P. (1994). Tolerance, danger, and the extended family. *Annual Review of Immunology, 12*, 991–1045. doi: 10.1146/annurev.iy.12.040194.005015.

Matzinger, P. (1998). An innate sense of danger. *Seminars in Immunology, 10*, 399–415. doi: 10.1006/smim.1998.0143.

Matzinger, P. (2002). The danger model: A renewed sense of self. *Science, 296*, 301–305. doi: 10.1126/science.1071059.

Matzinger, P. (2007). Friendly and dangerous signals: Is the tissue in control? *Nature Immunology, 8*, 11-13. doi: 10.1038/ni0107-11.

Medzhitov, R., & Janeway, C. A., Jr. (2002). Decoding the patterns of self and nonself by the innate immune system. *Science, 296*, 298–300. doi: 10.1126/science.1068883.

Medzhitov, R., Preston-Hurlburt, P., & Janeway, C. A., Jr. (1997). A human homologue of the *Drosophila* Toll protein signals activation of adaptive immunity. *Nature, 388*, 394–397. doi: 10.1038/41131.

Metchnikoff, E. (1883). Untersuchungen über die intracelluläre Verdauung bei wirbellosen Thieren (Research on the intracellular digestion of invertebrates). *Arbeiten aus den Zoologischen Instituten der Universität Wien und der Zoologischen Station in Triest, 5*, 141–168.

Metchnikoff, O. (1921). *Life of Elie Metchnikoff, 1845–1916*. Constable. 116–117.

Miller, J. F. A. P. (1961). Immunological function of the thymus. *Lancet, 278*, 748–749. doi: 10.1016/s0140-6736(61)90693-6.

Miller, J. F. A. P., & Mitchell, G. F. (1968). Cell to cell interaction in the immune response. I. Hemolysin-forming cells in neonatally thymectomized mice reconstituted with thymus or thoracic duct lymphocytes. *Journal of Experimental Medicine, 128*, 801–820. doi: 10.1084/jem.128.4.801.

Mitchell, G. F., & Miller, J. F. A. P. (1968a). Cell to cell interaction in the immune response. II. The source of hemolysin-forming cells in irradiated mice given bone marrow and thymus or thoracic duct lymphocytes. *Journal of Experimental Medicine, 128*, 821–837. doi: 10.1084/jem.128.4.821.

Mitchell, G. F., & Miller, J. F. A. P. (1968b). Immunological activity of the thymus and thoracic-duct lymphocytes. *Proceedings of the National Academy of Sciences of the United States of America, 59*, 296–303. doi: 10.1073/pnas.59.1.296.

Moulin, A. M. (1983a). De l'analyse au système: le développement de l'Immunologie (From analysis to system: Development of immunology). *Revue d'histoire des sciences, 36*, 53.

Moulin, A. M. (1983b). De l'analyse au système: le développement de l'Immunologie (From analysis to system: Development of immunology). *Revue d'histoire des sciences, 36*, 49–67.

Moulin, A. M. (1991a). *Le dernier langage de la médecine: Histoire de l'immunologie de Pasteur au Sida (The Last Language of Medicine: History of Immunology from Pasteur to AIDS)*. Presses Universitaires de France. 288.

Moulin, A. M. (1991b). *Le dernier langage de la médecine: Histoire de l'immunologie de Pasteur au Sida (The Last Language of Medicine: History of Immunology from Pasteur to AIDS)*. Presses Universitaires de France. 271.

Moulin, A. M. (1991c). *Le dernier langage de la médecine: Histoire de l'immunologie de Pasteur au Sida (The Last Language of Medicine: History of Immunology from Pasteur to AIDS)*. Presses Universitaires de France. 366–369.

Mudd, S. (1932). A hypothetical mechanism of antibody formation. *Journal of Immunology, 23*, 423–427. doi: 10.4049/jimmunol.23.6.423.

Nossal, G. J. V. (1995). Choices following antigen entry: Antibody formation or immunological tolerance? *Annual Review of Immunology, 13*, 1–27. doi: 10.1146/annurev.iy.13.040195.000245.

Nossal, G. J. V., Cunningham, A., Mitchell, G. F., & Miller, J. F. (1968). Cell to cell interaction in the immune response. III. Chromosomal marker analysis of single antibody-forming cells in reconstituted, irradiated, or thymectomized mice. *Journal of Experimental Medicine, 128*, 839–853. doi: 10.1084/jem.128.4.839.

Nossal, G. J. V., & Pike, B. L. (1980). Clonal anergy: persistence in tolerant mice of antigen-binding B lymphocytes incapable of responding to antigen or mitogen. *Proceedings of the National Academy of Sciences of the United States of America, 77*, 1602–1606. doi: 10.1073/pnas.77.3.1602.

Notarangelo, L. D., Bacchetta, R., Casanova, J. L., & Su, H. C. (2020). Human inborn errors of immunity: An expanding universe. *Science Immunology, 5*, eabb1662. doi: 10.1126/sciimmunol.abb1662.

Oldstone, M. B. A., Dixon, F. J., Mitchell, G. F., & McDevitt, H. O. (1973). Histocompatibility-linked genetic control of disease susceptibility. Murine lymphocytic choriomeningitis virus infection. *Journal of Experimental Medicine, 137*, 1201–1212. doi: 10.1084/jem.137.5.1201.

Oudin, J., & Michel, M. (1963). Une nouvelle forme d'allotypie des globulines γ du sérum de lapin, apparemment liée à la fonction et à la spécificité anticorps (A new form of allotypy of rabbit serum γ globulins, apparently related to antibody function and specificity). *Comptes Rendus Hebdomadaires des Séances de l'Acadéie des Sciences, 257*, 805–808.

Pauling, L. (1940). A theory of the structure and process of formation of antibodies. *Journal of American Chemical Society, 62*, 2643–2657. doi: 10.1021/ja01867a018.

Plato. (2009). *Phaedo*. Oxford University Press.

Porter, R. R. (1959). The hydrolysis of rabbit γ-globulin and antibodies with crystalline papaine. *Biochemical Journal, 73*, 119–126. doi: 10.1042/bj0730119.

Porter, R. R. (1963). Chemical structure of γ-globulin and antibodies. *British Medical Bulletin, 19*, 197–201. doi: 10.1093/oxfordjournals.bmb.a070056.

Pradeu, T., & Carosella, E. D. (2004). Analyse critique du modèle immunologique du soi et du non-soi et de ses fondements métaphysiques implicites (Critical analysis of the immunological model of self and nonself and its implicit metaphysical foundations). *Comptes Rendus Biologies, 327*, 481–492. doi: 10.1016/j.crvi.2004.04.003.

Pradeu, T., & Carosella, E. D. (2006). On the definition of a criterion of immunogenicity. *Proceedings of the National Academy of Sciences of the United States of America, 103*, 17858–17861. doi: 10.1073/pnas.0608683103.

Pradeu, T., Jaeger, S., & Vivier, E. (2013). The speed of change: Towards a discontinuity theory of immunity? *Nature Reviews Immunology, 13*, 764–769. doi: 10.1038/nri3521.

Pradeu, T., & Vivier, E. (2016). The discontinuity theory of immunity. *Science Immunology, 1*, aag0479. doi: 10.1126/sciimmunol.aag0479.

Prodi, G. (1988). Signs and codes in immunology. (E. E. Sercarz, F. Celada, N. A. Mitchison, & T. Tada, Eds.). *The Semiotics of Cellular Communication in the Immune System*. Springer-Verlag. 53–64.

Ribatti, D., Crivellato, E., & Vacca, A. (2006). The contribution of Bruce Glick to the definition of the role played by the bursa of Fabricius in the development of the B cell lineage. *Clinical and Experimental Immunology, 145*, 1–4. doi: 10.1111/j.1365-2249.2006.03131.x.

Rimer, J., Cohen, I. R., & Friedman, N. (2014). Do all creatures possess an acquired immune system of some sort? *Bioessays, 36*, 273–281. doi: 10.1002/bies.201300124.

Söderqvist, T. (2003a). *Science as Autobiography: The Troubled Life of Niels Jerne*. Yale University Press. 1–359.

Söderqvist, T. (2003b). *Science as Autobiography: The Troubled Life of Niels Jerne*. Yale University Press. 75–87.

Samelson, L. E., Harford, J. B., & Klausner, R. D. (1985). Identification of the components of the murine T cell antigen receptor complex. *Cell, 43*, 223–231. doi: 10.1016/0092-8674(85)90027-3.

Sender, R., Fuchs, S., & Milo, R. (2016). Are we really vastly outnumbered? Revisiting the ratio of bacterial to host cells in humans. *Cell, 164*, 337–340. doi: 10.1016/j.cell.2016.01.013.

Seong, S.-Y., & Matzinger, P. (2004). Hydrophobicity: An ancient damage-associated molecular pattern that initiates innate immune responses. *Nature Reviews Immunology, 4*, 469–478. doi: 10.1038/nri1372.

Sercarz, E. E., Celada, F., Mitchison, N. A., & Tada, T. (1988a). Editors' preface. (E. E. Sercarz, F. Celada, N. A. Mitchison, & T. Tada, Eds.). *The Semiotics of Cellular Communication in the Immune System*. Springer-Verlag. V–VIII.

Sercarz, E. E., Celada, F., Mitchison, N. A., & Tada, T. (Eds.) (1988b). *The Semiotics of Cellular Communication in the Immune System*. Springer-Verlag.

Silverstein, A. M. (1989a). *A History of Immunology*. Academic Press. 79.

Silverstein, A. M. (1989b). Background to the conflict. International politics. *A History of Immunology*. Academic Press. 44–46.

Silverstein, A. M. (1989c). *A History of Immunology*. Academic Press. 1–422.

Talmage, D. W. (1957). Allergy and immunology. *Annual Review of Medicine, 8*, 239–256. doi: 10.1146/annurev.me.08.020157.001323.

Talmage, D. W. (1959). Immunological specificity. Unique combinations of selected natural globulins provide an alternative to the classical concept. *Science, 129*, 1643–1648. doi: 10.1126/science.129.3364.1643.

Tauber, A. I. (1992). The birth of immunology. III. The fate of the phagocytosis theory. *Cellular Immunology, 139*, 505–530. doi: 10.1016/0008-8749(92)90089-8.

Taylor, R. L., Jr., & McCorkle, F. M., Jr. (2009). A landmark contribution to poultry science-Immunological function of the bursa of Fabricius. *Poultry Science, 88*, 816–823. doi: 10.3382/ps.2008-00528.

Thucydides. (1914a). *History of the Peloponnesian War*. (R. Crawley, Trans.). J. M. Dent & Sons. 132.

Thucydides. (1914b). *History of the Peloponnesian War*. (R. Crawley, Trans.). J. M. Dent & Sons. 1–614 (+ 5 pages of plans).

Tsukada, S., Saffran, D. C., Rawlings, D. J., Parolini, O., Allen, R. C., Klisak, I., Sparkes, R. S., Kubagawa, H., Mohandas, T., Quan, S., Belmont, J. W., Cooper, M. D., Conley, M. E., & Witte, O. N. (1993). Deficient expression of a B cell cytoplasmic tyrosine kinase in human X-linked agammaglobulinemia. *Cell, 72*, 279–290. doi: 10.1016/0092-8674(93)90667-f.

Vallery-Radot, R. (1919). *The Life of Pasteur*. (R. Devonshire, Trans.). Constable & Company. 332.

Vance, R. E. (2000). Cutting edge commentary: A Copernican revolution? Doubts about the danger theory. *Journal of Immunology, 165*, 1725–1728. doi: 10.4049/jimmunol.165.4.1725.

Vetrie, D., Vorechovský, I., Sideras, P., Holland, J., Davies, A., Flinter, F., Hammarström, L., Kinnon, C., Levinsky, R., Bobrow, M., Smith, C. I. E., & Bentley, D. R. (1993). The gene involved in X-linked agammaglobulinaemia is a member of the *src* family of protein-tyrosine kinases. *Nature, 361*, 226–233. doi: 10.1038/361226a0.

von Behring, E., & Kitasato, S. (1890). Über das Zustandekommen der Diphtherie-Immunität und der Tetanus-Immunität bei Thieren (On the establishment of diphtheria immunity and tetanus immunity in animals). *Deutsche Medizinische Wöchenschrift, 16*, 1113–1114. doi: 10.17192/eb2013.0164.

Watson, J. D., & Crick, F. H. C. (1953). Molecular structure of nucleic acids: A structure for deoxyribose nucleic acid. *Nature, 171*, 737–738. doi: 10.1038/171737a0.

Wiens, M., Korzhev, M., Perovic-Ottstadt, S., Luthringer, B., Brandt, D., Klein, S., & Müller, W. E. (2007). Toll-like receptors are part of the innate immune defense system of sponges (demospongiae: Porifera). *Molecular Biology and Evolution, 24*, 792–804. doi: 10.1093/molbev/msl208.

Wing, K., Onishi, Y., Prieto-Martin, P., Yamaguchi, T., Miyara, M., Fehervari, Z., Nomura, T., & Sakaguchi, S. (2008). CTLA-4 control over Foxp3+ regulatory T cell function. *Science, 322*, 271–275. doi: 10.1126/science.1160062.

Yakura, H. (2011). A "thought collective" around the idiotype network theory. *Bioessays, 33*, 552–554. doi: 10.1002/bies.201100041.

Yanagi, Y., Yoshikai, Y., Leggett, K., Clark, S. P., Aleksander, I., & Mak, T. W. (1984). A human T cell-specific cDNA clone encodes a protein having extensive homology to immunoglobulin chains. *Nature, 308*, 145–149. doi: 10.1038/308145a0.

Zinkernagel, R. M., & Doherty, P. C. (1973). Cytotoxic thymus-derived lymphocytes in cerebrospinal fluid of mice with lymphocytic choriomeningitis. *Journal of Experimental Medicine, 138*, 1266–1269. doi: 10.1084/jem.138.5.1266.

Zinkernagel, R. M., & Doherty, P. C. (1974a). Immunological surveillance against altered self components by sensitised T lymphocytes in lymphocytes choriomeningitis. *Nature, 251*, 547–548. doi: 10.1038/251547a0.

Zinkernagel, R. M., & Doherty, P. C. (1974b). Restriction of in vitro T cell-mediated cytotoxicity in lymphocytic choriomeningitis within a syngeneic or semiallogeneic system. *Nature, 248*, 701–702. doi: 10.1038/248701a0.

2 Autoimmunity, Symbiosis, and Organism

Autoimmunity is not merely a burden and an opportunity, it is a necessity.[1]

Irun Cohen

I is another.[2]

Arthur Rimbaud

In Chapter 1, we examined the development of theories concerning the fundamental issues surrounding immunity: the generation of specificity and diversity, the discrimination of self and nonself, the formation of immunological memory, and the mechanisms for the initiation of immune responses. Burnet's clonal selection theory emerged as the central theory of how the immune system operates, and we have viewed some of its modifications. We must now consider the physiological response to one's own components (autoimmunity) and symbiosis with others (microorganisms and fetuses). From Ehrlich to Burnet, the immune system has been theorized to be designed to either avoid recognizing the self or to suppress response to the self. However, symbiosis with microorganisms and the fact that a fetus with genes of paternal origin is not rejected by the mother do not appear to fit the currently supported theory of self–nonself discrimination. A central issue since the dawn of modern immunology and one that was theorized by Ehrlich is the inhibitory mechanism of autoimmunity along with the mechanism of diversity generation. Similarly, symbiosis with the gut microbiota has long been acknowledged, and a century ago, Metchnikoff considered the role of gut bacteria and tried to use them to improve our health. However, it is only recently that the significance of the microbiota has been understood and a series of intensive and extensive studies and important discoveries have been made.

When a phenomenon is found that does not fit a certain theory, there are at least two paths to take: one is to search for a new rule because the phenomenon does not conform to the rules governing the area of study at the time, and the other is to accept the phenomenon and search for a mechanism that can be explained within the framework of the current rules or to consider the raison d'être of the new phenomenon. The search for a raison d'être seems to be based on a Panglossian view that the world was created for the best, and everything that exists in it must thus have some meaning; however, such thinking can produce unexpected and interesting findings. In Chapter 2, I aim to investigate whether the phenomena of autoimmunity and symbiosis with microorganisms and fetuses are true deviations from current theories or physiological phenomena that can be explained within the framework of these theories. In addition, I will reflect on issues derived from these phenomena, such as the meaning of the term "organism."

2.1 AUTOIMMUNITY

2.1.1 *HORROR AUTOTOXICUS* OF PAUL EHRLICH

Autoimmunity is a condition in which autoreactive B cells, T cells, or free antibodies react with the body's components. At the turn of the 20th century, Jules Bordet (1870–1961; Nobel Prize in Physiology or Medicine 1919), who was born in Belgium and worked in the laboratory of Élie Metchnikoff at the Pasteur Institute in Paris, reported the presence of hemolytic antibodies in the sera of animals injected with erythrocytes (Bordet, 1898). Bordet also had important achievements

DOI: 10.1201/9781003486800-2

43

at the dawn of immunology, including the discovery of complement and the whooping cough bacterium, *Bordetella pertussis*, which was named after him. After reading Bordet's report, Paul Ehrlich initiated a series of experiments with his collaborator Julius Morgenroth on the assumption that the hemolytic antibodies produced in animals might be involved in the process of physiological destruction of effete red blood cells. They found that when goats were immunized with erythrocytes from animals of other species (heterologous) or other goats (homologous), they produced antibodies that lysed the erythrocytes used for immunization. However, goat never produced antibodies against its own red blood cells. Ehrlich named the phenomenon *horror autotoxicus*, meaning "the fear of self-toxicity or self-destruction," to indicate that the immune system somehow avoids autoaggression because it will lead to disastrous effects on the organism. This term is sometimes misinterpreted to refer to the horror of autoimmune disease, but Ehrlich's idea was that the body is equipped to avoid reactions that have a horrific effect on the self (Ehrlich and Morgenroth, 1900).

In 1900, following the publication of the paper of Ehrlich and Morgenroth, Sergei Métalnikoff (1870–1946), a Russian researcher working at the Pasteur Institute, reported that guinea pigs could produce antibodies to their own sperm (Métalnikoff, 1900). A closer examination of the original report by Arthur Silverstein revealed that Ehrlich did not completely rule out the production of autoantibodies but rather implied the internal regulatory mechanisms ("Einrichtung" in his words, meaning "contrivances"), whereby the autoantibodies were somehow prevented from acting on the body's constituents in the in vivo environment (Silverstein, 2001). Ehrlich also considered that the internal regulation for controlling or neutralizing the toxic activities of autoantibodies in vivo may be mediated by the interaction between autoantibodies and anti-autoantibodies. This idea of the regulation of antibody activity by an anti-antibody is reminiscent of Jerne's idiotypic network theory proposed more than 70 years later (Jerne, 1974). As described in Chapter 1, another theory advocated by Jerne, the natural selection theory of antibody formation (Jerne, 1955), shares similarities with Ehrlich's side-chain theory (Ehrlich, 1900). Returning to history to explain a newly emerged phenomenon may seem unusual in the field of science, but it may have been an approach that was comfortable for Jerne, who had a rich background outside of science. Unfortunately, none of Jerne's new theories were ever proven; however, it is interesting to note that his attitude of seeking the basis for new theories in the history of science seems to indicate consideration of the phenomena before us along with the heritage of humanity.

Despite Ehrlich's cautious reservation, the idea that autoimmunity does not inherently exist, together with the powerful dictum of *horror autotoxicus*, became a central theme in immunology. As mentioned above, in 1900, there was a report that antibodies against self-sperm could be produced in guinea pigs (Métalnikoff, 1900). In 1904, Julius Donath (1870–1850) and Karl Landsteiner discovered the mechanism for hemolysis in paroxysmal cold hemoglobinuria, which was the first human autoimmune disease but was not recognized as such (Donath and Landsteiner, 1904). Landsteiner, who discovered the ABO blood group system, demonstrated that individuals with group A antigens have anti-B agglutinin (antibody) in their sera, while individuals with group B have anti-A agglutinin (Landsteiner, 1900, 1901). Furthermore, in the 1930s, when he demonstrated that the immune system has an almost unlimited capacity to produce specific antibodies (Landsteiner, 1936), the production of self-reactive antibodies and their autoaggression was seen as a real threat. Despite the accumulation of similar findings, the concept of autoimmunity was not readily accepted in the scientific community at the time. During Ehrlich's influential years, experimental data indicating the existence of autoantibodies were dismissed or ignored (Silverstein, 1989, 2001), and the debate over whether autoimmune diseases existed continued into the 1950s and 1960s (Rose and Mackay, 2000; Rose, 2006). According to Arthur Silverstein, this phenomenon is indicative of the significant psychological effect that Ehrlich's dictum *horror autotoxicus* had on researchers, and the idea of autoimmunity may have disappeared from the collective consciousness (Silverstein, 2001). This is a characteristic of the "thought collective" referred to by Ludwig Fleck (discussed in Section 1.7.2, Chapter 1). Results that do not conform to the accepted framework of thought at the time are often ignored or dismissed, for example, as experimental errors or measurement noise. For adherents of Ehrlich's *horror autotoxicus*, the in vivo presence of autoantibodies would have been unacceptable. Although the possibility of autoimmunity certainly existed, the frequency of autoimmune diseases was relatively low, prompting immunologists to search for mechanisms to inhibit destructive immune responses to the self. In the late 1950s, the theory of immunological self-tolerance emerged.

2.1.2 The Forbidden Clone Hypothesis of Macfarlane Burnet

Interestingly, Burnet considered the strength of the clonal selection theory to be in its explanation of autoimmune disease. Compared with the instructive theory, the clonal selection theory could better explain the basis for the inhibition of the generation of self-reactive antibodies, B cells, and T cells. At the time, the genetic mechanism of antibody diversity generation was not yet clear, but Burnet understood that random mutations were constantly occurring in vivo and that self-reactive clones could emerge. Therefore, he assumed that there must be a mechanism that would prevent such clones from acting in vivo. He named such self-reactive clones "forbidden clones" to explain the mechanism of autoimmunity (Burnet, 1959a, 1959b). According to his hypothesis, forbidden clones are eliminated or inactivated by encountering antigenic determinants of the self; however, their cells sometimes proliferate, and the breakdown of self-tolerance is the true nature of the autoimmune disease. The factors that Burnet specified as contributing to the breakdown of self-tolerance and the activation of forbidden clones included genetic factors, namely somatic mutations that alter clonal specificity, the existence of a microenvironment that enables the proliferation of forbidden clones, and the ease of contact between self-antigen and autoreactive cells. It was these external or internal factors that lead to pathological conditions (Burnet, 1959a, 1959b, 1972). At the time, there was no other theory to explain the existence of autoantibodies other than the clonal selection theory, which attributed it to a breakdown of self-tolerance.

Later, as autoimmune phenomena were identified with non-negligible frequency, immunologists began to consider the implications of autoantibodies and autoreactive B and T cells in healthy individuals. The original Burnetian thesis assumes that autoreactive B cells are removed from the repertoire by a mechanism known as central tolerance in the bone marrow. However, autoantibodies or natural antibodies are observed in the blood of normal individuals (Coutinho et al., 1995). The majority of natural antibodies are often polyreactive and bind to a wide range of autoantigens (Coutinho et al., 1995; Wardemann et al., 2003). In mice, B cells that secrete natural antibodies belong to a subpopulation that expresses a differentiation antigen CD5 (B-1a cells) and resides primarily in the abdominal cavity. Remarkably, these self-reactive B cells are not eliminated; they are actively selected by self-antigens and form a pool of long-lived, self-renewing B cells that produce the majority of circulating natural IgM antibodies (Hardy, 2006; Baumgarth, 2011). Although this fact seems paradoxical for the tolerance of B cells, one should consider why natural autoantibodies have been selected throughout their long evolutionary history.

2.1.3 Inhibition Mechanisms of Autoimmunity

B cells mature in the bone marrow, where a special mechanism called gene rearrangement produces a group of antibodies with nearly infinite specificity. The specificity of an antibody is determined by the antigen-binding segment of the antibody or the variable region. The diversity of antibodies is produced by the random assembly of gene fragments that encode the variable region of the antibody molecule; the V (variable), D (diversity), and J (joining) gene fragments are randomly assembled in the antibody heavy chain (μ, δ, γ, α, ε), and the V and J gene fragments in the light chain (κ, λ). If there are $100\,V$ genes, $30\,D$ genes, and $6\,J$ genes in the human heavy chain, the random recombination of these gene fragments will result in 18,000 different specificities. The diversity further increases due to the imprecision of the binding of each gene fragment. The same phenomenon is observed for the V and J genes of the light chain. Furthermore, because the heavy and light chains are randomly joined, the diversity of antibodies becomes enormous. This diversity may include antibodies that can react with the self or with substances that do not currently exist. The same basic genetic mechanism is also involved in the process of generating the diversity of T cell receptors. Therefore, the clonal selection theory, which takes into account the possibility that autoreactive cells are produced in the primary lymphoid organs (bone marrow and thymus), assumes that autoreactive cells are eliminated in the primary lymphoid organs before migrating to the periphery, where they encounter self-antigens. At least five mechanisms for inhibiting autoreactivity have been identified to date (Goodnow et al., 1988; Nemazee and Bürki, 1989; Gay et al., 1993; Tiegs et al., 1993; Gauld et al., 2005).

The first mechanism is called the "central tolerance" or "clonal deletion" of autoreactive B cells. When autoreactive B cells are produced in the bone marrow and encounter self-antigens present in their microenvironment, they are driven to death by apoptosis and eliminated from the organism. Immature B cells are highly susceptible to this mechanism. The number of B cells eliminated in this manner varies between experimental systems, and the true number of cells lost during B cell maturation is unknown.

The second mechanism is called "anergy," which is a state of non-responsiveness where autoreactive cells enter an unresponsive state after encountering a self-antigen. This mechanism is maintained by chronic stimulation of the antigen and by inhibitory biochemical changes in the cell that occur after antigen stimulation. In other words, this unresponsiveness is not due to a lack of elements necessary for activation, but to the inhibition of intracellular biochemical processes initiated by the antigen receptor.

The third mechanism is called "receptor editing" and involves the generation of B cells in the bone marrow with antibodies on the cell surface that bind to self-antigens, causing a reorganization of the V and J genes of the antibody light chain, which acquire new antigen specificity toward nonself. Although not exactly, it is believed that about 25% of the antibody repertoire in mice is produced by receptor editing. Therefore, even if autoreactive cells are generated, there is a mechanism by which autoreactivity can be avoided by genetic ingenuity.

The fourth mechanism involves the lack of "co-stimulation," which is necessary for cell activation when cells are released to the periphery (see Section 1.6, Chapter 1). Cells that respond to their own components are present, but the lack of co-stimulation prevents their activation.

In the fifth mechanism, the involvement of Treg cells, which actively inhibit activation, has been demonstrated (Sakaguchi et al., 1995). These cells will be discussed further in the section on T cell tolerance (Section 2.1.4, Chapter 2).

How effective are these inhibitory mechanisms embedded in the immune system? It has been reported that normal human adults and mice have B cells that produce antibodies that react to a wide variety of self-antigens (Guilbert et al., 1982b, 1982a; Dighiero et al., 1983; Dighiero et al., 1985). For example, more than one-half (55%–75%) of the antibodies expressed by early immature B cells are self-reactive and polyreactive. This is thought to be due to the introduction of random mutations at specific sites in the heavy chain genes of antibodies (complementarity-determining region 3 involved in specificity determination) (Xu and Davis, 2000). Surprisingly, potentially harmful B cells account for more than one-half of the initial antibody repertoire; however, these cells can be said to be produced as a cost inherent in the immune system to generate the increased diversity and must be eliminated from the repertoire. According to a recent study on human B cells, there are two checkpoints for self-tolerance (Wardemann et al., 2003); one is at the stage of immature B cells in the bone marrow, where B cells are highly susceptible to cell death by antigen receptor stimulation, and self-reactive B cells are eliminated from the organism; the other is the stage in which B cells entering the periphery transition to mature B cells. However, approximately 20% of mature B cells circulating in the periphery after sorting at these two checkpoints remain autoreactive with low affinity, and 5% are polyreactive, reacting to a variety of self and nonself antigens. Despite the large proportion of autoreactive B cells among naïve B cells that have not encountered antigens, potentially harmful autoantibodies are not abundant in circulating blood because naïve B cells do not secrete a substantial number of autoantibodies. On the other hand, memory cells with IgM on their cell surface differentiate into antibody-producing cells independently of the antigen, making autoantibody production by these cells potentially harmful to the host. A subsequent study revealed a third checkpoint in the transition from naïve B cells to IgM-positive memory cells (Tsuiji et al., 2006). This checkpoint allows autoreactive and polyreactive antibodies present in naïve B cells to disappear when they become IgM-positive memory cells. However, because polyreactive antibodies respond to many different pathogens, it is assumed that they participate in the initial defense response. If this is true, autoreactive B cells likely play a physiological role because of their polyreactive nature.

2.1.4 T CELL TOLERANCE

Shifting the focus to T cells, I will outline their tolerance mechanism. As discussed in Section 1.5, Chapter 1, unlike the B cell receptor, which recognizes the tertiary structure of the antigen, the T cell receptor recognizes peptide fragments derived from the antigen that fits into a groove (pocket) at the tip of the MHC. The T cell receptor recognizes both the foreign antigen and its own MHC. Two types of MHCs are involved in antigen presentation: class I molecules, which are present on the surface of all nucleated cells, and class II molecules, which are expressed exclusively on cells like dendritic cells and B cells. Class I antigen presentation activates CD8$^+$ cytotoxic T cells (CTLs) that are responsible for defense against intracellular viruses, whereas class II antigen presentation on dendritic cells and B cells activates CD4$^+$ Th cells, which are involved in responding to soluble antigens and many microbes. CD4 and CD8 are glycoproteins that serve as co-receptors for the T cell receptor. While CD4 is expressed on the surface of Th cells, monocytes, and dendritic cells, CD8 is predominantly expressed on the surface of CTLs.

The maturation and differentiation of the T cell receptor repertoire occur in the thymus, the central organ of T cells, where central T cell tolerance occurs. The differentiation process in the thymus is complicated by a mechanism by which T cells recognize peptides bound to their own MHC class I or class II molecules. I will briefly discuss this mechanism here. Early immature thymocytes are called CD4$^-$CD8$^-$ double-negative cells because they express neither CD4 nor CD8 molecules. These cells undergo the following stages of differentiation within the thymic cortex. As thymocytes differentiate, they express an incomplete receptor called the pre-T cell receptor; by the time they differentiate into CD4$^+$CD8$^+$ double-positive cells, they express the full T cell receptor. These thymocyte receptors react with cortical thymic epithelial cells expressing MHC class I or class II that bind self-peptides. Because T cells recognize peptide-MHC complexes rather than the antigens alone, thymocytes that are unable to react adequately with self-MHC cannot function in the periphery and are destined to die.

Thymocytes with a sufficient affinity for the peptide-MHC complex are selected for further differentiation through a process called "positive selection." Cells undergoing positive selection migrate from the thymic cortex to the medulla, where they differentiate into single-positive cells expressing either CD4 or CD8. The repertoire of these cells is prepared to react to an almost infinite number of specificities, some of which are self-reactive. Therefore, self-reactive T cells must be eliminated before they enter the periphery through a process called "negative selection," where T cells that recognize self-peptides bound to the MHC with strong affinity are eliminated by apoptosis. The single-positive cells that survive this process are unresponsive to self-peptides but can recognize MHC and nonself peptides. They are delivered from the thymus for defense in the periphery.

For central tolerance to be complete, a repertoire of tissue-specific autoantigens covering the entirety of the self-component must be expressed within the thymus. For example, thousands of autoantigens (e.g., antigens of organs like lung, heart, testis, stomach, kidney, and various tissues) have been reported to be expressed in specialized cells called thymic medullary epithelial cells (Brennecke et al., 2015). This means that autoantigens that should be localized in peripheral organs and not in the thymus are ectopically expressed in the thymus. The process of ectopic autoantigen expression is regulated by an autoimmune regulator (AIRE) that controls the transcription process.

AIRE acts on areas of dense chromatin structure to induce the activation of repressed genes, contributing to the process of revealing the immunological self in the thymus. Mutations in the AIRE gene result in a rare inherited autoimmune disease called autoimmune polyendocrinopathy syndrome type 1, which is associated with candidiasis of the skin and mucosa, hypoparathyroidism, and adrenocortical insufficiency. This suggests that the transcription factor AIRE plays a critical role in establishing central tolerance within the thymus (Mathis and Benoist, 2007; Mathis and Benoist, 2009). However, as some autoantigens are not regulated by AIRE, the integrity of central tolerance is questionable. Recently, the existence of a transcription factor (Fezf2) involved in tissue-limited autoantigen expression in thymic medullary epithelial cells independent of AIRE was reported (Takaba et al., 2015). These results suggest that yet uncharacterized transcription factors may be involved to make tolerance in the thymus more complete; however, it remains possible that central tolerance mechanisms may not completely block the release of autoreactive T cells to the periphery.

At least three mechanisms have been identified that lead to T cell tolerance in the periphery; anergy, deletion, and regulation by Tregs. Anergy refers to a state in which autoreactive T cells are present but not activated. As mentioned earlier, the presence of co-stimulation is essential for the activation of T and B cells. In the absence of co-stimulatory signals from antigen-presenting cell (APCs), T cells are not activated and subsequently lose the ability to be activated. Alternatively, co-stimulation may react with inhibitory molecules on the T cell surface. In either case, in anergy, autoreactive T cells are present but remain functionally inactivated.

The second mechanism, deletion, involves the apoptosis-induced death of autoreactive T cells. Deletion occurs when T cells encounter very high concentrations of autoantigens or when T cells are excessively activated. This activation-induced cell death is caused by the activation of intracellular signaling pathways through the interaction of cell surface CD95 (Fas) with its ligand, CD95L (CD178).

The third mechanism is immunosuppression by T cells. In the 1970s, Richard Gershon (1932–1983) and colleagues of Yale University reported T cells that suppress immune responses (Gershon and Kondo, 1970, 1971). Until the early 1980s, the properties of these cells were studied from various angles by many groups, but their existence was not confirmed. Later, Shimon Sakaguchi (1951–) and his group identified a subset of T cells (Tregs) that suppress immune responses (Sakaguchi et al., 1995). These cells express CD4 and IL-2 receptor alpha chain (CD25) (Sakaguchi et al., 1995), and their differentiation is regulated by the transcription factor Foxp3 (Fontenot et al., 2003; Hori et al., 2003), a feature that made it possible to study its properties in detail. Although the transcription factor Foxp3 was initially believed to govern the induction of differentiation, subsequent studies have shown that Foxp3 expression alone is insufficient and that epigenetic changes in genes specific to Treg cells must be independently established (Ohkura et al., 2012; Kitagawa et al., 2017). Regarding Foxp3, loss of this transcription factor in humans results in a pathology called immunodysregulation, polyendocrinopathy, enteropathy, and X-linked (IPEX) syndrome (Bennett et al., 2001; Wildin et al., 2001), which is an X-chromosome-linked autoimmune disease that includes immune dysregulation with multiple endocrinopathies and intestinal disorders. In mice, a spontaneous mutant mouse (scurfy) discovered at the Oak Ridge National Laboratory in the United States in 1949 was shown to exhibit IPEX syndrome-like symptoms. The gene responsible was identified as *foxp3* and the mice lacked functional Treg cells (Khattri et al., 2003; Ramsdell and Ziegler, 2014).

The starting point for the identification of Tregs was the work of Yasuaki Nishizuka and Teruyo Sakakura that started in 1969 (Nishizuka and Sakakura, 1969; Sakakura and Nishizuka, 1972; Taguchi et al., 1980). The researchers assumed that removal of the thymus from 3-day-old mice would suppress the immune response due to a lack of T cells; in contrast, they observed an inflammatory response in organs such as the ovaries. The removal of T cells resulted in an autoimmune response. Using this model, Sakaguchi and colleagues found that autoimmune inflammation was suppressed by transplanting thymic tissue from normal mice into thymectomized mice and that the T cells in question expressed a molecule called Lyt-1 (then considered a marker for Th cells) on their cell surface (Sakaguchi et al., 1982). This finding initiated their focused research. Subsequently, Tregs were found to be involved in a wide range of biological regulation, not only in autoimmune diseases but also in infectious diseases, metabolic inflammation, allergy, microbiota regulation, cancer, and pregnancy (Sakaguchi et al., 2020). Recently, T cells with similar regulatory functions were discovered among CD8$^+$ cells (Nakagawa et al., 2018), and it will be interesting to see how they share their functions with CD4$^+$ Tregs.

Thus, unlike Th cells that enhance the effectiveness of immune responses and CTLs that kill target cells, Tregs exist as a third cell type that inhibits the immune response to achieve overall biological harmony. As discussed in Chapter 5, immunity by its very nature has the normative function of balancing biological polarity, and Treg cells can be seen to be deeply involved in this function.

2.1.5 PHYSIOLOGICAL AUTOIMMUNITY

Natural antibodies, including autoantibodies, are found not only in humans but also in antibody-producing species such as rabbits, mice, and rats. More than 60 years ago, Pierre Grabar (1898–1986), a Russian-born French biochemist working at the Pasteur Institute, hypothesized that antibodies to self and nonself have physiological functions (Grabar, 1947). The core of his hypothesis was that antibodies are not only involved in defense mechanisms but also play a physiological or maintenance role in the organism. In other words, autoantibodies are a normal component of the serum; they are involved in the transport of substances resulting from the metabolism and degradation of cellular and tissue constituents and augmenting the process of removing waste products from the organism through opsonization and phagocytosis. Therefore, his hypothesis suggests that autoantibodies reduce the risk of autoantigen circulation and use autoreactivity to maintain homeostasis (Cohen and Cooke, 1986; Avrameas, 1991; Coutinho et al., 1995; Avrameas et al., 2007). Homeostasis will be discussed in more detail in Section 3.4, Chapter 3. However, as Grabar stated 30 years later, it was extremely difficult to confront Ehrlich's idea of *horror autotoxicus* at the time, and reactions with autoantigens found in normal serum were often considered "nonspecific" (Grabar, 1983). Many reports on the physiological functions of natural autoantibodies were subsequently published. For example, the idea of "molecular mimicry" posits that if there is a structural similarity between a foreign antigen (especially a pathogen) and a self-component and a cross-reaction occurs between the two, the host immune system will respond to the self in the same way as it does to the pathogen, causing autoimmune disease (Oldstone, 1987). However, the presence of autoantibodies may prevent the host immune system from attacking itself by binding to antigenic determinants present in the microorganism (Cohen and Cooke, 1986; Avrameas, 1991; Coutinho et al., 1995; Avrameas et al., 2007). If we accept these hypotheses, the autoantibodies that are believed to cause autoimmunity are actually inhibiting the autoimmune response, and autoimmunity can be said to "bypass" autoimmunity.

Other hypotheses include the following. Spontaneous autoantibodies interact with self-components (molecules and cells) involved in the function of various systems in the organism to form an extensive dynamic network, thereby contributing to the maintenance of homeostasis in the organism rather than merely responding to nonself antigens from the external environment (Avrameas, 1991). The idea of the immune system reacting with self-components to form a systemic network is reminiscent of Jerne's idiotypic network theory and is also connected to Irun Cohen's immunological homunculus, which will be discussed in Section 2.1.6, Chapter 2. Furthermore, some reports indicate that autoreactive natural antibodies play a beneficial role in the defense against viral and bacterial infections. For example, an experiment was conducted in which mice unable to produce natural antibodies, including autoantibodies, were infected with vesicular stomatitis virus and *Listeria monocytogenes*, and the dynamics of the pathogens were examined (Ochsenbein et al., 1999a). According to this experiment, in normal mice, the spread of pathogens to major organs, such as the liver, kidney, and brain, was inhibited, and pathogens accumulated in the spleen, the secondary lymphoid organ where the response to infection defense occurs. However, in mice without natural antibodies, pathogen levels increased in the liver, kidney, and brain and decreased in the spleen, where the immune response should occur. This indicates that natural antibodies, including autoantibodies, suppress the spread of infection to important organs while directing pathogens to the spleen, the site where the immune response occurs. This process is dependent on complement activation for the formation of antigen–antibody complexes that are then delivered to secondary lymphoid organs such as the spleen (Ochsenbein et al., 1999b). Therefore, natural antibodies are involved not only in the maintenance function of the body but also in the defense function (Zavdy et al., 2014).

In T cells, there are reports that autoreactive cells play a key role in maintaining the functional integrity of tissues. In the central nervous system of mice and rats, autoreactive T cells have been considered harmful cells that target myelin basic protein (MBP) to destroy neural tissue and cause autoimmune encephalomyelitis. This experimentally induced autoimmune encephalomyelitis has been used in many studies as a model analogous to human multiple sclerosis. However, there are reports that the autoreactive T cells that induce the pathology are neuroprotective (Moalem et al., 1999; Yoles et al., 2001). After compression and injury of the optic nerve of rats, T cells reactive to MBP and T cells reactive to other antigens were administered, and their effects were compared. The results suggested that the recovery of optic nerve function was better when autoreactive T cells were administered. This indicates that autoreactive T cells do not always have a detrimental effect but in some cases have a beneficial effect on the host. Furthermore, as will be discussed in Chapter 4, the phenomenon of autoimmunity, in which cells react with their components, is widely observed not only in vertebrates but also in invertebrates, plants, and even bacteria, suggesting that autoimmunity is an inevitable necessity for any organism with an immune system—that is, all organisms.

2.1.6 IMMUNOLOGICAL HOMUNCULUS OF IRUN COHEN

According to the clonal selection theory, autoimmunity is a random and unfortunate event, so that it is assumed that no two autoimmune diseases are of the same type. However, the target antigens of autoimmunity are largely predictable. For example, systemic lupus erythematosus is characterized by the appearance of autoantibodies against nuclear and cell membrane phospholipid components (Riemekasten and Hahn, 2005), most patients with primary biliary cirrhosis have antibodies against an enzyme complex that is found in mitochondria (Invernizzi et al., 2005), and patients with insulin-dependent diabetes mellitus exhibit autoimmune T cell reactions and autoantibody formation against insulin and islet cell autoantigens (Roep, 1996; Pihoker et al., 2005). Therefore, autoantibody reactivity is biased. Furthermore, it has been observed that autoantigens targeted by autoimmune disease are also recognized by cells and antibodies of healthy individuals.

Given the biased self-reactivity of T cells and autoantibodies in patients and healthy individuals, Cohen speculated that autoimmune diseases are not random accidents, as the clonal selection theory suggests; instead, self-antigens targeted by autoimmune diseases are the self as the immune system routinely perceives it. He named this naturally occurring structure of autoimmunity the "immunological homunculus" (Cohen and Young, 1991; Cohen, 1992; Nobrega et al., 1993; Poletaev, 2002). The original meaning of a homunculus is a dwarf, and it is believed that alchemists aimed to manufacture them, but the immunological homunculus is derived from the homunculus of the cerebral cortex. The brain homunculus is a map that Canadian neurosurgeon Wilder Penfield (1891–1976) obtained by electrical stimulation during craniotomy surgery for the treatment of epilepsy (Penfield and Boldrey, 1937; Penfield and Rasmussen, 1950). It shows that the areas of the brain that control peripheral sensation and movement are reflected in the size of each body part that is controlled, and it is striking in that the proportions of the body part are grossly distorted (Figure 2.1).

According to Cohen's hypothesis, the immunological homunculus is the self as perceived by the immune system of a healthy person and represents the body's immune status. Specifically, the repertoire of the immune system in a healthy person includes T cells, B cells, and natural antibodies

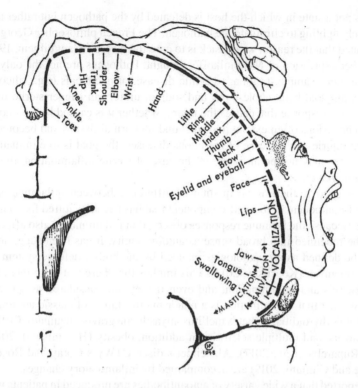

FIGURE 2.1 Penfield's homunculus of motor cortex. In the primary motor cortex of the cerebrum, the region that controls each body part is identified by Penfield. Penfield's homunculus is a small person depicted by converting the size of the area into the size of each body part. In particular, the size of the hands, fingers, lips, and mandible stand out. A similar drawing was made for the sensory cortex. (From Penfield, W. & Rasmussen, R. (1950). *The Cerebral Cortex of Man: A Clinical Study of Localization of Function.* Macmillan. Figure 115.)

that recognize a defined set of self-molecules, and as seen in the brain homunculus, these self-recognition receptors do not recognize any self-molecule equally but rather select and bind molecules that are important to the body (Cohen, 2007b). Because the recognized self-molecules include tissue antigens, stress proteins, and immunomodulatory molecules, they may serve as markers that indicate the parts of the body that are being altered and the extent of the alterations. In Burnet's clonal selection theory, autoreactive cells must either be eliminated from the system or inactivated, whereas, in Cohen's theory, autoreactivity is a physiological property that is positively selected for and embedded in the system. Because the antigens recognized during autoimmune disease overlap with physiologically recognized self-molecules, Cohen believes that from an evolutionary perspective, the benefits of autoimmunity in healthy individuals have more than outweighed the costs of autoimmune disease. Immunological homunculus-mediated autoreactivity regulates the physiological inflammation involved in the maintenance of the organism, such as tissue repair, cell proliferation and differentiation, elimination of senescent cells and cellular debris, and elimination of abnormal cells, such as tumors. Cohen also believes that disruption of this regulation leads to pathological inflammation and autoimmune diseases (Cohen, 2007b, 2007a). Attempts are being made to apply the findings of the immunological homunculus to the treatment of autoimmune diseases, such as type 1 diabetes, and tumors (Cohen, 2014).

2.1.7 AUTOIMMUNE DISEASES AND AUTOINFLAMMATORY DISEASES

Inflammation has long been regarded as a condition in which our bodies are attacked by pathogens. It was Metchnikoff who changed this view about a century ago. He argued that the essence of inflammation is not a state in which the host is defeated by the pathogen but rather a state in which the host is actively fighting to eliminate the pathogen. The French philosopher Georges Canguilhem (1904–1995) stated that the reason we get sick is to cure the disease (Canguilhem, 1991). This could be seen as another expression of Metchnikoff's thought. Pathogens are not the only major triggers of inflammation. For example, trauma, ischemic disease, or chemicals (e.g., silicon dioxide, calcium phosphate, amyloid beta, cholesterol, and sodium urate) can trigger sterile inflammation. It is the host's immune response that causes the injury, whether it is caused by a pathogen or a sterile inflammation. The lesions often extend into surrounding normal tissues and become a major problem as collateral injuries. In the case of infectious diseases, the goal is to eliminate the pathogen, so cost-effectiveness may not be an issue; in the case of sterile inflammation, the burden on the organism is much greater.

From this perspective, there is no qualitative difference between inflammation and immune response to a self-component or to a self-component that has been denatured for some other reasons (Boyden, 1964). Because the immune responses observed in inflammation also affect the self, these reactions may be redefined in a broad sense as autoimmunity. It has been suggested that autoimmune diseases be defined as all pathologies induced by the body's defense system that cannot be repaired by the organism (Kourilsky, 2014). This implies that there is a close relationship between autoimmune diseases and inflammation, and even if they are considered as separate categories, we must acknowledge that inflammation is a major manifestation of classic autoimmune diseases such as Hashimoto's thyroiditis, diabetes mellitus, myasthenia gravis, rheumatoid arthritis, systemic lupus erythematosus, and multiple sclerosis. In addition, obesity (Hotamisligil, 2006), cardiovascular disease (Ruparelia et al., 2017), Alzheimer's disease (Wyss-Coray and Rogers, 2012), and depression (Lee and Giuliani, 2019) are accompanied by inflammatory changes.

It has been reported that a wide variety of autoantibodies are produced in patients with COVID-19 caused by SARS-CoV-2 (Wang et al., 2021). In the study, a sample of 194 infected individuals was analyzed using a high-throughput system for the presence of antibodies to 2,770 extracellular and secreted proteins, and a dramatic increase in autoantibodies was found compared with non-infected individuals. These antibodies reacted with cytokines, chemokines, complement components, and cell surface proteins, which are proteins involved in immune regulation, suggesting that these autoantibodies interfere with the process of virus elimination. Furthermore, these autoantibodies were found to increase disease severity in the mouse model. These results suggest that COVID-19 may be considered an autoimmune disease. Furthermore, one can imagine that there is a close relationship between pathogen-induced inflammation and autoimmune disease, and that not a few lesions may not be due to a breakdown of self-tolerance, which Burnet postulated as a possible mechanism of autoimmune disease.

There are other inflammatory diseases for which the presence of pathogens cannot be confirmed. In 1999, Daniel Kastner's group at the National Institutes of Health reported a new autoinflammatory disease (McDermott et al., 1999). This disease presents with periodic fevers of unknown cause and is characterized by the absence of autoantibodies and autoreactive T cells, the hallmarks of classic autoimmunity. Instead, macrophages, dendritic cells, NK cells, and neutrophils, which are responsible for innate immunity, are abnormal, and mutations in the gene encoding the extracellular region of the tumor necrosis factor (TNF) receptor were responsible. The disease was found to have a variety of etiologies and is now classified into multiple categories, including transcription factor NF-κB activation disorders, protein-misfolding disorders, complement disorders, cytokine signaling diseases, and macrophage activation syndromes (Masters et al., 2009).

2.1.8 Physiological Autoimmunity and Self-Reflection

In the paradigm based on Burnet's clonal selection theory, autoreactivity or self-recognition was something to be avoided, and its positive significance for the organism was not considered. However, subsequent research has led to the view that autoimmunity is not an exception to the rule but rather an indispensable component of the immune system (Bendelac et al., 2001). If the immune system is viewed as an isolated cognitive machine, its role is to recognize elements in the environment surrounding the machine. If this is the case, then it would be natural for the machine to recognize the components in its surroundings when it enters a living organism. If the host is harmed by the reaction with its components, other mechanisms must be incorporated to avoid the destruction of the host. As will be discussed in more detail in Chapter 4, the phenomenon of immunity has been observed since the beginning of life, and the same is true of autoimmunity. For example, bacteria and archaea also have immune systems and autoimmunity, although the molecular mechanisms are quite different from those of vertebrates. Because no beneficial effects have been observed for autoimmunity in bacteria to date, it is assumed that they have taken the benefit of having an immune system while accepting the cost, but benefits may be discovered in the future. In any case, an adaptive mechanism has emerged to avoid self-destruction by autoimmunity in bacteria. In plants, hybrid necrosis, a phenomenon of dwarfing, tissue necrosis, malformation, and lethal changes in hybrids arising from normal parents, has been observed (Bomblies and Weigel, 2007). The cause was the recognition of self-components by receptors that recognize pathogens. When *Arabidopsis* was extensively studied, 2% of the plants exhibited the symptoms of hybrid necrosis, suggesting that autoimmunity is inevitably present even in plants. In animals, at least from the cnidarian level, a phenomenon has been observed that is equivalent to an autoimmune disease (Buss et al., 1985). For T cells to function properly, they must recognize the MHC as a self-component with appropriate strength. Furthermore, it has been proposed that self-recognizing antibodies produced by B cells eliminate cells and tissues that are no longer needed (Grabar, 1983). Although strong autoimmunity leading to pathology must be avoided, the immune system must be equipped with the ability to recognize the self in order to maintain homeostasis in the body (Avrameas, 1991).

While Burnet's central focus was on B cells, some of the revised theories that have since been proposed in the course of broadening the view argue that it is changes in the environment surrounding immune cells that determine the initiation of immune responses (see Chapter 1). As will be discussed in Chapter 3, to broaden the perspective even further, immunity can be viewed as a systemic response involving many elements in the body. Although never proven, Jerne's idiotypic network theory can be reinterpreted as a theory of systemic homeostasis maintenance based on autoimmunity in the sense that immune molecules (antibodies) recognize their own molecules (antibodies). The influence of Jerne's theory can be seen in Irun Cohen's immunological homunculus theory of monitoring and maintaining the internal condition of an organism through recognition of the self-components. Such a maintenance function of the organism, unlike the immune response to a stimulus, is difficult to capture externally. Because immunology has concentrated on looking at responses to stimuli, it is fair to say that in many cases stimulus-independent functions have been out of view. To maintain the survival of an organism, it is essential that baseline functions are working properly. Therefore, physiological autoimmunity may play an important role in the organism, and this point will be discussed again in Section 2.4, Chapter 2.

Expanding the imagination regarding the self-referential nature of immunity recalls "know thyself" (*Gnothi seauton*) as a human mission. It is Socrates' teaching that life without self-examination is not worth living. To become a better person and maintain a peaceful inner life, we must repeat self-reflection; we must continue to reflect on ourselves and turn our gaze inward throughout our lives. Such a function is built into human beings, and only by fully utilizing this function can mental homeostasis be ensured. Aristotle stated that the highest things in man are intellect and philosophic wisdom, and contemplation is the activity that is most in line with these concepts because that is the most effective, most continuous, and most self-sufficient. If a person can continue this activity to the end of their life, there is something divine that transcends the human being, and their life is the happiest (Aristotle, 1925).

When I entered philosophy from science, I realized that self-reflection is not structurally embedded in the activities of science. Of course, historically speaking, there have been scientists who have conducted deep reflection, but their mental activities are largely due to their personal qualities.

If self-reflection were structurally embedded in science, then all scientists would be aware of philosophy. The reality is rather the opposite: science ignores or eliminates philosophy, and its influence is so pervasive in modern society that not only is the reflection on science and the self by scientists neglected, but also those outside of science are no longer practicing the teachings of Socrates. According to Martin Heidegger (1889–1976), there are two modes of thinking: one is calculating thought with a set objective, as science does, and the other is reflective thought that questions the meaning of existence (Heidegger, 1990). In the modern age, the prevalence of calculation-based thinking prevents us from realizing the importance of self-reflection or autocriticism. From this perspective, it could be said that the immune system is more faithful to self-examination than our minds.

2.2   SYMBIOSIS WITH MICROORGANISMS

In the late 19th century, Robert Koch (1842–1910) and Louis Pasteur discovered the involvement of microorganisms in the pathogenesis of multiple diseases, marking the advent of the germ theory of the disease. This theory has since had a profound influence on medical science, and the view that microorganisms and pathogens are almost synonymous has become fixed. Furthermore, antibiotics and vaccines were developed to fight infectious diseases based on this paradigm, and the improvement of hygienic conditions, which was especially important, has saved many lives and significantly extended our lifespan. The life expectancy of the global population in 1900 was about 30 years, and it more than doubled to over 70 years by 2020 (Roser et al., 2019). However, recent technological advances in microbiology and molecular biology have produced a major shift in the "microbe=pathogen" view that has prevailed for a century. The image of microorganisms as indispensable for our survival, rather than always leading to disease, has emerged. Technological advances include high-throughput sequencing and the analysis of the 16S ribosomal RNA gene that makes up the small ribosomal unit of the microbe. The sequence of this gene is conserved in all prokaryotes, and it can be used to amplify microbial gene fragments. These fragments contain variable regions containing species-specific sequences and are useful for studying evolutionary phylogeny. Moreover, because this analysis does not require in vitro culture, it allows us to analyze microorganisms in their entirety, including those that exist in special locations and were previously impossible to culture.

2.2.1   Inseparable Relationship Between Human Physiology and Microbiota

Over the past two decades, a vast amount of data has accumulated on the microorganisms present in humans. For example, more than 1,000 species of microorganisms have been identified in the intestine, at least almost as many as adult somatic cells (Luckey, 1972; Savage, 1977; Sender et al., 2016). The bacterial number per gram of colon content is 10^{11}–10^{12} bacteria, which constitutes 60% of the fecal mass. Although there are 55 bacterial phyla and 13 branches of archaea on Earth (Rappe and Giovannoni, 2003), only a relatively limited number of phyla are found among the intestinal microbiota. The adult gut microbiota is dominated by the phyla Firmicutes (60%–80%), which includes the genera *Clostridium* and *Eubacteria*, Bacteroidetes (20%–40%) among the bacteria, and only one member of Archaea (Bäckhed et al., 2005; Ley et al., 2006; Dethlefsen et al., 2007). This finding suggests that there is strong selection pressure in the gut environment and that the host and microbes have coevolved.

If one accepts the Burnetian paradigm, the following question arises: why does the immune system accept these foreign microorganisms? If there is a significant number of microorganisms that are at least equivalent to somatic cells, there are many more antigenic determinants. Does our immune system miss them? Or is there a mechanism by which the immune system recognizes them but prevents a strong reaction from occurring? Second, if the presence of microorganisms in our bodies is the result of a long coevolutionary process, then we can imagine that their symbiosis has beneficial effects. What are those effects and what mechanisms support them? With these questions in mind, I will examine the reality of symbiosis in our bodies.

The term symbiosis originally refers to people "living together." In 1877, German botanist Albert Bernhard Frank (1839–1900) proposed the term symbiosis (Symbiotismus) to describe the mutualistic (beneficial to both) relationship of lichens, where algae are symbiotic with fungi that cannot photosynthesize. He was also the first to use the term "mycorrhiza" in 1885 to describe symbionts between roots and fungi. Against Frank's definition, in 1879, Heinrich Anton de Barry (1831–1888), a German surgeon and botanist, provided a more inclusive definition of symbiosis (Symbiose) as any association between different species, in which the organisms are in persistent contact, but the relationship need not be advantageous to all the participants (Douglas, 2010). This definition has long been a source of confusion because it differs from Frank's exclusive view. However, de Bary's definition is widely accepted today, and it has the advantage of promoting broader research in the field. Symbiosis can take the following forms: parasitism, in which one species survives at the expense of the other; commensalism, in which one species benefits while the other does not; and mutualism, which corresponds to Frank's definition, in which both species are beneficiaries.

First, I will outline how our gut microbiota is formed. Two hypotheses have been proposed to explain this phenomenon. One is the vertical transmission of the microbiota from mother to child. The argument is that the composition of the gut microbiota overlaps among family members and that this effect can be observed over several generations (Ley et al., 2006). The second hypothesis is the horizontal transmission of microbiota, which claims that the newborn acquires its initial microbiota from the vagina and feces of the mother (Mändar and Mikelsaar, 1996). This is based on the observation that different microorganisms are established in newborns born by cesarean section compared with normal delivery (Grönlund et al., 1999). The assumption is that the uterus is sterile and that the fetus is born sterile (Funkhouser and Bordenstein, 2013). However, over the past decade, studies have been conducted to determine whether the uterus is truly sterile. Some studies have drawn the conventional conclusion that the uterus is sterile (Perez-Muñoz et al., 2017; de Goffau et al., 2019); in contrast, there are reports that the uterus is not necessarily sterile. Although there are differences between individuals, microorganisms are present in the intestines (Younge et al., 2019; Rackaityte et al., 2020) or lungs (Al Alam et al., 2020) of the fetus, as bacterial, archaeal, fungal, and viral DNA and microorganisms are found in the placenta, amniotic fluid, and feces. A recent study has found that the genetic signals of microorganisms in addition to bacteria-like morphologies are present in the intestine, skin, lungs, and placenta of human fetuses in the second trimester of pregnancy (Mishra et al., 2021). Treg cells and memory T cells were also identified, indicating pre-sensitization by antigens. In vitro stimulation of T cells in mesenteric lymph nodes with bacteria found in fetuses induces the formation of memory cells. These results strongly suggest that the fetus may be sensitized by bacteria before birth. Large-scale studies with strict control of microbial contamination and other factors may be necessary to reach a conclusion.

Considering the classification of symbiosis, most relationships between humans and intestinal microorganisms are either mutualistic or commensal. For example, humans cannot break down polysaccharides such as cellulose and pectin found in plant cell walls, which are broken down by gut microorganisms that use them for their growth. In return, gut microorganisms produce substances, such as butyrate, that function as an important source of energy for the host (Flint et al., 2007) and inhibit pathogens or detoxify substances that are harmful to the host (Bäumler and Sperandio, 2016). This increases the survival rate of the host, which in turn increases the opportunity for the microorganism to survive and multiply. Interestingly, mutualistic symbiosis can also be observed between different microorganisms living in the gut. For example, microorganisms that lack the enzymes needed to break down polysaccharides consume the sugars produced by other microorganisms and in return provide growth factors to the sugar-producing microorganisms (Flint, 2004).

I will now more closely examine the mechanisms that support this symbiotic relationship. The surface area of the lumen of the intestine, where the largest volume of microbiota resides, is the largest interface between the host and the external environment, reaching approximately $200 \, \text{m}^2$

if the villi are included. Therefore, the intestine contains the largest number of immune cells. Furthermore, not only does the immune system control the growth of microorganisms, but it has been shown that the gut microbiota influences the maturation and function of the immune system (Rakoff-Nahoum et al., 2004; Kelly et al., 2005; Mazmanian et al., 2005; Mazmanian and Kasper, 2006; Mazmanian et al., 2008; Round and Mazmanian, 2009). It is fascinating to observe such a close bidirectional relationship supported by exquisite interactions. I will now examine some specific examples.

In sterile animals, immune tissues and cells are reduced, and immune responses are attenuated. When the composition of the microbiota is disturbed by antibiotics or changes in diet, pathologies such as autoimmune diseases, inflammatory diseases, and even allergies can occur. This suggests that the microbiota is involved in the regulation of the immune response, and a scenario in which deviations from the homeostasis created by the steady interaction of the microbiota and the immune system produce pathology becomes possible. Like the APCs mentioned in Section 1.6, Chapter 1, PRRs are present on intestinal epithelial cells and recognize MAMPs. This response is important for biological defense and essential for maintaining intestinal homeostasis and protecting against intestinal injury (Rakoff-Nahoum et al., 2004). When mice deficient in PRRs (TLR2 and TLR4) or a molecule (MyD88) essential for signaling through TLRs to induce inflammatory cytokine production were orally administered a toxic agent to the intestinal epithelium (sodium dextran sulfate), more mice died rather than their inflammatory lesions were attenuated. However, this was not due to microbial growth, but to intestinal hemorrhage and anemia. The results of this experiment suggest that TLR-mediated interactions with the microbiota may be involved in the protective action of the intestinal epithelium through the production of humoral factors (e.g., IL-6 and KC-1) that protect the intestinal epithelium from injury (Rakoff-Nahoum et al., 2004).

The gut also possesses mechanisms to maintain homeostasis in the intestine by minimizing contact between the microbiota and host immune cells. These include mucus that suppresses microbial migration, epithelial cells that produce antimicrobial peptides (e.g., C-type lectins and defensins), macrophages that kill microbes that enter through epithelial cells, antigen-specific Treg cells, dendritic cells that induce IgA-producing B cells, and proinflammatory Th17 cells that secrete IL-17 and IL-22. IL-22 plays a versatile function in enhancing the production of antimicrobial peptides and epithelial regeneration. In addition, Th17 cells induce IgA production. Microbe-specific IgA forms dimers that pass through the epithelial cells and bind to microorganisms in the intestinal lumen, inhibiting their entry. Although the interplay between these defense elements is complex, these protective barriers (i.e., "firewalls") are not perfect, and B and T cells that react to symbiotic microorganisms or metabolites of symbiotic microorganisms are recognized in the blood. In other words, because the immune system does indeed recognize symbiotic microorganisms, it builds a firewall to keep them as separated as possible. However, the protective wall is not perfect, and a reaction is triggered, although, under normal conditions, it does not develop into pathology. The relationship between the immune system and symbiotic microorganisms is controlled such that it does not always develop into pathology.

The microbiota acts on diverse immune cells. In germ-free animals, abnormalities of the intestinal epithelium, maturation of intestinal lymphoid tissue, and the whole immune system have been observed, indicating that the microbiota supports the maturation and differentiation of the immune system (Hooper, 2004). In 2005, Sarkis Mazmanian (1972–) and colleagues identified a type of symbiotic bacterium involved in immune system maturation (Mazmanian et al., 2005). It belonged to the genus *Bacteroides* (*Bacteroides fragilis*), and the polysaccharide A (PSA) produced by this bacterium increased T cells throughout the body, promoted the formation of lymphoid organs, and corrected the pathology-causing imbalance between Th1 cells (which produce interferon-gamma [IFN-γ] and Il-2 and are involved in cellular immunity) and Th2 cells (which produce IL-4, IL-5, IL-13, etc., and are involved in humoral immunity). In germ-free mice, Th2 cells predominate, enhancing IL-4 production and conversely decreasing IFN-γ production; however, PSA produced by *B. fragilis* reverses this profile. When PSA is presented by MHC class II on dendritic cells,

CD4+ cells are activated and induce the production of the appropriate cytokines. These effects are absent when a PSA mutant of *B. fragilis* is introduced into germ-free mice. This report is the first to demonstrate that the product of a single symbiotic bacterium is essential for the maturation of the immune system.

Treg cells, which are involved in the maintenance of immune tolerance and homeostasis in the intestinal mucosa, can be induced by 17 strains from the genus *Clostridium*, which comprises anaerobic endospore-forming rod-shaped bacteria (Atarashi et al., 2011; Atarashi et al., 2013). Furthermore, when these bacteria were orally administered to mice and were processed to develop colitis or allergic diarrhea, both symptoms were milder in the *Clostridium*-treated group than in the control group. These results indicate that a specific group of bacteria induces Treg cells and may subsequently suppress the inflammatory response. A similar relationship was observed between symbiotic microorganisms and Th17 cells (Ivanov et al., 2009). No Th17 cells were found in mice without microbiota, but Th17 cells appeared when microorganisms were returned to the intestinal tract, suggesting that the microbiota is involved in the maturation process of Th17 cells. However, it is not clear whether it is an unspecified number of microorganisms or specific bacteria that induce the maturation of Th17 cells. A subsequent investigation revealed that a single genus of commensal microbes, segmented filamentous bacteria (SFB), is sufficient for this process. SFB adhere strongly to the epithelial cells of the ileum and induce local production of serum amyloid A protein, which in turn acts on dendritic cells in the mucosal lining to induce the differentiation of Th17 cells, thereby enhancing the defense against pathogens. Moreover, the presence of SFB increases resistance to the pathogen *Citrobacter rodentium* in mice. In addition to SFB, the induction of Th17 cells in the small intestine has been observed with *Citrobacter* and enterohemorrhagic *Escherichia coli*, where adhesion to small intestinal epithelial cells is reported to be important (Atarashi et al., 2015). In humans, it is not the SFB that are involved, but a symbiotic bacterium *Bifidobacterium adolescentis*, which alone induces an increase in the number of Th17 cells in the small intestine of mice (Tan et al., 2016). These results suggest that a limited number of symbiotic bacteria influence the host immune system. If such a relationship with symbiotic bacteria is confirmed for a wider variety of immune cells in the future, it would provide evidence for the role of symbiotic bacteria in regulating the maturation and differentiation of immune cells with considerable selectivity, thereby regulating the composition of the immune system. Therefore, the bacteria, which were originally strangers to the host, would create a state of readiness so that the host can appropriately respond to internal and external changes. The identification of such a process might allow for a fine-tuned approach to managing a wide variety of immune abnormalities.

The effects of this type of symbiosis are not limited to the host-microbe interactions and immune function that occur locally, such as in the gut. As mentioned above, bacteria comprising the gut microbiota break down dietary fiber, which is difficult for the host to digest, to produce short-chain fatty acids (e.g., butyrate, acetate, and propionate). These short-chain fatty acids are transferred into the bloodstream; their levels are correlated with the amount of dietary fiber and are undetectable in germ-free animals lacking microbiota. G protein-coupled receptors (e.g., Gpr41, Gpr43, and Olfr78) have been identified as receptors for short-chain fatty acids. The olfactory receptor Olfr78 is located in the afferent arterioles of the kidney, coinciding with the site where the enzyme renin, which catalyzes substances involved in blood pressure elevation, is stored. Interestingly, mice lacking Olfr78 have lower blood pressure, and conversely, mice lacking Gpr41 have higher blood pressure (Pluznick et al., 2013; Natarajan et al., 2016). These findings indicate that metabolites produced by the microbiota are involved in the regulation of kidney physiology, especially blood pressure; however, it would not be surprising if they also affected the function of other organs and cells. In fact, the generation of Treg cells in the intestine is affected by short-chain fatty acids (Arpaia et al., 2013; Furusawa et al., 2013; Smith et al., 2013).

The effects of the microbiota on systemic physiological functions are diverse, and the research is extensive (Hooper and Gordon, 2001; Ley et al., 2005; Wen et al., 2008). I will examine the relationship between the gut and the central nervous system, also known as the "microbiota-gut-brain axis," as a representative example. Studies on germ-free mice and humans have shown that the absence of gut microbiota is correlated with hyperactivity, anxious behavior, impaired learning and memory abilities, the development of autism spectrum disorders, and increased permeability of the blood-brain barrier. Therefore, it has been suggested that the gut microbiota may influence neurological function. The two are intricately intertwined, as abnormal cognitive function affects not only the immune system but also the gut microbiota. Reports have suggested a role for the gut microbiota in pathological conditions of the nervous system, such as schizophrenia, Parkinson's disease, and Alzheimer's disease (Sharon et al., 2016; Cryan et al., 2019; Morais et al., 2021). These results indicate a close relationship between the immune system, nervous system, and microbiota. It will take time to identify the causative microorganisms or elucidate the mechanisms by which they are related, but it would not be surprising if a causal relationship is revealed from these studies.

Ivan Pavlov (1849–1936; Nobel Prize in Physiology or Medicine 1904) established a system of conditioned reflexes, or classical conditioning. Because the research using this system will be covered later, I will briefly summarize it here. In his experiments on the digestive process in dogs, Pavlov noticed that the salivation of dogs increased when a laboratory assistant who provided them with food was present. Based on this observation, if the dogs were made to learn that food is served after the sound of a bell, salivation would be enhanced simply by hearing the bell, a stimulus that is normally unrelated to salivation (Pavlov, 1927). Classical conditioning refers to a phenomenon in which the animal learns the relationship between the food (a stimulus that induces an unconditioned response) and the neutral stimulus (the sound of a bell, which by itself cannot induce a response), and a neutral stimulus becomes a conditioned stimulus and induces a change in response or behavior. Using this system, four metabolites produced by gut microorganisms (phenyl sulfate, pyrocatechol sulfate, 3-(3-sulfooxyphenyl)propanoic acid, and indoxyl sulfate) have been shown to influence recovery from fear. Mice conditioned with a sound and pain stimulus, having learned that the sound is followed by pain, typically forget the sound/stimulus association after about 3 days of being exposed to the non-stimulus sound. However, when the gut microbiota is removed with antibiotics, the mice are unable to escape the fear (Chu et al., 2019). When this phenomenon occurs in humans, it can lead to post-traumatic stress disorder (PTSD) and chronic anxiety disorders, which are important medical problems. When the brains of mice treated with antibiotics were compared with control mice, changes were observed in a specific region, called the medial prefrontal cortex. The change is a reduction in the formation of spines protruding from the dendrites of excitatory neurons involved in learning and memory. In addition, the four metabolites are reduced in mice without symbiotic bacteria, and the authors surmise that these substances are involved in the communication with the brain and affect mental function. Interestingly, two of the four identified substances (a derivative of 3-(3-sulfooxyphenyl)propanoic acid) and indoxyl sulfate) have been implicated in schizophrenia and autism (Shaw, 2010). In addition, the involvement of the microbiota has been investigated in obesity and diabetes (Gurung et al., 2020), asthma (Hufnagl et al., 2020), inflammatory bowel diseases such as Crohn's disease and ulcerative colitis (Round and Mazmanian, 2009), and cancer (Helmink et al., 2019; Sepich-Poore et al., 2021).

Coevolution usually occurs at the intersection of different species. As a result of repeated coevolution of humans with microorganisms, our existence is not a mere collection of different species, but an ecosystem in which each component forms an interconnected network. The boundary between the organism and environment has blurred, and in a sense, the inside and outside have merged into one. This perspective is markedly different from Jerne's idiotype network theory, which views the immune system as enclosed. As Joshua Lederberg proposed 20 years ago, we may need to rethink our attitude toward microbes through the elucidation of the microbial gene cluster (microbiome), including shifting our attitude toward microbes from the previous metaphor of war to that of ecology (Lederberg, 2000). However, even as we have been watching news reports since the COVID-19 pandemic began, our relationship with microorganisms has been rife with war metaphors. While this is understandable given the severity of the pandemic, we should actively adopt an ecological perspective to accurately reflect on organisms, individuals, and ultimately life.

This type of reflection has the potential to reveal what lurks deep within phenomena and is difficult to see as reality.

2.2.2 Symbioses with Microorganisms Ubiquitously Present in the Living World

The gut microbiota is not merely a regulator of the immune system; it is closely intertwined with metabolism and nervous system function. Our bodies regard the gut microbiota not as a stranger but as an essential component. This relationship extends beyond humans and is widespread in the biological world, and symbiosis is the rule rather than the exception. It is easy to imagine that when new organisms appear on the Earth, they have to compete with pre-existing organisms. This is especially true when there are limited places to live and limited sources of nutrients. It is understandable that they would choose to work together to complement each other, rather than to exclude each other. Symbiosis is the solution chosen as a result of the struggle, rather than the default mechanism.

Symbiosis with microorganisms found in the living world is recognized from the stage of sponges, which are considered to be the oldest animals, existing for about 580 million years (Li et al., 1998; Hentschel et al., 2012; Webster and Taylor, 2012). Sponges are mostly marine, although some freshwater sponges exist, and they filter large amounts of seawater using a filtration apparatus. Most marine sponges contain about 30 phyla of bacteria, archaea, fungi, and algae, and large numbers of viruses, which reside in an extracellular mesohyl (gelatin-like matrix). These other organisms sometimes comprise up to 40% of the sponge. Sponges obtain nutrients and metabolites effective against pathogens from microorganisms, while providing them with a place to survive. Interestingly, symbiotic microorganisms can be transmitted horizontally by uptake from the surrounding environment or vertically across generations (Bright and Bulgheresi, 2010; Webster and Thomas, 2016). In the former case, there is a risk of pathogen uptake; however, it may be advantageous from the perspective of natural selection, as the organisms are dependent on the surrounding environment for acquiring new microorganisms. The latter has the advantage of ensuring that the microorganisms necessary for adaptation are transmitted from the parent, but the number of transmitted symbiotic microorganisms is limited and diversity may be lost over time.

Symbiosis with bacteria, archaea, fungi, and viruses has also been observed in cnidarians such as corals, sea anemones, and jellyfish, but the mutualism with the protist dinoflagellate is more prominent (Davy et al., 2012). In this case, the symbiont is not extracellular but is present within the cells of the gastric layer that covers the inner surface of the stomach cavity and is integrated with the host. Involved in this integration process is the recognition of MAMPs by the host's PRRs, which play a central role in innate immunity. The symbiont supports host metabolism, growth, reproduction, and survival in nutrient-poor environments by providing the products of photosynthesis. In contrast, the host protects the symbiont from predators, ensures access to light, and provides nutrients in its waste products. One well-known example of a characteristic relationship is the symbiosis between the Hawaiian bobtail squid and the luminescent bacterium *Vibrio fischeri*. These squids have organs that contain luminescent bacteria; at night, they emerge from the sand where they hide during the day to pursue their prey. The light emitted by the luminescent bacteria hides the shadows that form under the squid on moonlit nights, protecting the host from attacks by foreign enemies. At dawn, the squid expels the bacteria, and the remaining bacteria multiply as the squid burrows back under the sand for the night. The host squid provides nutrients such as sugars and amino acids to the bacteria and helps them multiply in a mutualistic relationship.

Plants have been living in water since their origin, but they began to live on land 450 million years ago. An important part of this process was symbiosis with a fungus that attached itself to the roots and assisted in the intake of nutrients and water, a form of symbiosis that has been confirmed in fossils dating back 400 million years. The fungus, called arbuscular mycorrhiza, not only supplies plants with phosphorus, water, and micronutrients but also confers resistance to plant pathogens and environmental stressors, such as intense light, high temperature, and drought. Nutrients are transported by structures called arbuscules that form in the roots. The host plant provides carbon compounds (e.g., sucrose and glucose) produced by photosynthesis to arbuscular mycorrhizal fungi to establish a mutualistic relationship. Such symbiosis occurs in more than 80% of terrestrial plants (Parniske, 2008). In addition, the roots of leguminous plants such as soybeans are symbiotic with a soil bacterium called rhizobium. The bacteria colonize plant cells to form root nodules where they fix atmospheric nitrogen into ammonia, which is then supplied to the plant. The host specificity of legumes is high; for example, soybeans have soybean rhizobia, and alfalfa has alfalfa rhizobia. Rhizobial symbiosis is thought to have been established based on symbiosis with arbuscular mycorrhizal fungi, and both use a common gene network (Parniske, 2008). Similarly, orchids form root-specific orchid mycorrhiza, and the specificity is so strict that germination will not occur unless symbiosis with a specific symbiotic bacterium is established.

Diverse symbioses have also been established in other organisms. Here, I will mention a problem related to the COVID-19 pandemic that originated in Wuhan, China, in the fall of 2019. Examining the past few decades, such emerging infectious disease pandemics have included Marburg hemorrhagic fever caused by the Marburg virus, Ebola hemorrhagic fever caused by the Ebola virus, SARS caused by the SARS-CoV, the Middle East respiratory syndrome (MERS) caused by the MERS coronavirus (MERS-CoV), and COVID-19. These infections are considered to be caused by viruses of zoonotic origin. For SARS-CoV-2, the causative virus of COVID-19, it has been suggested that the natural host bat, which serves as a reservoir, infects humans via another animal. Bats are the only mammals equipped with flight; they have a low tumor incidence rate and account for 18 of 19 mammalian species with a life span per body size longer than that of humans (Austad, 2010). For this reason, bats are considered a research model for cancer and longevity. Furthermore, bats can retain viruses without presenting clinical symptoms, and the mechanisms behind this are under investigation.

Bats harbor more viruses than other mammals (Luis et al., 2013; Brook and Dobson, 2015; Olival et al., 2017) and rarely develop disease when infected with Ebola virus or MERS-CoV (Swanepoel et al., 1996; Munster et al., 2016). A hypothesis was proposed that the high metabolism and high body temperature caused by flight are detrimental to viral replication (O'Shea et al., 2014). However, subsequent studies have predominantly suggested that rather than an active protective response by suppressing viral replication, there is a mechanism that prevents disease onset despite viral replication (Pavlovich et al., 2018; Ahn et al., 2019). This can be considered a tolerance for viruses, and bats may be symbiotic with viruses. Specifically, IFNs with antiviral activity, which are normally induced only by a viral infection, and genes induced by IFNs are expressed at a steady state in bats. In addition, an increase in autophagy, which is involved in the elimination of pathogens, and an increase in the expression of heat shock proteins, which are beneficial for cell survival under stress, have been observed in bats. There is a series of intracellular signaling pathways that begin with the recognition of MAMPs by PRRs as part of innate immunity against infection. An important element involved in this pathway is an intracellular protein complex called the inflammasome, which induces the secretion of inflammatory cytokines (IL-1β and IL-18). This complex contains intracellular sensors (e.g., NLRP3) that are involved in the recognition of endogenous DAMPs, MAMPs, adaptor proteins (apoptosis-associated speck-like protein containing a caspase activation and recruitment domain: ASCs), and an enzyme (caspase 1) that converts precursors of IL-1β and IL-18 to their mature forms. The complex is not only involved in the induction of inflammation but also in metabolic (obesity, atherosclerosis, and type 2 diabetes) and neurodegenerative (multiple sclerosis, Alzheimer's disease, and Parkinson's disease) diseases. It has been suggested that in bats, the inflammatory response to viruses is attenuated and immune tolerance may be established due to the reduced function of the NLRP3 sensor, IL-1β or caspase-1 (Ahn et al., 2016; Xie et al., 2018; Goh et al., 2020; Irving et al., 2021). Considering these peculiarities, there remains a risk that human infectious viruses will continue to emerge from bats, and preventing this process will represent a future challenge.

2.3 SYMBIOSIS WITH THE FETUS

People in the past did not find the phenomena of pregnancy and delivery particularly strange, and we imagine that they hoped for the uneventful passage of 40 weeks and safe delivery. However, the British immunologist Peter Medawar (1915–1987; Nobel Prize in Physiology or Medicine 1960) believed that the survival of the fetus within the mother for a certain period was a mysterious phenomenon that must be explained and found immunological significance in it. In his 1953 paper, *Some immunological and endocrinological problems raised by the evolution of viviparity in vertebrates*, Medawar drew on the results of his experimental transplantation studies to explain why the fetus is not rejected by the maternal immune system despite containing genes derived from the father that are almost certain to differ from those of the mother (Medawar, 1953). The fetus was viewed as an allogeneic graft, which provided the foresight to get to the essence of the matter. Since then, various possibilities have been discussed as to why the fetus can coexist with the mother.

Initially, Medawar considered three possibilities: first, the fetus and mother are anatomically isolated; second, the fetus is antigenically immature; and third, the mother's immunity is compromised during pregnancy. Medawar considered the first possibility the most important. In 1964, his colleague Rupert Billingham (1921–2002) offered a fourth possibility: the uterus, like the brain, testes, and anterior chamber of the eye, was an immunologically privileged site beyond the reach of the host's immune system (Billingham, 1964b, 1964a). However, none of Medawar's hypotheses were ever proven. For example, the fetus encounters and invades the endometrium via placental cells called extravillous trophoblasts, but Medawar believed that these cells are not exposed to the maternal immune system due to a perfect barrier. In reality, there is traffic between mother and child, with cells of fetal origin in the maternal blood and cells of maternal origin in the fetus. Furthermore, the hypothesis that low fetal antigenicity and weak maternal immunity prevent an immune response was not substantiated. It was found that cells and antibodies recognizing fetal antigens of paternal origin were present in the mother. It also became clear that the uterus was not necessarily an immunologically privileged site, as transplantation immunity can be elicited in a normal manner within this organ (Billington, 2003). Instead, it was believed that although an immune response occurs in the mother, a mechanism operates to suppress it.

I will now discuss the bidirectional exchanges between the mother and fetus. Fetal-derived trophoblasts were observed in maternal pulmonary vessels by German pathologist Georg Schmorl (1861–1932) in 1893 (Lapaire et al., 2007). Subsequent studies have shown that immune cells and mesenchymal stem cells of fetal origin are not only found in maternal blood but are also incorporated into tissues such as the mammary gland, heart, pancreas, and brain and are present long after birth. Similarly, cells of maternal origin are found in the fetus and are in a state of mutual microchimerism (Nelson, 2003; Boddy et al., 2015; Gammill and Harrington, 2017). Whether this is a phenomenon associated with pregnancy or a mechanism selected for adaptation by the organism remains unclear. However, maternal microchimerism has been implicated in lactation, wound healing, tissue regeneration, autoimmune diseases such as type 1 diabetes, Hashimoto's thyroiditis, and breast cancer. To further complicate matters, a pregnant woman not only receives cells from her fetus, but she may also transmit cells that she received from her mother when she was a fetus, or from her older siblings. As we saw in the case of symbiosis with microorganisms, "I is another," as Rimbaud said. What physical and mental effects does microchimerism have on the organism? This is a matter of unending interest.

As mentioned above, while none of Medawar's hypotheses were confirmed, was it not meaningful to redefine pregnancy within the new framework of allogeneic transplantation and to provide a reason for the establishment of pregnancy or the absence of rejection? As mentioned in Section 1.8, Chapter 1, the importance of a hypothesis is not whether it is proven, but whether it provides a new direction, a new perspective, a connection to other fields, or a concept that advances our knowledge (Cooper, 1997; Galison, 2007). If it is more important whether or not the hypothesis paves the way for the future, then Medawar's proposal may have served well as a hypothesis. This hypothesis has stimulated subsequent research with the participation of related fields, and has led to the development of the new field of reproductive immunology.

Let us consider the mechanisms of maternal immunological tolerance that establish pregnancy that reproductive immunology has revealed to date. First is the role of the MHC, which is important in transplantation. In humans, this is called HLA, which encodes several classes of molecules: class I is expressed on all cell surfaces; class II is expressed on special cells such as APCs; and class III (e.g., complement), which, unlike class I and class II, is not involved in antigen presentation. Initially, HLA class I was not detectable on trophoblasts, which was thought to explain the establishment of pregnancy (i.e., the absence of fetal rejection). However, subsequent studies revealed that HLA class I molecules include the classical class Ia molecules (HLA-A, -B, and -C), which are expressed on all cells and are highly polymorphic, in addition to the non-classical class Ib molecules (HLA-E, -F, and -G), which are more localized and less polymorphic. Human extravillous trophoblasts that invade the mother do not express HLA-A, -B, or class II molecules but do express HLA-C and class Ib molecules. Maternal and paternal HLA-C are present in extravillous trophoblasts, and paternally derived HLA-C can be recognized by NK cells (killer lymphocytes in innate immunity) and T cells in the maternal decidua and may induce rejection. NK cells are predominant in early pregnancy and have killer cell Ig-like receptors (KIRs) on their cell surface that use HLA-C expressed on extravillous trophoblasts as a ligand. There are inhibitory (A) and active (B) forms of KIR, and if the mother is homozygous (AA) for inhibitory KIR, there is a risk of abnormal pregnancy (e.g., preeclampsia) due to binding with fetal HLA-C (Hiby et al., 2004). Therefore, the interaction between NK cells in the decidua and HLA-C expressed on the extravillous trophoblasts may determine the extent of trophoblastic cell invasion and local vascular remodeling, which are essential for fetal growth.

Another MHC that plays an important role in immune tolerance in pregnancy is HLA-G, which belongs to the non-classical MHC class Ib (Ferreira et al., 2017). The gene was first identified about 40 years ago (Orr et al., 1982) and was named HLA-G in 1990 (Bodmer et al., 1990). HLA-G is expressed exclusively on extravillous trophoblasts (Kovats et al., 1990). This strict localization was sufficient to suspect the involvement of HLA-G in fetal immune tolerance. Studies in the 1990s revealed that the expression of HLA-G in NK cell lines that specifically respond to HLA-C suppressed the killing ability of the NK cells (Pazmany et al., 1996) and experiments with peripheral blood NK cells demonstrated that HLA-G is an inhibitory ligand for NK cells (Rouas-Freiss et al., 1997). Furthermore, a KIR molecule (KIR2DL4) expressed on all NK cells was reported to be a receptor for HLA-G (Rajagopalan and Long, 1999). These results suggest that HLA-G expressed on extravillous trophoblasts may induce immune tolerance against the fetus by suppressing the activity of all maternal NK cells.

Another mechanism by which HLA-G confers suppressive properties on NK cells is trogocytosis. The term is derived from the Greek word *trogo*, meaning "to gnaw" or "to cut off little by little." As the name implies, trogocytosis is a mechanism by which fragments of the cell membrane are transferred to other cells in a gnawing manner to alter their functions. At the mother–infant interface, maternal NK cells nibble HLA-G from the fetus' extravillous trophoblasts and suppress their ability to kill, thereby inducing immune tolerance in the mother. Here we see an interesting synergy between mother and child that makes pregnancy possible. The process of trogocytosis is widely recognized, and it has been suggested that trogocytosis may have operated early in evolution as a symbiotic principle to nourish other cells (Joly and Hudrisier, 2003).

I will now discuss the involvement of Treg cells (CD4+, CD25+, and Foxp3+) in the immunosuppression of pregnancy. Tregs were introduced as cells that suppress autoimmunity (Section 2.1, Chapter 2). However, according to a 2004 study, in mice in which CD4+ and CD25+ cells were removed, fetuses conceived from genetically identical inbred parents had no abnormalities, but those from allogeneic (between different strains) parents aborted (Aluvihare et al., 2004). There are reports that Tregs can suppress immunity in a fetal-specific or -nonspecific manner, that they are increased in the decidua during pregnancy, and some become memory cells and remain present postpartum, and that Tregs are decreased in infertility, recurrent miscarriage, and pre-eclampsia

(Tilburgs et al., 2008; Erlebacher, 2013; La Rocca et al., 2014; Green et al., 2021). These results suggest that Tregs may be involved in immune tolerance during pregnancy.

Other diverse factors have been reported to be involved in immune tolerance, including PD-1, PD-L1, and indoleamine oxygenase, which degrades tryptophan, one of the essential amino acids. One can imagine that many of these factors play their respective roles in maintaining pregnancy. Recently, beyond the conventional framework of attributing successful pregnancy to the immunosuppression of graft rejection, a more dynamic view that includes the involvement of the microbiota has emerged (Mor et al., 2017). Although 70 years have passed since Medawar raised the issue, the whole picture of pregnancy has not yet been revealed, and it continues to be a phenomenon full of mystery.

2.4 PROBLEMS POSED BY SYMBIOSIS

We have examined autoimmunity and symbiosis with others, and it has become clear that many organisms are so dependent on others that they routinely incorporate microorganisms and cannot exist without symbionts. This view is now predominant, and symbiosis can be considered an inevitable principle in the evolution of plants and animals (McFall-Ngai et al., 2013; Douglas, 2014). When new organisms appeared on the Earth, microorganisms were already there; at first, they likely killed each other intensely, but over the course of evolution, they were selected to live together when mutually favorable conditions were established. This framework would apply to species that are completely dependent on the microbiota, such as humans, squids, and corals, but would exclude organisms that do not have symbiotic relationships, such as ants and caterpillars. To explain this phenomenon, one view posits that there are species that depend on the microbiota (e.g., humans) and species that do not have a microbiota, and there is not a discontinuity between the two, but rather a continuum of different species with varying degrees of dependence on the microbiota (Hammer et al., 2019). According to this view, if the microorganisms are transiently present in the organism and their presence does not contribute to the adaptive capacity of the host, it is merely a passing presence. In addition, certain species perform functions such as digestion of plant fiber and luminescence using their own systems without the help of symbiotic microorganisms. The authors highlight that symbiosis is not inevitable just because we live in a world full of microorganisms and not all organisms have been examined for their microbiota thus far (Hammer et al., 2019).

On the other hand, there is the position that the essence of nature is not symbiosis but rather savage combat and competition for survival. This idea has had strong supporters to the present day. For example, Herbert Spencer (1820–1903) erroneously described Darwin's evolution by natural selection as the "survival of the fittest" (Spencer, 1864), which has spread to the general public and has influenced the way we face social problems. Joseph de Maistre (1753–1821), an anti-revolutionary and anti-enlightenment French diplomat, described the world as follows:

> There is no moment in time when one living being is not devoured by another. Above these many types of animals is placed man, whose destructive hand spares nothing that lives; he kills to feed, dress, adorn, attack, defend, instruct, amuse, and kill. A superb and terrible king, he needs everything, and nothing resists him.
>
> **de Maistre (2007a)**

Or,

> This is how the great law of the violent destruction of living beings is fulfilled without ceasing, from the mite to the man. The whole Earth, continually soaked in blood, is but an immense altar where every living thing must be immolated endlessly, without measure, without respite, until the consummation of things, the extinction of evil, and the death of death.
>
> **de Maistre (2007b)**

This represents a clear belief that reflects the cruel reality that killing each other rules the biological world and nothing else. However, in the struggle for survival, there is one perspective in which anthropocentrism is at the forefront, and it assumes that humans, who reign at the top, are safe.

We are reminded of the epic experience of the Australian ecofeminist philosopher Val Plumwood (1939–2008) and the ideas that emerged from it. She criticized the viewpoint of superiority or domination in the dualistic elements found in Western thought—for example, nature and culture, human and nature (as a non-human entity), universal and particular, mind and body, reason and bestial nature, subject and object, self and other, master and slave, and man and woman. She advocated a repositioning of the human being in an ecological context and of non-human beings in ethical relations (Plumwood, 1993). One important event caused a radical change in her thinking.

On February 19, 1985, while exploring the lagoons of Kakadu National Park in northern Australia, she was attacked and nearly devoured by a crocodile (Plumwood, 1995). This event triggered a shift from the de Maistre view, in which man is master and the individual can do anything to protect himself, to the view of Heraclitus (c. 540–c. 480 BC). In the Heraclitean world, human beings are mere lumps of meat like other animals and can become prey for other animals in the food chain of nature. Like other animals, when they disappear, the world moves on as if nothing had happened to them. With this realization, one is forced to conclude that the anthropocentric view does not reflect reality. Parasitism seems to conform to this view, and the phenomena of commensalism and mutualism can also be established under the condition that they do not mutually prey on each other.

I would like to consider this conflict of struggle or symbiosis more broadly and apply it to the workings of science. For example, there is the idea that the pursuit of truth by individuals out of sheer curiosity is what brings about scientific progress. On the other hand, there is the view that the combative instinct, which seems to be built into human nature, is what brings about scientific and technological progress. The former argument seems to be formed from a wish that it should be so and demands that we must learn to control our human nature in order to do so. In the latter argument, the raw, primitive human instincts are triggered and may spontaneously appear when our routine inhibitions are released. Perhaps both elements are at work in real research, but one or the other has sometimes been emphasized at different times.

Another conflict can be considered. At one extreme is the position that the essence of science is only competition and that it is meaningless unless it is first discovered. However, as this would make the existence of any other scientist worthless, the idea has emerged that science should be viewed as a community activity, and within that community, people should seek others who can work with them to jointly make discoveries. Richard Roberts (1943–; Nobel Prize in Physiology or Medicine 1993) takes the latter position and advocates for "community-based projects" (Roberts, 2004). In 1997, he reported that not all DNA becomes protein but that there is a segment of DNA called an intron that is cut off before it becomes transcribed (Chow et al., 1977). Roberts finally received the Nobel Prize 16 years after his discovery, against his expectations. According to Roberts, James Watson (1928–; Nobel Prize in Physiology or Medicine 1962), his boss at the Cold Spring Harbor Laboratory, liked to go out and compete aggressively in highly competitive areas where important discoveries were likely to be made. It is clear that Watson viewed science as competition. These two poles in nature and human society will always exist. As with the two poles of pathology and physiology, disease and health, discussed in Chapter 5, the question will continue to be how to strike a balance between them.

Michel Serre (1930–2019), a philosopher who is sometimes called a modern encyclopedist, developed his own speculations on symbiosis and parasitism. In his book *The Parasite*, he explains the three meanings of the French word "parasite" (Serres, 1980). The first is that of a person who lives in idleness and is dependent on others and society, an existence that can be described in terms such as "parasite of society." To explain this, he cites "The Town Rat and the Country Rat" in *The Fables* by La Fontaine (1621–1695) (La Fontaine, 1886). It is the parasite who enters a person's house and eats what is there, and the meal is interrupted by the noise of the houseowner. The parasite takes but gives nothing, and the host gives but takes nothing. Both parties engage in one-way acts, and this is the basis of the relationship, reflecting that there is no exchange in society. This is incompatible with the idea that giving is the basis of the relationship. The second meaning is parasitism in the biological sense, in which one organism expropriates nourishment from the other, and this is the most basic strategy applied in the biological world. These two forms of parasitisms are characterized by the unidirectional nature of taking without giving. The third parasite is a relationship found in the realm of the physical sciences: noise that impairs the reception of radio signals (i.e., noise that masks a meaningful signal). This is always found in communication systems, and there is no communication without this interference, no conversation without misunderstanding, and no nature without background noise. An important aspect of noise is its potential to create new complexity and diversity in a system. Serres states the following regarding the parasitism that lies at the foundation of the relationship:

> Background noise is perhaps the foundation of existence. Existence is neither resting nor moving. It is being shaken. The background noise never stops. It is unlimited, continuous, endless, and unchangeable.
>
> **Serres (1982)**

However, mutualism and commensalism are widely recognized in the biological world. Some people say that the biological world is founded on symbiosis. If we accept this fact, then we should say that rather than parasitism, symbiosis including parasitism is the foundation of the relationship. In contrast, if we adopt Plumwood's view, the symbiosis found in the biological world assumes that one's existence is guaranteed. In this sense, there is a certain truth in Serres' formula that "parasitism is the essence of existence." However, if we refer to his later work, such as *The Natural Contract* (Serres, 2018), it is clear that he did not ignore symbiosis altogether. He proceeds with the following logic on ecological issues that will be important for the future of humankind. Looking back through history, the subject of the rights acquired in human society has been the humans, but as these rights have gradually extended to nature as a whole, we are entering an era in which contracts are formed between nature and objects, including humans, and between nature and society/state. He highlights that it is important that the contract be a bidirectional "contract of symbiosis." With the increasing number of difficult problems facing humanity, it is hoped that people with this new awareness will be born to solve them. Metaphorically speaking, what is needed for this is not the conventional education that consists of two linear elements—the traveler and the destination—but a third place in between that is uncertain and difficult to balance. To learn is to expose oneself to this situation.

Here I would like to discuss the view that background noise is the basis of existence. For example, there is an ongoing interaction between the gut microbiota and the host that does not lead to pathological changes. However, this does not mean that nothing is happening; changes are occurring that should be referred to as physiological inflammation. It could be said that this constitutes the background noise of existence. The noise is not meaningless; it is related to the maturation of immune cells and the construction of barriers against pathogens. Physiological inflammation plays a maintenance function that supports the baseline of vital activities and prepares the body to respond to internal and external changes that are about to occur. Therefore, when this function is abnormal, various immune abnormalities occur. Furthermore, in the phenomenon known as physiological autoimmunity, self-recognition at a steady state may be involved in certain processes such as tissue repair, cell proliferation and differentiation, elimination of senescent cells, or killing of tumor cells (Cohen, 2007b), and when it is disrupted, pathological inflammation or autoimmune diseases develop (Cohen, 2007b, 2007a). In this case, self-recognition (i.e., binding of self-antigen to antigen receptor) sends signals into the cell and causes fluctuations in the cell, but it does not lead to the destruction of the self. Even in the immune system, where seemingly nothing is happening, there is ongoing activity that generates the background noise that is essential for host survival.

When considering the functions that support such a baseline, the default mode network (DMN) in the nervous system comes to mind (Raichle et al., 2001; Raichle, 2006, 2015). According to Marcus Reichle (1937–) of Washington University in St. Louis, our brains are permanently active even when we are not focusing our attention on the external world or when we are in a daze and removed from purposeful thinking. The energy consumed far exceeds that of doing something with a purpose. The DMN is the connection between the areas involved in this baseline activity. Let us take a brief look back at the history of the DMN. When the German psychiatrist Hans Berger (1873–1941) first recorded brain waves in 1929, he observed that the brain was active even in a steady state of doing nothing consciously. However, his findings were ignored for many years. In science, the pre- and post-stimulus conditions are often compared, and the changes observed before the stimulus are generally subtracted as noise to be used as a control. Therefore, it is not surprising that attention was not paid to the baseline condition before the stimulus. Positron emission tomography was introduced in the late 1970s, and functional magnetic resonance imaging (fMRI) in the 1990s, and brain activity could be observed as changes in glucose metabolism and blood flow. During this period, Reichle's group noticed that certain regions were active not only when facing a task but also in the baseline state, or conversely, certain regions were less active when performing a task, leading to the discovery of the DMN. Close examination revealed that 60%–80% of the brain's total energy is expended at baseline, and the brain's energy expenditure during a task is only 5% higher than the baseline.

Although there is no consensus on the function of the DMN, it is believed to be related to inward mental activity. For example, the DMN is activated when we are dreaming, when we are thinking independently of stimuli, when we retrieve memories, when we imagine the thoughts and feelings of third parties, when we are thinking about the future, and when we are conscious of what we are thinking. Anatomically, the medial prefrontal cortex, posterior cingulate cortex, precuneus, and lower parietal lobe are believed to be involved. According to an international collaborative study conducted in 2008, fMRI observation of the brain of a person performing a task on a computer revealed that the state of the DMN could predict whether the person would make a mistake 30 seconds before performing the task (Eichele et al., 2008). Therefore, the DMN is involved in preparation for upcoming situations, which is reminiscent of physiological inflammation functioning to prepare for the future in the immune system. It has also been suggested that activating the DMN may enhance the ability to reflect on the past and future, which in turn may foster imagination and creativity. Conversely, being in a state of mind that is not focused anywhere else will strengthen the ability to move toward imagination and creation. To move toward creation, one must become accustomed to being in a state of inaction. On a personal note, my experience of spending over 10 years in France in which I did not focus my consciousness on any specific things provided me with a concrete understanding of the concept behind the DMN. In addition, abnormalities in areas overlapping with the DMN have been observed in Alzheimer's disease, depression, autism, and schizophrenia, indicating the importance of the DMN in maintaining physiological function. In the two higher functioning systems, nervous and immune, sufficient attention has not been given to stimulus-independent baseline activity. To understand more fully the function of a single system, it would be impossible to ignore baseline activities that function in a stimulus-independent manner, because the system's unexpected essence may be hidden in the baseline activities.

2.5   WHAT DOES "ORGANISM" MEAN?

As we have already seen, the microorganisms present in our intestines, skin, oral cavity, and vagina are not to be dismissed as strangers but are inseparably linked to human physiology and deeply involved in many processes from birth to death. One's view of organism will change depending on how one interprets this symbiosis with microorganisms. This raises the scientific and philosophical question of what "organism" means. This issue was debated even before it became clear that symbiosis with microorganisms was a rule of life. However, depending on the area in which the term is used (e.g., evolution, embryology, physiology, ecology, immunology, or cognitive science), its connotations are not always consistent, so clearly defining organism has not been easy. For example, the issue of identity in organisms in which cells are constantly replaced was a subject of debate. There is a thought experiment from ancient Greece called the Ship of Theseus. The question is whether a ship can be said to be the same even if parts of it are repaired over time and the original materials used are eventually no longer present. At the biological level, it may be possible to discuss identity by defining the values that must be maintained to be considered identical, but in general this is difficult. From a psychological point of view, this leads to the question of whether the person I was when I was younger is the same as the person I am now. When I reread my writings from my youth, I find it difficult to believe that we are the same person. This can be attributed to the process of growing up; however, even comparing the time when I seemed to have settled down, I sometimes question the identity of the two persons. Upon closer observation, there is a difference between the self of yesterday and the self of today. Therefore, it is difficult to determine the identity of the self within a certain frame of time.

The issue of the organism has also been discussed in relation to biological individuals. Specific definitions and theories are needed to solve this problem. The theory of evolution, which forms the basis of biology, can be useful. This theory is based on mutation, natural selection, and reproductive success or failure. Darwin believed that natural selection operates through the phenomenal organism, which we usually recognize as such. From this theory emerged the trend to define the biological individual as a "unit of natural selection," which remains a powerful view today (Hull, 1978). According to this view, the biological individual, also called the Darwinian individual, includes not only a gene or cell that is unlikely to be accepted as a phenomenal organism but also groups as a set of organisms and even species as the basic taxonomic unit. As gene centrism gained strength in the late 20th century, Richard Dawkins (1941–) expressed the view that genes are the target of natural selection and that so-called organisms are mere containers that carry genes (Dawkins, 1976). So-called organisms represent only one level of the hierarchy of biological individuals.

Some objections have been raised to this definition from an evolutionary perspective. One of these objections recommends considering the biological individual from a physiological perspective rather than an evolutionary one. Ernst Mayr (1904–2005) categorized biology into functional biology and evolutionary biology (Mayr, 1961). Functional biologists examine how molecules, organs, and other components work in a given system; they isolate the components, control the experimental conditions, and repeat the experiment until they believe that they have revealed the function of the target. Their research addresses "how" a phenomenon occurs. In contrast, evolutionary biologists believe that all organisms—both as individuals and as members of a species—are the product of a long history of about four billion years, and we cannot understand their current function without taking that historical background into account. In addition, they aim to understand the reason for the existence of the organisms and "for what purpose" they are equipped with these functions. In this classification, the physiological perspective corresponds to the position of functional biology. For example, a physiological view of an organism can be described as a functionally integrated and coherent whole composed of causally connected elements that are constantly changing (Sober, 2000). For further clarification regarding functional integration, a definition has been proposed that it is linked locally by the biochemical interactions of different elements and is subject to systemic control by the immune system (Pradeu, 2010). Many other criteria have been considered concerning the biological individual, including autonomy, reproduction, heredity, separation of somatic and embryonic cells, and adaptability (Clarke, 2010). However, there is still a lack of consensus on the criteria that can define all organisms.

Finally, I will consider the question of how organisms that can be confirmed to symbiotically coexist with microorganisms should be viewed. Half a century ago, the American biologist Lynn Margulis (1938–2011) proposed the theory of intracellular symbiosis, which postulates that intracellular organelles such as mitochondria and chloroplasts are the result of bacterial symbiosis (Margulis, 1967). Although this theory was initially considered heretical and subjected to intense criticism, it eventually settled into its rightful place in orthodoxy. If we accept this theory, it is not surprising that our bodies are composed of numerous organisms and their components. An ecological perspective will become increasingly important when considering not only the immune system, but also what an organism is. In 1991, Margulis considered this situation and proposed the concept of the "holobiont" as an ecological unit that goes beyond the classical organism or individual and includes the host and all its associated microorganisms (Margulis and Fester, 1991). This term was coined from the ancient Greek word *holos*, meaning whole, and *biont*, meaning unit of life. However, it should be noted that this concept was previously reported by the German theoretical biologist Adolf Meyer-Abig (1893–1971) in 1943 (Baedke et al., 2020).

In 2008, Ilana Zilber-Rosenberg and Eugene Rosenberg of Tel Aviv University submitted a theory of hologenomic evolution that posits that the holobiont and its genetic information (hologenome) are the unit of natural selection (Zilber-Rosenberg and Rosenberg, 2008). The theory states that symbionts are transmitted across generations, that the host-microbe relationship affects the holobiont's adaptability to its environment, and that hologenomic changes occur in both the host and the microbe, with the more rapidly mutating microbe playing a more central role than the host. The condition presented in this paper—the transmission of microorganisms acquired from parents and the environment to the next generation—is reminiscent of the theory of Jean-Baptiste Lamarck (1744–1829).

In his *Zoological Philosophy* (1809), Lamarck proposed the first law on "use and disuse" and the second law on "inheritance of acquired characteristics" (Lamarck, 1809). Furthermore, in the first volume of his *Natural History of Animals without Vertebrae* (1815), he summarized the framework of his theory as four laws (Lamarck, 1815). According to Lamarck, the first three laws relate to the process of organization of organisms and the formation of organs, and they correspond to the first law outlined in the *Zoological Philosophy*. The fourth law is explained as follows:

> Everything that has been acquired, traced or changed in the organization of individuals during the course of their lives is preserved by generation, and transmitted to the new individuals who come from those who have undergone these changes.

Lamarck (1815)

Lamarck's ideas, which came to be known as the "inheritance of acquired characteristics," were the subject of intense criticism during his lifetime. Translated from a modern perspective, the ideas may be summarized as follows: first, environmental factors cause genetic changes; second, these changes target certain genes; and third, the resulting genetic changes are adaptations to the original environmental factors (Koonin and Wolf, 2009).

Darwin proposed the pangenesis hypothesis in Chapter 27 of *The Variation of Animals and Plants under Domestication* (Darwin, 1868). This hypothesis asserts that cells throughout the body release microscopic particles (which he named "gemmules"), and when collected from all parts of the body, the particles become the elements of reproduction and are transmitted to the next generation. The hypothesis may be classified as a Lamarckian mode of inheritance in that it postulates that somatic cells affected by the environment contribute to inheritance (although the mechanism has not been clarified) and environmental influences are transmitted to the next generation. However, his joint experiments with his half-cousin Francis Galton (1822–1911), a proponent of social Darwinism and eugenics, failed to substantiate Darwin's hypothesis, and Darwin never mentioned the pangene hypothesis again. He was ultimately unable to clarify the mechanism of heredity.

The concept of the hologenome, which recalls Lamarck's mode of inheritance, has attracted much attention. However, critics of the concept question whether the evidence is sufficient. Symbiotic microorganisms are functionally integrated with their hosts, but it is hard to see a physical relationship between them, such as that of mitochondria or chloroplasts. However, 10 years after submitting their theory of hologenomic evolution, the Rosenbergs acknowledged that vertical transmission, which is a prerequisite for the theory that the hologenome is the unit of evolutionary selection, is the most controversial aspect, but that there are animals that exhibit such a mode of inheritance. (Rosenberg and Zilber-Rosenberg, 2018). It will be interesting to see how this theory develops in the future.

While some believe that the microorganisms that make up the microbiota existed as symbionts from the beginning, others believe that they were initially pathogens. In the latter case, one can imagine that our ancestors who survived the attack of pathogens took the path of coevolution with these microorganisms and became inextricably linked with them. The result is an ecological condition that embraces the external within itself. One century ago, the German obstetrician and gynecologist Albert Döderlein (1860–1941) demonstrated that lactic acid bacteria, which he named the Döderlein bacillus, constituted a bacterial flora in the vagina that maintained an acidic environment and contributed to biological defense (Döderlein, 1892). In addition, Metchnikoff suggested that bacterial intake has a positive effect on intestinal microflora and that lactobacilli and fermented foods are important for human health and longevity (Metchnikoff, 1910). We are now entering an era in which this relationship can be analyzed at the molecular level. All the evidence collected to date indicates that we cannot imagine our life or existence without considering the microorganisms in our body, not only from the immunological point of view but also from the philosophical perspective.

From a broader perspective, what has become clear is that all organisms need others for their existence, that is, we must accept others to live fully. This requirement can be found in the very beginning of the evolution of life. Notably, bacteria always exchange their genetic material between cells by horizontal gene transfer, which is critical to the generation of novelty and diversity (see Section 4.1.1, Chapter 4), which remains a source of creativity in life. The immune system understands the deeper meaning of the need for others.

NOTES

1 Cohen, I. (1992). The cognitive paradigm and the immunological homunculus. *Immunology Today* 13: 493.

2 Rimbaud. A. (1871). « Je est un autre » in French. Letter to Paul Demeny (May 15).

REFERENCES

Ahn, M., Anderson, D. E., Zhang, Q., Tan, C. W., Lim, B. L., Luko, K., Wen, M., Chia, W. N., Mani, S., Wang, L. C., Ng, J. H. J., Sobota, R. M., Dutertre, C.-A., Ginhoux, H., Shi, Z.-L., Irving, A. T., & Wang, L.-F. (2019). Dampened NLRP3-mediated inflammation in bats and implications for a special viral reservoir host. *Nature Microbiology, 4*, 789–799. doi: 10.1038/s41564-019-0371-3.

Ahn, M., Cui, J., Irving, A. T., & Wang, L.-F. (2016). Unique loss of the PYHIN gene family in bats amongst mammals: Implications for inflammasome sensing. *Scientific Reports, 6*, 21722. doi: 10.1038/srep21722.

Al Alam, D., Danopoulos, S., Grubbs, B., Ali, N. A. B. M., MacAogain, M., Chotirmall, S. H., Warburton, D., Gaggar, A., Ambalavanan, N., & Lal, C. V. (2020). Human fetal lungs harbor a microbiome signature. *American Journal of Respiratory and Critical Care Medicine, 201*, 1002–1006. doi: 10.1164/rccm.201911-2127LE.

Aluvihare, V. R., Kallikourdis, M., & Betz, A. G. (2004). Regulatory T cells mediate maternal tolerance to the fetus. *Nature Immunology, 5*, 266–271. doi: 10.1038/ni1037.

Aristotle. (1925). Book X. Pleasure, happiness. (D. Ross, Trans.). *The Nicomachean Ethics of Aristotle*. Oxford University Press. 248–278.

Arpaia, N., Campbell, C., Fan, X., Dikiy, S., an der Veeken, J., deRoos, P., Liu, H., Cross, J. R., ., Pfeffer, K., Coffer, P. J., & Rudensky, A. Y. (2013). Metabolites produced by commensal bacteria promote peripheral regulatory T-cell generation. *Nature, 504*, 451–455. doi: 10.1038/nature12726.

Atarashi, K., Tanoue, T., Ando, M., Kamada, N., Nagano, Y., Narushima, S., Suda, W., Imaoka, A., Setoyama, H., Nagamori, T., Ishikawa, E., Shima, T., Hara, T., Kado, S., Jinnohara, T., Ohno, H., Kondo, T., Toyooka, K., Watanabe, E., Yokoyama, S., et al. (2015). Th17 cell induction by adhesion of microbes to intestinal epithelial cells. *Cell, 163*, 367–380. doi: 10.1016/j.cell.2015.08.058.

Atarashi, K., Tanoue, T., Oshima, K., Suda, W., Nagano, Y., Nishikawa, H., Fukuda, S., Saito, T., Narushima, S., Hase, K., Kim, S., Fritz, J. V., Wilmes, P., Ueha, S., Matsushima, K., Ohno, H., Olle, B., Sakaguchi, S., Taniguchi, T., Morita, H., et al. (2013). Treg induction by a rationally selected mixture of *Clostridia* strains from the human microbiota. *Nature, 500*, 232–236. doi: 10.1038/nature12331.

Atarashi, K., Tanoue, T., Shima, T., Imaoka, A., Kuwahara, T., Momose, Y., Cheng, G., Yamasaki, S., Saito, T., Ohba, Y., Taniguchi, T., Takeda, K., Hori, S., Ivanov, I. I., Umesaki, Y., Itoh, K., & Honda, K. (2011). Induction of colonic regulatory T cells by indigenous *Clostridium* species. *Science, 331*, 337–341. doi: 10.1126/science.1198469.

Austad, S. N. (2010). Methusaleh's Zoo: How nature provides us with clues for extending human health span. *Journal of Comparative Pathology, 142*, S10–S21. doi: 10.1016/j.jcpa.2009.10.024.

Avrameas, S. (1991). Natural autoantibodies: From 'horror autotoxicus' to 'gnothi seauton'. *Immunology Today, 12*, 154–159. doi: 10.1016/S0167-5699(05)80045-3.

Avrameas, S., Ternynck, T., Tsonis, I. A., & Lymberi, P. (2007). Naturally occurring B-cell autoreactivity: A critical overview. *Journal of Autoimmunity, 29*, 213–218. doi: 10.1016/j.jaut.2007.07.010.

Bäckhed, F., Ley, R. E., Sonnenburg, J. L., Peterson, D. A., & Gordon, J. I. (2005). Host-bacterial mutualism in the human intestine. *Science, 307*, 1915–1920. doi: 10.1126/science.1104816.

Bäumler, A. J., & Sperandio, V. (2016). Interactions between the microbiota and pathogenic bacteria in the gut. *Nature, 535*, 85–93. doi: 10.1038/nature18849.

Baedke, J., Fábregas-Tejeda, A., & Nieves Delgado, A. (2020). The holobiont concept before Margulis. *Journal of Experimental Zoology Part B: Molecular Developmental Evolution, 334*, 149–155. doi: 10.1002/jez.b.22931.

Baumgarth, N. (2011). The double life of a B-1 cell: Self-reactivity selects for protective effector functions. *Nature Reviews Immunology, 11*, 34–46. doi: 10.1038/nri2901.

Bendelac, A., Bonneville, M., & Kearney, J. F. (2001). Autoreactivity by design: Innate B and T lymphocytes. *Nature Reviews Immunology, 1*, 177–186. doi: 10.1038/35105052.

Bennett, C. L., Christie, J., Ramsdell, F., Brunkow, M. E., Ferguson, P. J., Whitesell, L., Kelly, T. E., Saulsbury, F. T., Chance, P. F., & Ochs, H. D. (2001). The immune dysregulation, polyendocrinopathy, enteropathy, X-linked syndrome (IPEX) is caused by mutations of *FOXP3*. *Nature Genetics, 27*, 20–21. doi: 10.1038/83713.

Billingham, R. E. (1964a). Transplantation immunity and the maternal-fetal relation. *New England Journal of Medicine, 270*, 720–725. doi: 10.1056/NEJM196404022701406.

Billingham, R. E. (1964b). Transplantation immunity and the maternal-fetal relation. *New England Journal of Medicine, 270*, 667–672. doi: 10.1056/NEJM196403262701306.

Billington, W. D. (2003). The immunological problem of pregnancy: 50 years with the hope of progress. A tribute to Peter Medawar. *Journal of Reproductive Immunology, 60*, 1–11. doi: 10.1016/s0165-0378(03)00083-4.

Boddy, A. M., Fortunato, A., Wilson Sayres, M., & Aktipis, A. (2015). Fetal microchimerism and maternal health: A review and evolutionary analysis of cooperation and conflict beyond the womb. *Bioessays, 37*, 1106–1018. doi: 10.1002/bies.201500059.

Bodmer, J. G., Marsh, S. G. E., Parham, P., Erlich, H. A., Albert, E., Bodmer, W. F., Dupont, B., Mach, B., Mayr, W. R., Sasazuki, T., Schreuder, G. M. T., Strominger, J. L., Svejgaard, A., & Terasaki, P. I. (1990). Nomenclature for factors of the HLA system, 1989. *Tissue Antigens, 35*, 1–8. doi: 10.1111/j.1399-0039.1990.tb01749.x

Bomblies, K., & Weigel, D. (2007). Hybrid necrosis: Autoimmunity as a potential gene-flow barrier in plant species. *Nature Reviews Genetics, 8*, 382–393. doi: 10.1038/nrg2082.

Bordet, J. (1898). Sur l'agglutination et la dissolution des globules rouges par le sérum d'animaux injectés de sang défibriné (On the agglutination and dissolution of red blood cells by the serum of animals injected with defibrinated blood). *Annales de l'Institut Pasteur, 12*, 688–695.

Boyden, S. (1964). Autoimmunity and inflammation. *Nature, 201*, 200–201. doi: 10.1038/201200a0.

Brennecke, P., Reyes, A., Pinto, S., Rattay, K., Nguyen, M., Küchler, R., Huber, W., Kyewski, B., & Steinmetz, L. M. (2015). Single-cell transcriptome analysis reveals coordinated ectopic gene-expression patterns in medullary thymic epithelial cells. *Nature Immunology, 16*, 933–941. doi: 10.1038/ni.3246.

Bright, M., & Bulgheresi, S. (2010). A complex journey: Transmission of microbial symbionts. *Nature Reviews Microbiology, 8*, 218–230. doi: 10.1038/nrmicro2262.

Brook, C. E., & Dobson, A. P. (2015). Bats as 'special' reservoirs for emerging zoonotic pathogens. *Trends in Microbiology, 23*, 172–180. doi: 10.1016/j.tim.2014.12.004.

Burnet, F. M. (1959a). Auto-immune disease: I. Modern immunological concepts. *British Medical Journal, 2*, 645–650. doi: 10.1136/bmj.2.5153.645.

Burnet, F. M. (1959b). Auto-immune disease: II. Pathology of the immune response. *British Medical Journal, 2*, 720–725. doi: 10.1136/bmj.2.5154.720.

Burnet, F. M. (1972). A reassessment of the forbidden clone hypothesis of autoimmune disease. *Australian Journal of Experimental Biology and Medical Science, 50*, 1–9. doi: 10.1038/icb.1972.1.

Buss, L. W., Moore, J. L., & Green, D. R. (1985). Autoreactivity and self-tolerance in an invertebrate. *Nature, 313*, 400–402. doi: 10.1038/313400a0.

Canguilhem, G. (1991). *The Normal and the Pathological*. (C. R. Fawcett & R. S. Cohen, Trans.). Zone Books. 41.

Chow, L. T., Gelinas, R. E., Broker, T. R., & Roberts, R. J. (1977). An amazing sequence arrangement at the 5' ends of adenovirus 2 messenger RNA. *Cell, 12*, 1–8. doi: 10.1016/0092-8674(77)90180-5.

Chu, C., Murdock, M. H., Jing, D., Won, T. H., Chung, H., Kressel, A. M., Tsaava, T., Addorisio, M. E., Putzel, G. G., Zhou, L., Bessman, N. J., Yang, R., Moriyama, S., Parkhurst, C. N., Li, A., Meyer, H. C., Teng, F., Chavan, S. S., Tracey, K. J., Regev, A., et al. (2019). The microbiota regulate neuronal function and fear extinction learning. *Nature, 574*, 543–548. doi: 10.1038/s41586-019-1644-y.

Clarke, E. (2010). The problem of biological individuality. *Biological Theory, 5*, 312–325. doi: 10.1162/BIOT_a_00068.

Cohen, I. R. (1992). The cognitive paradigm and the immunological homunculus. *Immunology Today, 13*, 490–494. doi: 10.1016/0167-5699(92)90024-2.

Cohen, I. R. (2007a). Biomarkers, self-antigens and the immunological homunculus. *Journal of Autoimmunity, 29*, 246–249. doi: 10.1016/j.jaut.2007.07.016.

Cohen, I. R. (2007b). Real and artificial immune systems: Computing the state of the body. *Nature Reviews Immunology, 7*, 569–574. doi: 10.1038/nri2102.

Cohen, I. R. (2014). Activation of benign autoimmunity as both tumor and autoimmune disease immuno-therapy: A comprehensive review. *Journal of Autoimmunity, 54*, 112–117.

Cohen, I. R., & Cooke, A. (1986). Natural autoantibodies might prevent autoimmune disease. *Immunology Today, 7*, 363-364. doi: 10.1016/0167-5699(86)90026-5.

Cohen, I. R., & Young, D. B. (1991). Autoimmunity, microbial immunity and the immunological homunculus. *Immunology Today, 12*, 105–110. doi: 10.1016/0167-5699(91)90093-9.

Cooper, G. (1997). Clever Bunny. *The Independent*. https://www.independent.co.uk/life-style/clever-bunny-1267594.html.

Coutinho, A., Kazatchkine, M. D., & Avrameas, S. (1995). Natural autoantibodies. *Current Opinion in Immunology, 7*, 812–818. doi: 10.1016/0952-7915(95)80053-0.

Cryan, J. F., O'Riordan, K. J., Cowan, C. S. M., Sandhu, K. V., Bastiaanssen, T. F. S., Boehme, M., Codagnone, M. G., Cussotto, S., Fulling, C., Golubeva, A. V., Guzzetta, K. E., Jaggar, M., Long-Smith, C. M., Lyte, J. M., Martin, J. A., Molinero-Perez, A., Moloney, G., Morelli, E., Morillas, E., O'Connor, R., et al. (2019). The microbiota-gut-brain axis. *Physiological Reviews, 99*, 1877–2013. doi: 10.1152/physrev.00018.2018.

Döderlein, A. (1892). *Das Scheidensekret und seine Bedeutung für das Puerperalfieber (Vaginal Secretions and Their Significance for Puerperal Fever)*. Eduard Basold.

Darwin, C. (1868). *The Variation of Animals and Plants under Domestication. Vol. 2*. John Murray. 349–399.

Davy, S. K., Allemand, D., & Weis, V. (2012). Cell biology of cnidarian-dinoflagellate symbiosis. *Microbiology and Molecular Biology Reviews, 76*, 229–261. doi: 10.1128/mmbr.05014-11.

Dawkins, R. (1976). *The Selfish Gene*. Oxford University Press.

de Goffau, M. C., Lager, S., Sovio, U., Gaccioli, F., Cook, E., Peacock, S. J., Parkhill, J., Charnock-Jones, S., & Smith, G. C. S. (2019). Human placenta has no microbiome but can contain potential pathogens. *Nature, 572*, 329–334. doi: 10.1038/s41586-019-1451-5.

de Maistre, J. (2007a). *Joseph de Maistre Œuvre (Joseph de Maistre's Work)*. (H. Yakura, Trans.) Robert Laffont. 659–660.

de Maistre, J. (2007b). *Joseph de Maistre Œuvre (Joseph de Maistre's Work)*. (H. Yakura, Trans.) Robert Laffont. 661.

Dethlefsen, L., McFall-Ngai, M., & Relman, D. A. (2007). An ecological and evolutionary perspective on human-microbe mutualism and disease. *Nature, 449*, 811–818. doi: 10.1038/nature06245.

Dighiero, G., Lymberi, P., Holmberg, D., Lundquist, I., Coutinho, A., & Avrameas, S. (1985). High frequency of natural autoantibodies in normal newborn mice. *Journal of Immunology, 134*, 765–771. doi: 10.4049/jimmunol.134.2.765.

Dighiero, G., Lymberi, P., Mazié, J. C., Rouyre, S., Butler-Browne, G. S., Whalen, R. G., & Avrameas, S. (1983). Murine hybridomas secreting natural monoclonal antibodies reacting with self antigens. *Journal of Immunology, 131*, 2267–2272. doi: 10.4049/jimmunol.131.5.2267.

Donath, J., & Landsteiner, K. (1904). Über paroxysmale Hämoglobinurie (On paroxysmal hemoglobinuria). *Münchener Medizinische Wochenschrift, 51*, 1590–1593.

Douglas, A. E. (2010). *The Symbiotic Habit*. Princeton University Press. 5.

Douglas, A. E. (2014). Symbiosis as a general principle in eukaryotic evolution. *Cold Spring Harbor Perspectives in Biology, 6*, a016113. doi: 10.1101/cshperspect.a016113.

Ehrlich, P. (1900). Croonian lecture. On immunity with special reference to cell life. *Proceedings of the Royal Society of London, 66*, 424–448. doi: 10.1098/rspl.1899.0121.

Ehrlich, P., & Morgenroth, J. (1900). Über haemolysine. Dritte Mittheilung. (On hemolysis. Third communication). *Berliner Klinische Wochenschrift, 37*, 453–458.

Eichele, T., Debener, S., Calhoun, V. D., Specht, K., Engel, A. K., Hugdahl, K., von Cramon, D. Y., & Ullsperger, M. (2008). Prediction of human errors by maladaptive changes in event-related brain networks. *Proceedings of the National Academy of Sciences of the United States of America, 105*, 6173–6178. doi: 10.1073/pnas.0708965105.

Erlebacher, A. (2013). Immunology of the maternal-fetal interface. *Annual Review of Immunology, 31*, 387–411. doi: 10.1146/annurev-immunol-032712-100003.

Ferreira, L. M. R., Meissner, T. B., Tilburgs, T., & Strominger, J. L. (2017). HLA-G: At the interface of maternal-fetal tolerance. *Trends in Immunology, 38*, 272–286. doi: 10.1016/j.it.2017.01.009.

Flint, H. J. (2004). Polysaccharide breakdown by anaerobic microorganisms inhabiting the mammalian gut. *Advances in Applied Microbiology, 56*, 89–120. doi: 10.1016/S0065-2164(04)56003-3.

Flint, H. J., Duncan, S. H., Scott, K. P., & Louis, P. (2007). Interactions and competition within the microbial community of the human colon: Links between diet and health. *Environmental Microbiology, 9*, 1101–1111. doi: 10.1111/j.1462-2920.2007.01281.x.

Fontenot, J. D., Gavin, M. A., & Rudensky, A. Y. (2003). Foxp3 programs the development and function of CD4+CD25+ regulatory T cells. *Nature Immunology, 4*, 330–336. doi: 10.1038/ni904.

Funkhouser, L. J., & Bordenstein, S. R. (2013). Mom knows best: The universality of maternal microbial transmission. *PLoS Biology, 11*, e1001631. doi: 10.1371/journal.pbio.1001631.

Furusawa, Y., Obata, Y., Fukuda, S., Endo, T. A., Nakato, G., Takahashi, D., Nakanishi, Y., Uetake, C., Kato, K., Kato, T., Takahashi, M., Fukuda, N. N., Murakami, S., Miyauchi, E., Hino, S., Atarashi, K., Onawa, S., Fujimura, Y., Lockett, T., Clarke, J. M., et al. (2013). Commensal microbe-derived butyrate induces the differentiation of colonic regulatory T cells. *Nature, 504*, 446–450. doi: 10.1038/nature12721.

Galison, P. (2007). Sur quels critères juger une Théorie? (What are the criteria for judging a theory?). *La Recherche, 411*, 42.

Gammill, H. S., & Harrington, W. E. (2017). Microchimerism: Defining and redefining the prepregnancy context - A review. *Placenta, 60*, 130–133. doi: 10.1016/j.placenta.2017.08.071.

Gauld, S. B., Benschop, R. B., Merrell, K. T., & Cambier, J. C. (2005). Maintenance of B cell anergy requires constant antigen receptor occupancy and signaling. *Nature Immunology, 6*, 1160–1167. doi: 10.1038/ni1256.

Gay, D., Saunders, T., Camper, S., & Weigert, M. (1993). Receptor editing: An approach by autoreactive B cells to escape tolerance. *Journal of Experimental Medicine, 177*, 999–1008. doi: 10.1084/jem.177.4.999.

Gershon, R. K., & Kondo, K. (1970). Cell interactions in the induction of tolerance: The role of thymic lymphocytes. *Immunology, 18*, 723–737.

Gershon, R. K., & Kondo, K. (1971). Infectious immunological tolerance. *Immunology, 21*, 903–914.

Goh, G., Ahn, M., Zhu, F., Lee, L. B., Luo, D., Irving, A. T., & Wang, L.-F. (2020). Complementary regulation of caspase-1 and IL-1β reveals additional mechanisms of dampened inflammation in bats. *Proceedings of the National Academy of Sciences of the United States of America, 117*, 28939–28949. doi: 10.1073/pnas.2003352117.

Goodnow, C. C., Crosbie, J., Adelstein, S., Lavoie, T. B., Smith-Gill, S. J., Brink, R. A., Pritchard-Briscoe, H., Wotherspoon, J. S., Loblay, R. H., Raphael, K., Trent, R. J., & Basten, A. (1988). Altered immunoglobulin expression and functional silencing of self-reactive B lymphocytes in transgenic mice. *Nature, 334*, 676–682. doi: 10.1038/334676a0.

Grönlund, M. M., Lehtonen, O. P., Eerola, E., & Kero, P. (1999). Fecal microflora in healthy infants born by different methods of delivery: Permanent changes in intestinal flora after cesarean delivery. *Journal of Pediatric Gastroenterology and Nutrition, 28*, 19–25. doi: 10.1097/00005176-199901000-00007.

Grabar, P. (1947). *Les Globulines du sérum sanguin (Globulins in blood serum).* Desoer.

Grabar, P. (1983). Autoantibodies and the physiological role of immunoglobulins. *Immunology Today, 4*, 337–340. doi: 10.1016/0167-5699(83)90169-X.

Green, S., Politis, M., Rallis, K. S., Saenz de Villaverde Cortabarria, A., Efthymiou, A., Mureanu, N., Dalrymple, K. V., Scottà, C., Lombardi, G., Tribe, R. M., Nicolaides, K. H., & Shangaris, P. (2021). Regulatory T cells in regnancy adverse outcomes: A systematic review and meta-analysis. *Frontiers in Immunology, 12*, 737862. doi: 10.3389/fimmu.2021.737862.

Guilbert, B., Dighiero, G., & Avrameas, S. (1982a). Naturally occurring antibodies against nine common antigens in human sera. I. Detection, isolation and characterization. *Journal of Immunology, 128*, 2779–2787. doi: 10.4049/jimmunol.128.6.2779.

Guilbert, B., Dighiero, G., & Avrameas, S. (1982b). Naturally occurring antibodies against nine common antigens in human sera. II. High incidence of monoclonal Ig exhibiting antibody activity against actin and tubulin and sharing antibody specificities with natural antibodies. *Journal of Immunology, 128*, 2788–2792. doi: 10.4049/jimmunol.128.6.2788.

Gurung, M., Li, Z., You, H., Rodrigues, R., Jump, D. B., Morgun, A., & Shulzhenko, N. (2020). Role of gut microbiota in type 2 diabetes pathophysiology. *EBioMedicine, 51*, 102590. doi: 10.1016/j.ebiom.2019.11.051.

Hammer, T. J., Sanders, J. G., & Fierer, N. (2019). Not all animals need a microbiome. *FEMS Microbiology Letters, 366*, fnz117. doi: 10.1093/femsle/fnz117.

Hardy, R. R. (2006). B-1B cell development. *Journal of Immunology, 177*, 2749–2754. doi: 10.4049/jimmunol.177.5.2749.

Heidegger, M. (1990). Sérénité. (A. Préau, Trans.). *Questions III et IV*. Gallimard. (Originally published 1959). 136–137.

Helmink, B. A., Khan, M. A. W., Hermann, A., Gopalakrishnan, V., & Wargo, J. A. (2019). The microbiome, cancer, and cancer therapy. *Nature Medicine, 25*, 377–388. doi: 10.1038/s41591-019-0377-7.

Hentschel, U., Piel, J., Degnan, S. M., & Taylor, M. W. (2012). Genomic insights into the marine sponge microbiome. *Nature Reviews Microbiology, 10*, 641–654. doi: 10.1038/nrmicro2839.

Hiby, S. E., Walker, J. J., O'Shaughnessy, K. M., Redman, C. W. G., Carrington, M., Trowsdale, J., & Moffett, A. (2004). Combinations of maternal KIR and fetal HLA-C genes influence the risk of preeclampsia and reproductive success. *Journal of Experimental Medicine, 200*, 957–965. doi: 10.1084/jem.20041214.

Hooper, L. V. (2004). Bacterial contributions to mammalian gut development. *Trends in Microbiology, 12*, 129–134. doi: 10.1016/j.tim.2004.01.001.

Hooper, L. V., & Gordon, J. J. (2001). Commensal host-bacterial relationships in the gut. *Science, 292*, 1115–1118. doi: 10.1126/science.1058709.

Hori, S., Nomura, T., & Sakaguchi, S. (2003). Control of regulatory T cell development by the transcription factor *Foxp3*. *Science, 299*, 1057–1061. doi: 10.1126/science.1079490.

Hotamisligil, G. S. (2006). Inflammation and metabolic disorders. *Nature, 444*, 860–867. doi: 10.1038/nature05485.

Hufnagl, K., Pali-Schöll, I., Roth-Walter, F., & Jensen-Jarolim, E. (2020). Dysbiosis of the gut and lung microbiome has a role in asthma. *Seminars in Immunopathology, 42*, 75–93. doi: 10.1007/s00281-019-00775-y.

Hull, D. L. (1978). A matter of individuality. *Philosophy of Science, 45*, 335–360. doi: 10.1086/288811.

Invernizzi, P., Selmi, C., Ranftler, C., Podda, M., & Wesierska-Gadek, J. (2005). Antinuclear antibodies in primary biliary cirrhosis. *Seminars in Liver Disease, 25*, 298–310. doi: 10.1055/s-2005-916321.

Irving, A. T., Ahn, M., Goh, G., Anderson, D. E., & Wang, L.-F. (2021). Lessons from the host defences of bats, a unique viral reservoir. *Nature, 589*, 363–370. doi: 10.1038/s41586-020-03128-0.

Ivanov, I. I., Atarashi, K., Manel, N., Brodie, E. L., Shima, T., Karaoz, U., Wei, D., Goldfarb, K. C., Santee, C. A., Lynch, S. V., Tanoue, T., Imaoka, A., Itoh, K., Takeda, K., Umesaki, Y., Honda, K., & Littman, D. R. (2009). Induction of intestinal Th17 cells by segmented filamentous bacteria. *Cell, 139*, 485–498. doi: 10.1016/j.cell.2009.09.033.

Jerne, N. K. (1955). The natural-selection theory of antibody formation. *Proceedings of the National Academy of Sciences of the United States of America, 41*, 849–857. doi: 10.1073/pnas.41.11.849.

Jerne, N. K. (1974). Toward a network theory of the immune system. *Annales d'Immunologie, 125C*, 373–389.

Joly, E., & Hudrisier, D. (2003). What is trogocytosis and what is its purpose? *Nature Immunology, 4*, 815. doi: 10.1038/ni0903-815.

Kelly, D., Conway, S., & Aminov, R. (2005). Commensal gut bacteria: Mechanisms of immune modulation. *Trends in Immunology, 26*, 326–333. doi: 10.1016/j.it.2005.04.008.

Khattri, R., Cox, T., Yasayko, S. A., & Ramsdell, F. (2003). An essential role for Scurfin in CD4+CD25+ T regulatory cells. *Nature Immunology, 4*, 337–342. doi: 10.1038/ni909.

Kitagawa, Y., Ohkura, N., Kidani, Y., Vandenbon, A., Hirota, K., Kawakami, R., Yasuda, K., Motooka, D., Nakamura, S., Kondo, M., Taniuchi, I., Kohwi-Shigematsu, T., & Sakaguchi, S. (2017). Guidance of regulatory T cell development by Satb1-dependent super-enhancer establishment. *Nature Immunology, 18*, 173–183. doi: 10.1038/ni.3646.

Koonin, E. V., & Wolf, Y. I. (2009). Is evolution Darwinian or/and Lamarckian? *Biology Direct, 4*, 42. doi: 10.1186/1745-6150-4-42.

Kourilsky, P. (2014). *Le Jeu du hasard et de la complexité: La nouvelle science de l'immunologie (The Game of Chance and Complexity: The New Science of Immunology)*. Odile Jacob. 231.

Kovats, S., Main, E. K., Librach, C., Stubblebine, M., Fisher, S. J., & DeMars, R. (1990). A class I antigen, HLA-G, expressed in human trophoblasts. *Science, 248*, 220–223. doi: 10.1126/science.2326636.

La Fontaine, J. (1886). The Town Rat and the Country Rat. (W. Thornbury, Trans.). *The Fables of La Fontaine*. Cassell, Petter & Galpin. (Originally published 1668). 27–28.

La Rocca, C., Carbone, F., Longobardi, S., & Matarese, G. (2014). The immunology of pregnancy: Regulatory T cells control maternal immune tolerance toward the fetus. *Immunology Letters, 162*, 41–48. doi: 10.1016/j.imlet.2014.06.013.

Lamarck, J. B. (1809). *Philosophie zoologique (Zoological Philosophy)*. Duminil-Lesueur. 235.

Lamarck, J. B. (1815). *Histoire naturelle des animaux sans vertèbres, Tome 1 (Natural History of the Invertebrate Animals, Volume 1)*. (H. Yakura, Trans.). Abel Lanoë. 181–182.

Landsteiner, K. (1900). Zur Kenntnis der antifermentativen, lytischen und agglutinierenden Wirkungen des Blutserums und der Lymphe (For knowledge of the antifermentative, lytic and agglutinating effects of blood serum and lymph). *Zentralblatt für Bakteriologie. Originale, 27*, 357–362.

Landsteiner, K. (1901). Über Agglutinationserscheinungen normalen menschlichen Blutes (On agglutination phenomena of normal human blood). *Wiener klinische Wochenschrift, 14*, 1132–1134.

Landsteiner, K. (1936). *The Specificity of Serological Reactions*. Charles C. Thomas.

Lapaire, O., Holzgreve, W., Oosterwijk, J. C., Brinkhaus, R., & Bianchi, D. W. (2007). Georg Schmorl on trophoblasts in the maternal circulation. *Placenta, 28*, 1–5. doi: 10.1016/j.placenta.2006.02.004.

Lederberg, J. (2000). Infectious history. *Science, 288*, 287–293. doi: 10.1126/science.288.5464.287.

Lee, C.-H., & Giuliani, F. (2019). The role of inflammation in depression and fatigue. *Frontiers in Immunology, 10*, 1696. doi: 10.3389/fimmu.2019.01696.

Ley, R. E., Bäckhed, F., Turnbaugh, P., Lozupone, C. A., Knight, R. D., & Gordon, J. I. (2005). Obesity alters gut microbial ecology. *Proceedings of the National Academy of Sciences of the United States of America, 102*, 11070–11075. doi: 10.1073/pnas.0504978102.

Ley, R. E., Peterson, D. A., & Gordon, J. I. (2006). Ecological and evolutionary forces shaping microbial diversity in the human intestine. *Cell, 124*, 837–848. doi: 10.1016/j.cell.2006.02.017.

Li, C. W., Chen, J. Y., & Hua, T. E. (1998). Precambrian sponges with cellular structures. *Science, 279*, 879–882. doi: 10.1126/science.279.5352.879.

Luckey, T. D. (1972). Introduction to intestinal microecology. *American Journal of Clinical Nutrition, 25*, 1292–1294. doi: 10.1093/ajcn/25.12.1292.

Luis, A. D., Hayman, D. T. S., O'Shea, T. J., Cryan, P. M., Gilbert, A. T., Pulliam, J. R. C., Mills, J. N., Timonin, M. E., Willis, C. K. R., Cunningham, A. A., Fooks, A. R., Rupprecht, C. E., Wood, J. L. N., & Webb, C. T. (2013). A comparison of bats and rodents as reservoirs of zoonotic viruses: are bats special? *Proceedings of the Royal Society B: Biological Sciences, 280*, 20122753. doi: 10.1098/rspb.2012.2753.

Mändar, R., & Mikelsaar, M. (1996). Transmission of mother's microflora to the newborn at birth. *Biology of the Neonate, 69*, 30–35. doi: 10.1159/000244275.

Métalnikoff, S. (1900). Étude sur la spermotoxine (Study on spermotoxin). *Annales de l'Institut Pasteur, 14*, 577–589.

Margulis, L. (1967). On the origin of mitosing cells. *Journal of Theoretical Biology, 14*, 225–274. doi: 10.1016/0022-5193(67)90079-3.

Margulis, L., & Fester, R. (Eds.) (1991). *Symbiosis as a Source of Evolutionary Innovation: Speciation and Morphogenesis*. MIT Press.

Masters, S. L., Simon, A., Aksentijevich, I., & Kastner, D. L. (2009). Horror autoinflammaticus: The molecular pathophysiology of autoinflammatory disease. *Annual Review of Immunology, 27*, 621–668. doi: 10.1146/annurev.immunol.25.022106.141627.

Mathis, D., & Benoist, C. (2007). A decade of AIRE. *Nature Reviews Immunology, 7*, 645–650. doi: 10.1038/nri2136.

Mathis, D., & Benoist, C. (2009). Aire. *Annual Review of Immunology, 27*, 287–312. doi: 10.1146/annurev.immunol.25.022106.141532.

Mayr, E. (1961). Cause and effect in biology. *Science, 134*, 1501–1506. doi: 10.1126/science.134.3489.1501.

Mazmanian, S. K., & Kasper, D. L. (2006). The love-hate relationship between bacterial polysaccharides and the host immune system. *Nature Reviews Immunology, 6*, 849–858. doi: 10.1038/nri1956.

Mazmanian, S. K., Liu, C. H., Tzianabos, A. O., & Kasper, D. L. (2005). An immunomodulatory molecule of symbiotic bacteria directs maturation of the host immune system. *Cell, 122*, 107–118. doi: 10.1016/j.cell.2005.05.007.

Mazmanian, S. K., Round, J. L., & Kasper, D. L. (2008). A microbial symbiosis factor prevents intestinal inflammatory disease. *Nature, 453*, 620–625. doi: 10.1038/nature07008.

McDermott, M. F., Aksentijevich, I., Galon, J., McDermott, E. M., Ogunkolade, B. W., Centola, M., Mansfield, E., Gadina, M., Karenko, L., Pettersson, T., McCarthy, J., Frucht, D. M., Aringer, M., Torosyan, Y., Teppo, A. M., Wilson, M., Karaarslan, H. M., Wan, Y., Todd, I., Wood, G., et al. (1999). Germline mutations in the extracellular domains of the 55 kDa TNF receptor, TNFR1, define a family of dominantly inherited autoinflammatory syndromes. *Cell, 97*, 133–144. doi: 10.1016/s0092-8674(00)80721-7.

McFall-Ngai, M., Hadfield, M. G., Bosch, T. C., Carey, H. V., Domazet-Lošo, T., Douglas, A. E., Dubilier, N., Eberl, G., Fukami, T., Gilbert, S. F., Hentschel, U., King, N., Kjelleberg, S., Knoll, A. H., Kremer, N., Mazmanian, S. K., Metcalf, J. L., Nealson, K., Pierce, N. E., Rawls, J. F., et al. (2013). Animals in a bacterial world, a new imperative for the life sciences. *Proceedings of the National Academy of Sciences of the United States of America, 110*, 3229–3236. doi: 10.1073/pnas.1218525110.

Medawar, P. B. (1953). Some immunological and endocrinological problems raised by the evolution of viviparity in vertebrates. *Symposia of the Society for Experimental Biology, 7*, 320–328.

Metchnikoff, E. (1910). Études sur la flore intestinale. Deuxième mémoire (Studies on intestinal flora. Second report). *Annales de l'Institut Pasteur, 24*, 755–770.

Mishra, A., Lai, G. C., Yao, L. J., Aung, T. T., Shental, N., Rotter-Maskowitz, A., Shepherdson, E., Singh, G. S. N., Pai, R., Shanti, A., Wong, R. M. M., Lee, A., Khyriem, C., Dutertre, C. A., Chakarov, S., K.G., S., Shadan, N. B., Zhang, X. M., Khalilnezhad, S., Cottier, F., et al. (2021). Microbial exposure during early human development primes fetal immune cells. *Cell, 184*, 3394–3409. doi: 10.1016/j.cell.2021.04.039.

Moalem, G., Leibowitz-Amit, R., Yoles, E., Mor, F., Cohen, I. R., & Schwartz, M. (1999). Autoimmune T cells protect neurons from secondary degeneration after central nervous system axotomy. *Nature Medicine, 5*, 49–55. doi: 10.1038/4734.

Mor, G., Aldo, P., & Alvero, A. (2017). The unique immunological and microbial aspects of pregnancy. *Nature Reviews Immunology, 17*, 469–482. doi: 10.1038/nri.2017.64.

Morais, L. H., Schreiber IV, H. L., & Mazmanian, S. K. (2021). The gut microbiota-brain axis in behaviour and brain disorders. *Nature Reviews Microbiology, 19*, 241–255. doi: 10.1038/s41579-020-00460-0.

Munster, V. J., Adney, D. R., van Doremalen, N., Brown, V. R., Miazgowicz, K. L., Milne-Price, S., Bushmaker, T., Rosenke, R., Scott, D., Hawkinson, A., de Wit, E., Schountz, T., & Bowen, R. A. (2016). Replication and shedding of MERS-CoV in Jamaican fruit bats (*Artibeus jamaicensis*). *Scientific Reports, 6*, 21878. doi: 10.1038/srep21878.

Nakagawa, H., Wang, L., Cantor, H., & Kim, J. (2018). New insights into the biology of CD8 regulatory T cells. *Advances in Immunology, 140*, 1–20. doi: 10.1016/bs.ai.2018.09.001.

Natarajan, N., Hori, D., Flavahan, S., Steppan, J., Flavahan, N. A., Berkowitz, D. E., & Pluznick, J. L. (2016). Microbial short chain fatty acid metabolites lower blood pressure via endothelial G protein-coupled receptor 41. *Physiological Genomics, 48*, 826–834. doi: 10.1152/physiolgenomics.00089.2016.

Nelson, J. L. (2003). Microchimerism in human health and disease. *Autoimmunity, 36*, 5–9. doi: 10.1080/0891693031000067304.

Nemazee, D. A., & Bürki, K. (1989). Clonal deletion of B lymphocytes in a transgenic mouse bearing anti-MHC class I antibody genes. *Nature, 337*, 562–566. doi: 10.1038/337562a0.

Nishizuka, Y., & Sakakura, T. (1969). Thymus and reproduction: Sex-linked dysgenesis of the gonad after neonatal thymectomy in mice. *Science, 166*, 753–755. doi: 10.1126/science.166.3906.753.

Nobrega, A., Haury, M., Grandien, A., Malanchère, E., Sundblad, A., & Coutinho, A. (1993). Global analysis of antibody repertoires. II. Evidence for specificity, self-selection and the immunological "homunculus" of antibodies in normal serum. *European Journal of Immunology, 23*, 2851–2859. doi: 10.1002/eji.1830231119.

O'Shea, T. J., Cryan, P. M., Cunningham, A. A., Fooks, A. R., Hayman, D. T., Luis, A. D., Peel, A. J., Plowright, R. K., & Wood, J. L. (2014). Bat flight and zoonotic viruses. *Emerging Infectious Diseases, 20*, 741–745. doi: 10.3201/eid2005.130539.

Ochsenbein, A. F., Fehr, T., Lutz, C., Suter, M., Brombacher, F., Hengartner, H., & Zinkernagel, R. M. (1999a). Control of early viral and bacterial distribution and disease by natural antibodies. *Science, 286*, 2156–2159. doi: 10.1126/science.286.5447.2156.

Ochsenbein, A. F., Pinschewer, D. D., Odermatt, B., Carroll, M. C., Hengartner, H., & Zinkernagel, R. M. (1999b). Protective T cell-independent antiviral antibody responses are dependent on complement. *Journal of Experimental Medicine, 190*, 1165–1174. doi: 10.1084/jem.190.8.1165.

Ohkura, N., Hamaguchi, M., Morikawa, H., Sugimura, K., Tanaka, A., Ito, Y., Osaki, M., Tanaka, Y., Yamashita, R., Nakano, N., Huehn, J., Fehling, H. J., Sparwasser, T., Nakai, K., & Sakaguchi, S. (2012). T cell receptor stimulation-induced epigenetic changes and Foxp3 expression are independent and complementary events required for Treg cell development. *Immunity, 37*, 785–799. doi: 10.1016/j.immuni.2012.09.010.

Oldstone, M. B. A. (1987). Molecular mimicry and autoimmune disease. *Cell, 50*, 819-820. doi: 10.1016/0092-8674(87)90507-1.

Olival, K. J., Hosseini, P. R., Zambrana-Torrelio, C., Ross, N., Bogich, T. L., & Daszak, P. (2017). Host and viral traits predict zoonotic spillover from mammals. *Nature, 546*, 646–650. doi: 10.1038/nature22975.

Orr, H. T., Bach, F. H., Ploegh, H. L., Strominger, J. L., Kavathas, P., & DeMars, R. (1982). Use of HLA loss mutants to analyse the structure of the human major histocompatibility complex. *Nature, 296*, 454–456. doi: 10.1038/296454a0.

Parniske, M. (2008). Arbuscular mycorrhiza: The mother of plant root endosymbioses. *Nature Reviews Microbiology, 6*, 763–775. doi: 10.1038/nrmicro1987.

Pavlov, I. P. (1927). *Conditioned Reflexes: An Investigation of the Physiological Activity of the Cerebral Cortex.* (G. V. Anrep, Trans.). Oxford University Press.

Pavlovich, S. S., Lovett, S. P., Koroleva, G., Guito, J. C., Arnold, C. E., Nagle, E. R., Kulcsar, K., Lee, A., Thibaud-Nissen, F., Hume, A. J., Mühlberger, E., Uebelhoer, L. S., Towner, J. S., Rabadan, R., Sanchez-Lockhart, M., Kepler, T. B., & Palacios, G. (2018). The Egyptian rousette genome reveals unexpected features of bat antiviral immunity. *Cell, 173*, 1098–1110. doi: 10.1016/j.cell.2018.03.070.

Pazmany, L., Mandelboim, O., Valés-Gómez, M., Davis, D. M., Reyburn, H. T., & Strominger, J. L. (1996). Protection from natural killer cell-mediated lysis by HLA-G expression on target cells. *Science, 274*, 792–795. doi: 10.1126/science.274.5288.792.

Penfield, W., & Boldrey, E. (1937). Somatic motor and sensory reporesentation in the cerebral cortex of man as studied by electrical stimulation. *Brain, 60*, 389–443. doi: 10.1093/brain/60.4.389.

Penfield, W., & Rasmussen, R. (1950). *The Cerebral Cortex of Man: A Clinical Study of Localization of Function.* Macmillan.

Perez-Muñoz, M. E., Arrieta, M., Ramer-Tait, A. E., Ramer-Tait, A. E., & Walter, J. (2017). A critical assessment of the "sterile womb" and "in utero colonization" hypotheses: Implications for research on the pioneer infant microbiome. *Microbiome, 5*, 48. doi: 10.1186/s40168-017-0268-4.

Pihoker, C., Gilliam, L. K., Hampe, C. S., & Lernmark, A. (2005). Autoantibodies in diabetes. *Diabetes, 54 Suppl 2*, 552–561. doi: 10.2337/diabetes.54.suppl_2.s52.

Plumwood, V. (1993). *Feminism and the Mastery of Nature.* Routledge.

Plumwood, V. (1995). Human vulnerability and the experience of being prey. *Quadrant, 29*, 29–34.

Pluznick, J. L., Protzko, R. J., Gevorgyan, H., Peterlin, Z., Sipos, A., Han, J., Brunet, I., Wan, L. X., Rey, F., Wang, T., Firestein, S. J., Yanagisawa, M., Gordon, J. I., Eichmann, A., Peti-Peterdi, J., & Caplan, M. J. (2013). Olfactory receptor responding to gut microbiota-derived signals plays a role in renin secretion and blood pressure regulation. *Proceedings of the National Academy of Sciences of the United States of America, 110*, 4410–4415. doi: 10.1073/pnas.1215927110.

Poletaev, A. B. (2002). The immunological homunculus (immunculus) in normal state and pathology. *Biochemistry (Mosc), 67*, 600–608. doi: 10.1023/a:1015514732179.

Pradeu, T. (2010). What is an organism? An immunological answer. *History and Philosophy of the Life Sciences, 32*, 247–267.

Rackaityte, E., Halkias, J., Fukui, E. M., Mendoza, V. F., Hayzelden, C., Crawford, E. D., Fujimura, K. E., Burt, T. D., & Lynch, S. V. (2020). Viable bacterial colonization is highly limited in the human intestine in utero. *Nature Medicine, 26*, 599–607. doi: 10.1038/s41591-020-0761-3.

Raichle, M. E. (2006). The brain's dark energy. *Science, 314*, 1249–1250. doi: 10.1126/science.113440.

Raichle, M. E. (2015). The brain's default mode network. *Annual Review of Neuroscience, 38*, 433-447. doi: 10.1146/annurev-neuro-071013-014030.

Raichle, M. E., MacLeod, A. M., Snyder, A. Z., Powers, W. J., Gusnard, D. A., & Shulman, G. L. (2001). A default mode of brain function. *Proceedings of the National Academy of Sciences of the United States of America, 98*, 676–682. doi: 10.1073/pnas.98.2.676.

Rajagopalan, S., & Long, E. O. (1999). A human histocompatibility leukocyte antigen (HLA)-G-specific receptor expressed on all natural killer cells. *Journal of Experimental Medicine, 189*, 1093–1100. doi: 10.1084/jem.189.7.1093.

Rakoff-Nahoum, S., Paglino, J., Eslami-Varzaneh, F., Edberg, S., & Medzhitov, R. (2004). Recognition of commensal microflora by toll-like receptors is required for intestinal homeostasis. *Cell, 118*, 229–241. doi: 10.1016/j.cell.2004.07.002.

Ramsdell, F., & Ziegler, S. F. (2014). FOXP3 and scurfy: How it all began. *Nature Reviews Immunology, 14*, 343–349. doi: 10.1038/nri3650.

Rappe, M. S., & Giovannoni, J. I. (2003). The uncultured microbial majority. *Annual Review of Microbiology, 57*, 369–394. doi: 10.1146/annurev.micro.57.030502.090759.

Riemekasten, G., & Hahn, B. H. (2005). Key autoantigens in SLE. *Rheumatology, 44*, 975–982. doi: 10.1093/rheumatology/keh688.

Roberts, R. J. (2004). Identifying protein function-a call for community action. *PLoS Biology, 2*, e42. doi: 10.1371/journal.pbio.0020042.

Roep, B. O. (1996). T-cell responses to autoantigens in IDDM. The search for the Holy Grail. *Diabetes, 45*, 1147–1156. doi: 10.2337/diab.45.9.1147.

Rose, N. R. (2006). Life amidst the contrivances. *Nature Immunology, 7*, 1009–1011. doi: 10.1038/ni1006-1009.

Rose, N. R., & Mackay, I. R. (2000). *The Autoimmune Diseases*. Academic Press. iv.

Rosenberg, E., & Zilber-Rosenberg, I. (2018). The hologenome concept of evolution after 10 years. *Microbiome, 6*, 78. doi: 10.1186/s40168-018-0457-9.

Roser, M., Ortiz-Ospina, E., & Ritchie, H. (2019). Life Expectancy. How did life expectancy change over time? (Originally published 2013). https://ourworldindata.org/life-expectancy#how-did-life-expectancy-change-over-time.

Rouas-Freiss, N., Marchal, R. E., Kirszenbaum, M., Dausset, J., & Carosella, E. D. (1997). The α1 domain of HLA-G1 and HLA-G2 inhibits cytotoxicity induced by natural killer cells: Is HLA-G the public ligand for natural killer cell inhibitory receptor? *Proceedings of the National Academy of Sciences of the United States of America, 94*, 5249–5254. doi: 10.1073/pnas.94.10.5249.

Round, J. L., & Mazmanian, S. K. (2009). The gut microbiota shapes intestinal immune responses during health and disease. *Nature Reviews Immunology, 9*, 313–323. doi: 10.1038/nri2515.

Ruparelia, N., Chai, J. T., Fisher, E. A., & Choudhury, R. P. (2017). Inflammatory processes in cardiovascular disease: A route to targeted therapies. *Nature Reviews Cardiology, 14*, 133–144. doi: 10.1038/nrcardio.2016.185.

Sakaguchi, S., Mikami, N., Wing, J. B., Tanaka, A., Ichiyama, K., & Ohkura, N. (2020). Regulatory T cells and human disease. *Annual Review of Immunology, 26*, 541–566. doi: 10.1146/annurev-immunol-042718-041717.

Sakaguchi, S., Sakaguchi, N., Asano, M., Itoh, M., & Toda, M. (1995). Immunologic self-tolerance maintained by activated T cells expressing IL-2 receptor α-chains (CD25): Breakdown of a single mechanism causes various autoimmune diseases. *Journal of Immunology, 155*, 1151–1164. doi: 10.4049/jimmunol.155.3.1151.

Sakaguchi, S., Takahashi, T., & Nishizuka, Y. (1982). Study on cellular events in post-thymectomy autoimmune oophoritis in mice. II. Requirement of Lyt-1 cells in normal female mice for the prevention of oophoritis. *Journal of Experimental Medicine, 156*, 1577–1586. doi: 10.1084/jem.156.6.1577.

Sakakura, T., & Nishizuka, Y. (1972). Thymic control mechanism in ovarian development: Reconstitution of ovarian dysgenesis in thymectomized mice by replacement with thymic and other lymphoid tissues. *Endocrinology, 90*, 431–437. doi: 10.1210/endo-90-2-431.

Savage, D. C. (1977). Microbial ecology of the gastrointestinal tract. *Annual Review of Microbiology, 31*, 107–133. doi: 10.1146/annurev.mi.31.100177.000543.

Sender, R., Fuchs, S., & Milo, R. (2016). Are we really vastly outnumbered? Revisiting the ratio of bacterial to host cells in humans. *Cell, 164*, 337–340. doi: 10.1016/j.cell.2016.01.013.

Sepich-Poore, G. D., Zitvogel, L., Straussman, R., Hasty, J., Wargo, J. A., & Knight, R. (2021). The microbiome and human cancer. *Science, 371*, eabc4552. doi: 10.1126/science.abc4552.

Serres, M. (1980). *Le Parasite (The Parasite)*. Grasset. 9–24.

Serres, M. (1982). *Genèse (Genesis)*. (H. Yakura, Trans.) Bernard Grasset. 32.

Serres, M. (2018). *Le Contrat naturel (The Natural Contract)*. Le Pommier. (Originally published 1990).

Sharon, G., Sampson, T. R., Geschwind, D. H., & Mazmanian, S. K. (2016). The central nervous system and the gut microbiome. *Cell, 167*, 915–932. doi: 10.1016/j.cell.2016.10.027.

Shaw, W. (2010). Increased urinary excretion of a 3-(3-hydroxyphenyl)-3-hydroxypropionic acid (HPHPA), an abnormal phenylalanine metabolite of Clostridia spp. in the gastrointestinal tract, in urine samples from patients with autism and schizophrenia. *Nutritional Neuroscience, 13*, 135–143. doi: 10.1179/147683010X12611460763968.

Silverstein, A. M. (1989). *A History of Immunology*. Academic Press. 160–163.

Silverstein, A. M. (2001). Autoimmunity versus *horror autotoxicus*: The struggle for recognition. *Nature Immunology, 2*, 279–281. doi: 10.1038/86280.

Smith, P. M., Howitt, M. R., Panikov, N., Michaud, M., Gallini, C. A., Bohlooly -Y, M., Glickman, J. N., & W.S., G. (2013). The microbial metabolites, short-chain fatty acids, regulate colonic Treg cell homeostasis. *Science, 341*, 569–573. doi: 10.1126/science.1241165.

Sober, E. (2000). *Philosophy of Biology*. (Second Ed.). Westview Press. 8.

Spencer, H. (1864). *Principles of Biology. Vol. I.* Williams and Norgate. 444–445.

Swanepoel, R., Leman, P. A., Burt, F. J., Zachariades, N. A., Braack, L. E., Ksiazek, T. G., Rollin, P. E., Zaki, S. R., & Peters, C. J. (1996). Experimental inoculation of plants and animals with Ebola virus. *Emerging Infectious Diseases, 2*, 321–325. doi: 10.3201/eid0204.960407.

Taguchi, O., Nishizuka, Y., Sakakura, T., & Kojima, A. (1980). Autoimmune oophoritis in thymectomized mice: Detection of circulating antibodies against oocytes. *Clinical & Experimental Immunology, 40*, 540–553.

Takaba, H., Morishita, Y., Tomofuji, Y., Danks, L., Nitta, T., Komatsu, N., Kodama, T., & Takayanagi, H. (2015). Fezf2 orchestrates a thymic program of self-antigen expression for immune tolerance. *Cell, 163*, 975–987. doi: 10.1016/j.cell.2015.10.013.

Tan, T. G., Sefik, E., Geva-Zatorsky, N., Kua, L., Naskar, D., Teng, F., Pasman, L., Ortiz-Lopez, A., Jupp, R., Wu, H. J., Kasper, D. L., Benoist, C., & Mathis, D. (2016). Identifying species of symbiont bacteria from the human gut that, alone, can induce intestinal Th17 cells in mice. *Proceedings of the National Academy of Sciences of the United States of America, 113*, E8141–E8150. doi: 10.1073/pnas.1617460113.

Tiegs, S. L., Russell, D. M., & Nemazee, D. (1993). Receptor editing in self-reactive bone marrow B cells. *Journal of Experimental Medicine, 177*, 1009–1020. doi: 10.1084/jem.177.4.1009.

Tilburgs, T., Roelen, D. L., van der Mast, B. J., de Groot-Swings, G. M., Kleijburg, C., Scherjon, S. A., & Claas, F. H. (2008). Evidence for a selective migration of fetus-specific CD4+CD25bright regulatory T cells from the peripheral blood to the decidua in human pregnancy. *Journal of Immunology, 180*, 5737–5745. doi: 10.4049/jimmunol.180.8.5737.

Tsuiji, M., Yurasov, S., Velinzon, K., Thomas, S., Nussenzweig, M. C., & Wardemann, H. (2006). A checkpoint for autoreactivity in human IgM+ memory B cell development. *Journal of Experimental Medicine, 203*, 393–400. doi: 10.1084/jem.20052033.

Wang, E. Y., Mao, T., Klein, J., Dai, Y., Huck, J. D., Jaycox, J. R., Liu, F., Zhou, T., Israelow, B., Wong, P., Coppi, A., Lucas, C., Silva, J., Oh, J. E., Song, E., Perotti, E. S., Zheng, N. S., Fischer, S., Campbell, M., Fournier, J. B., et al. (2021). Diverse functional autoantibodies in patients with COVID-19. *Nature, 595*, 283–288. doi: 10.1038/s41586-021-03631-y.

Wardemann, H., Yurasov, S., Schaefer, A., Young, J. W., Meffe, E., & Nussenzweig, M. C. (2003). Predominant autoantibody production by early human B cell precursors. *Science, 301*, 1374–1377. doi: 10.1126/science.1086907.

Webster, N. S., & Taylor, M. W. (2012). Marine sponges and their microbial symbionts: Love and other relationships. *Enviornmental Microbiology, 14*, 335–346. doi: 10.1111/j.1462-2920.2011.02460.x.

Webster, N. S., & Thomas, T. (2016). The sponge hologenome. *mBio, 7*, e00135–00116. doi: 10.1128/mBio.00135-16.

Wen, L., Ley, R. E., Volchkov, P. Y., Stranges, P. B., Avanesyan, L., Stonebraker, A. C., Hu, C., Wong, F. S., Szot, G. L., Bluestone, J. A., Gordon, J. I., & Chervonsky, A. V. (2008). Innate immunity and intestinal microbiota in the development of type 1 diabetes. *Nature, 455*, 1109–1113. doi: 10.1038/nature07336.

Wildin, R. S., Ramsdell, F., Peake, J., Faravelli, F., Casanova, J. L., Buist, N., Levy-Lahad, E., Mazzella, M., Goulet, O., Perroni, L., Bricarelli, F. D., Byrne, G., McEuen, M., Proll, S., Appleby, M., & Brunkow, M. E. (2001). X-linked neonatal diabetes mellitus, enteropathy and endocrinopathy syndrome is the human equivalent of mouse scurfy. *Nature Genetics, 27*, 18–20. doi: 10.1038/83707.

Wyss-Coray, T., & Rogers, J. (2012). Inflammation in Alzheimer disease--A brief review of the basic science and clnical literature. *Cold Spring Harbor Perspectives in Medicine, 2*, a006346. doi: 10.1101/cshperspect.a006346.

Xie, J., Li, Y., Shen, X., Goh, G., Zhu, Y., Cui, J., Wang, L. F., Shi, Z. L., & Zhou, P. (2018). Dampened STING-dependent interferon activation in bats. *Cell Host & Microbe, 23*, 297–301. doi: 10.1016/j.chom.2018.01.006.

Xu, J. L., & Davis, M. M. (2000). Diversity in the CDR3 region of V(H) is sufficient for most antibody specificities. *Immunity, 13*, 37–45. doi: 10.1016/s1074-7613(00)00006-6.

Yoles, E., Hauben, E., Palgi, O., Agranov, E., Gothilf, A., Cohen, A., Kuchroo, V., Cohen, I. R., Weiner, H., & Schwartz, M. (2001). Protective autoimmunity is a physiological response to CNS trauma. *Journal of Neuroscience, 21*, 3740–3748. doi: 10.1523/jneurosci.21-11-03740.2001.

Younge, N., McCann, J. R., Ballard, J., Plunkett, C., Akhtar, S., Araújo-Pérez, F., Murtha, A., Brandon, D., & Seed, P. C. (2019). Fetal exposure to the maternal microbiota in humans and mice. *JCI Insight, 4*, e127806. doi: 10.1172/jci.insight.127806.

Zavdy, O., Shoenfeld, Y., & Amital, H. (2014). Natural autoantibodies--Homeostasis, autoimmunity and therapeutic potential. (Third Ed.). *Autoantibodies*. Elsevier. 21–32.

Zilber-Rosenberg, I., & Rosenberg, E. (2008). Role of microorganisms in the evolution of animals and plants: The hologenome theory of evolution. *FEMS Microbiology Reviews, 32*, 723–735. doi: 10.1111/j.1574-6976.2008.00123.x.

3 The Immune System at the Organism Level

We must therefore carefully avoid every species of system, because systems are not in nature, but only in the mind of man.[1]

Claude Bernard

As we have seen, modern immunology, which began at the end of the 19th century, has gathered a vast amount of information on the structure of the immune system and its physiological functions and sought order in it. This effort has contributed significantly to our understanding of pathological conditions, and the research momentum has accelerated. Much research has concentrated on highly evolved organisms, especially mice. However, since these results are often not applicable to humans, a growing body of research focuses on humans. As we have already seen, Ernst Mayr divided biology into functional and evolutionary biology, leading to two major functional divisions. The first is "etiological function" from an evolutionary perspective, a historical concept that addresses what it is for (Wright, 1973). The second is "systemic function," which addresses the mechanisms within the system as it currently exists (Cummins, 1975). In the following, I will consider these perspectives and review immunity from two aspects. In other words, in Chapter 3, I will analyze the immune system at the organismal level, especially in mice and humans, where a vast amount of research has been accumulated. In Chapter 4, I will conduct a diachronic analysis following the evolutionary phylogenetic tree. In doing so, I would like to prepare to approach the essence of immunity.

3.1 BLURRED BOUNDARIES WITHIN THE IMMUNE SYSTEM

From a textbook perspective, there are two immunity mechanisms (innate and acquired) that have long been studied as separate areas. Let us summarize the characteristics of these two types of immunity. Innate immunity responds quickly to microorganisms but lacks specificity or memory for incoming microorganisms. It is a universal defense mechanism recognized from early evolutionary times, and in humans and mice involves dendritic cells, monocytes, macrophages, granulocytes, innate lymphoid cells (ILCs)—including natural killer (NK) cells—and other cells. In contrast, acquired immunity is limited to jawed vertebrates (Gnathostomata) and takes longer to respond but is highly specific and has immunological memory. T and B cells are involved in this type of immunity. In other words, while innate immunity is widely found in the living world but lacks specificity and memory, acquired immunity is found only in a limited number of organisms but has specificity and memory. However, recent studies have shown that there are cases that do not fit into this clearly defined category (Sun et al., 2009; Paust and von Andrian, 2011; Sun et al., 2014; Lee et al., 2015; O'Sullivan et al., 2015; Reeves et al., 2015; Hammer et al., 2018). For example, some cells responsible for innate immunity have immunological memory and specificity. Conversely, some T cells constituting acquired immunity have characteristics reminiscent of rapidly responding innate immune cells.

Before going into specific examples, I would like to reflect on immunological memory, which separates the two immune mechanisms. As already stated above, immunological memory is a fundamental function of immunity recognized since ancient Greece. While it underlies the effectiveness of vaccines, many points remain to be clarified (Kurosaki et al., 2015).

The first point is the diversity of memory cells. The B cells' surface bears different classes of antibodies: IgM, IgD, IgG, IgA, and IgE. In the secondary response that occurs when the immune

DOI: 10.1201/9781003486800-3

system reencounters the same antigen or microorganism, mutations in the B cell receptor gene (somatic hypermutation) cause affinity maturation that increases affinity for the antigen. Long-lived memory B cells are generated after a class switch from IgM to IgG, providing a more effective defense response. However, recent studies have shown that long-lived memory B cells emerge independent of the germinal center, which has been regarded as the site of memory B cell production (Kaji et al., 2012; Taylor et al., 2012) or that there are memory cells that keep expressing IgM with different functions than IgG memory cells (Dogan et al., 2009; Pape et al., 2011). Furthermore, factors different from the transcription factors involved in IgG memory cells are involved in maintaining IgA memory cells (Wang et al., 2012), indicating the existence of subpopulations within memory B cells.

Similarly, heterogeneity is observed within memory T cells. For example, two types of memory cells with different localization and function have been identified based on differences in cell surface molecules (Sallusto et al., 1999). One type resides in tissues other than the lymphoid organs and immediately functions as an effector upon secondary stimulation. The other type resides in the lymphoid organs and differentiates into effector memory cells after secondary stimulation. It has also been reported that CD8+ T cells (Usherwood et al., 1999) and CD4+ T cells (Ahmadzadeh et al., 2001) have two types of memory cells, one in an effector state and the other in a quiescent state, which can be distinguished by cell surface markers.

The second point is the localization of memory cells. Memory T cells that do not enter the circulatory system after the initial infection but remain localized and respond immediately upon reinfection have been demonstrated (Gebhardt et al., 2009; Teijaro et al., 2011; Masopust and Picker, 2012). Similarly, cells of the B cell lineage have been found to exhibit specific localization. In mice, transplantation experiments showed that antibody-producing cells (plasma cells) are present in the spleen and bone marrow for over a year (Slifka et al., 1998). In humans, long-lived plasma cells are present in the bone marrow, suggesting they may be involved in infection defense (Halliley et al., 2015). These results call for caution in judging the status of immunological memory based solely on cells present in the blood.

The third point is the antigen dependence of memory maintenance. There is an interesting record of a survey of experts on immunological memory in 2016 (Farber et al., 2016). While some experts define memory cells as "cells that survive for a long time independently of antigenic stimulation or antigen persistence," Zinkernagel noted the following: for a long time, immunological memory was thought to be the ability to defend against reinfection, but about 80 years ago, immunological memory came to be considered a "faster and stronger" response than the primary response. He further emphasized that the high-affinity neutralizing antibodies involved in defense rapidly diminish if the antigen is absent or there is no reinfection. In other words, the immunological memory of a "faster and stronger" secondary immune response elicited with a non-pathogenic antigen in the laboratory is different from the immunological memory involved in actual defense against infection. Zinkernagel reiterates that the maintenance of a memory that functions as protective immunity requires frequent infections or sustained reactions with antigens that remain as immune complexes in the body (Zinkernagel, 2000, 2002, 2012, 2018).

What, then, are the implications of the existence of memory cells with such diverse localizations and functions? Moreover, through what pathways do each of them, alone or in concert, ultimately produce effective defense responses? Many of the details remain a mystery. If awakening memory cells in local tissues is also essential for defense, then the heterogeneity of memory cells will be an important topic to consider for effective vaccine development.

More recently, accumulating reports suggest that immunological memory, thought to be the exclusive property of acquired immunity, also exists in cells responsible for innate immunity. Let us now examine some specific examples. First, NK cells were identified in 1975 as cells that can kill tumor cells without pretreatment (Herberman et al., 1975a; Herberman et al., 1975b; Kiessling et al., 1975a; Kiessling et al., 1975b). These cells have been thought to be responsible for innate immunity because of their rapid response and the fact that they do not have receptors for various antigens like T and B cells and, therefore, can only assume nonspecific responses. However, it has been reported that NK cells also have antigen specificity and immunological memory (O'Leary et al., 2006; Cooper and Yokoyama, 2010; Paust and von Andrian, 2011; Vivier et al., 2011; O'Sullivan et al., 2015). For example, reports have examined contact hypersensitivity reactions in mice lacking T and B cells, because the genes for the enzymes involved in recombining the antigen receptor genes, recombination-activating genes (*RAG-1* and *RAG-2*), have been deleted. This reaction occurs when a chemical (hapten) is applied to the skin (e.g., abdomen) and then to another area (auricle), causing inflammation and swelling. The intensity of the reaction is assessed by the thickness of the ear, and it is believed to be mediated by T and B cells (Tsuji et al., 2002). However, contact hypersensitivity can be induced in mice without T and B cells, and no reaction occurs unless the same hapten is used for the second stimulation. Furthermore, immunological memory persists for a month after sensitization, and memory cells are found in the liver. Importantly, it was shown that contact hypersensitivity is no longer observed when NK cells are deleted from mice lacking T and B cells and that the liver cells that confer memory to mice in this condition have the characteristics of NK cells (O'Leary et al., 2006).

The antigen specificity and immunological memory of NK cells shown in the system using non-immunogenic small molecules have been confirmed for pathogens of greater physiological significance. In a mouse model of cytomegalovirus infection, NK cells, like T cells, responded in a four-step process: first proliferating, then decreasing in number through apoptosis, from which memory cells are induced and respond to renewed infection. The trigger is the binding of a cytomegalovirus-specific protein to an activating receptor (Ly49H) expressed on a subpopulation of NK cells. Because of their self-renewal capacity, they persist in non-lymphoid and lymphoid tissues over the following months to prepare for future reactions (Sun et al., 2009). Furthermore, in a human model of cytomegalovirus infection, it was shown that NK cells differentiate into long-lived memory cells by epigenetic mechanisms and that memory NK cells are immediately activated upon re-infection (Lee et al., 2015). Epigenetic changes are alterations in gene expression due to chemical modifications without changing the DNA sequence itself, such as the methylation of DNA and methylation or acetylation of histones around which DNA winds to create nucleosomes. These properties of immunological memory have also been demonstrated in models of infection by vaccinia virus (Gillard et al., 2011), influenza virus (van Helden et al., 2012), and herpes simplex virus (Abdul-Careem et al., 2012). Therefore, while considered to belong to innate immunity, NK cells also have antigen specificity and the capacity for immunological memory.

Immunological memory has also been observed in monocytes and macrophages, which are thought to be responsible for innate immunity. In mice, infection with a sublethal dose of *Candida albicans* (a species of fungus) protected against subsequent lethal doses of *C. albicans* infection (Quintin et al., 2012). Interestingly, this effect was also observed in mice lacking T and B cells but was abolished in mice lacking monocytes, meaning that the effect depends on monocytes rather than T and B cells. In addition, histone methylation was observed in monocytes stimulated with fungal membrane component β-glucans.

Similar results are evident from studies on the Bacillus Calmette–Guérin (BCG) attenuated live vaccine used to prevent tuberculosis (Kleinnijenhuis et al., 2012). Since its initial use, the BCG vaccine has been reported to reduce the overall mortality rate in children and protect against diseases other than tuberculosis. According to the latest study, when blood samples were taken from individuals two weeks and three months after BCG vaccination and stimulated with *Mycobacterium tuberculosis*, the production of humoral factors (e.g., IFN-γ, TNF-α, and IL-1β) was elevated compared to non-vaccinated individuals at both time points. Interestingly, similar changes were observed when the cells were stimulated with *Staphylococcus aureus* and *C. albicans* other than *M. tuberculosis*. Vaccination has been shown to increase subpopulations of monocytes and enhance histone methylation in monocytes. Furthermore, BCG-vaccinated mice lacking T and B cells showed significant survival compared to the control group when injected with lethal doses of *C. albicans*. These results suggest that immunological memory is also observed in monocytes, which is mediated through epigenetic changes, and its defensive activity is effective not only against the original pathogen but also against unrelated pathogens (Kleinnijenhuis et al., 2012; Quintin et al., 2012).

Mihai Netea (1968–) and others have proposed the concept of "trained immunity" for this phenomenon (Netea et al., 2011; Netea et al., 2016). This is a type of immunity in which, independent of T and B cells, innate immune cells undergo epigenetic changes under the influence of stimuli such as pathogens encountered in the past and use their memory for future nonspecific defense. Regarding nonspecific cross-protection by infection, George Mackaness (1922–2007) reported the following in the 1960s (Mackaness, 1964). When animals sensitized with BCG were reinjected with BCG, they showed a protective response to *Listeria monocytogenes* infection. In addition, animals sensitized and reinoculated with *L. monocytogenes* showed resistance to *Brucella abortus*. Moreover, animals sensitized and reinoculated with *B. abortus* showed activity against *Listeria* infection. While the mechanism's details are unclear, one would imagine that changes similar to trained immunity are likely occurring. This type of immunity could be actively used to induce epigenetic changes by appropriately stimulating (or training) innate immunity cells with live vaccines such as BCG or measles, which could then protect against a wide range of invading pathogens. Netea et al. also argued that providing temporary protection against diseases for which vaccines have not yet been prepared may be possible. They also discussed the possibility that activation of trained immunity by the BCG vaccine might reduce COVID-19 severity (Netea et al., 2020; O'Neill and Netea, 2020). While vaccines against COVID-19 have been developed at an alarming rate, they showed in a randomized controlled trial on elderly patients with an average age of 80 years a lower frequency of new COVID-19 infections in those given the BCG vaccine than a placebo (Giamarellos-Bourboulis et al., 2020). The previously hidden and formidable power of innate immunity appears to be beginning to emerge.

Other findings regarding immune memory are also evident in ILCs. These cells, like T and B cells, differentiate and mature from common lymphocyte progenitors but do not have antigen receptors on their cell surface, nor do they have the characteristics of myeloid cells (e.g., granulocytes and monocytes). ILCs comprise three groups of cells (ILC1, ILC2, and ILC3) differentiated by their cytokine secretion patterns and NK and other cells (Spits et al., 2013; Artis and Spits, 2015; Eberl et al., 2015). ILC1 is a group of cells that produces IFN-γ. The ILC2 group comprises cells that produce type 2 cytokines (e.g., IL-4, IL-5, IL-9, and IL-13) involved in allergic inflammation or infection with helminth parasites. The ILC3 group comprises cells that produce IL-17 and IL-22. Among these groups, in addition to the previously mentioned NK cells, immunological memory has been reported in ILC1 (Wang et al., 2018) and ILC2 cells (Martinez-Gonzalez et al., 2018).

As we have seen, it is evident that memory exists in innate immunity. However, it is important to note that how "immunological memory" is implemented differs significantly between innate and acquired immunity. If we define memory as the ability to respond faster and stronger to a second encounter for effective defense, we can state that the two immune arms have a memory function. However, this does not mean that their mechanisms are the same. Specifically, unlike acquired immunity, in which T and B cells survive and function as memory cells, innate immunity involves epigenetic processes that alter gene expression without altering the DNA sequence. From the discussion in Chapter 4, it will become clear that immunological memory exists in animals, plants, and even bacteria, which do not have T or B cells, and its modalities will be even more diverse. This situation is also true for the concept of "immunity," the theme of this book. In other words, "immunity" refers to a wide range of different things depending on the species. With that in mind, this book will take the position of accepting that variety of contents within a single term.

In his book *The Game of Chance and Complexity: The New Science of Immunology*, Philippe Kourilsky states that any cell possesses some sort of memories (Kourilsky, 2014). For example, if a cell transitions from state A to state B, it is assumed that the regulatory molecules characteristic of state A do not disappear immediately after the cell enters into state B and that the cell may still have memories of state A when it transitions to state C. Considering the moment-to-moment struggle for survival, the ability of diverse cells to support memory through various mechanisms should be an important prerequisite for the survival of any organism. If this logic is accepted, it would not be beneficial to the organism to exclude innate immunity or any other cells from this role, and the memory shown by innate immunity should not be surprising.

A similar situation is seen in cells responsible for acquired immunity. Some T cells have a memory cell phenotype and are effector-like cells that respond more rapidly than normal T cells and secrete large amounts of cytokines. Examples include natural killer T (NKT) cells, which have T cell receptors and NK cell markers, or mucosal-associated invariant T cells, which, like NKT cells, have T cell receptors and NK cell markers and localize to the intestinal mucosa and Peyer's patches. Therefore, cells that do not necessarily fit into the classical classification of acquired and innate immunity are being progressively revealed. In addition to the blurred boundary between innate and acquired immunity, the activation of innate immunity and its appropriate communication with acquired immunity is necessary to initiate an immune response (Iwasaki and Medzhitov, 2015). The issue of innate and acquired immunity will be further explored in Chapter 4 by examining the immunity of invertebrates, plants, and bacteria in more detail.

3.2   AN IMMUNE SYSTEM THAT PERMEATES THE WHOLE ORGANISM

In his Nobel Prize lecture in 1984, Niels Jerne described the immune system as an organ composed of approximately 10^{12} lymphocytes (Jerne, 1985). As Jerne also noted, the immune system does not have clear boundaries like the liver or the heart, which the word "organ" implies. However, because it has long been considered independent and isolated, thought about this system has necessarily been limited to within it. However, as the examination of the role of the microbiota in Chapter 2 has made clear, the immune system interacts closely with other systems in the body, such as the nervous, endocrine, and metabolic systems, and appears to function as if it were integrated into the organismal whole. Such systemic effects of immunity were noted even before studying the microbiota became common. For example, cells and humoral factors derived from tissues and organs outside the immune system in the classical sense are involved in immune function, while immune cells and humoral factors affect the functions of the nervous and endocrine systems. These results blur the boundaries between the various systems and stimulate the idea that immunity should be redefined as the action of the entire organism. In that case, the boundaries of the immune system would coincide with those of the organism. Such thoughts raise fundamental questions about what constitutes the immune system, how to define the totality of the immune system in multicellular organisms, and, more importantly, whether there is such a thing as an immune system in the first place.

As indicated in the epigraph, Claude Bernard (1813–1878), the founder of modern physiology and experimental medicine, persistently cautioned in his magnum opus, *An Introduction to the Study of Experimental Medicine*, in 1865 that we must avoid any systems created by the human mind (Bernard, 1949a). His discussion seems to concentrate on personal doctrines and philosophical systems, arguing that the experimental medical scientist must deal with phenomena and facts, not words, and that experimental medicine is the negation of all systems. However, if we elaborate on this argument a little further, could we not also consider that no natural entity, including living organisms, is compartmentalized by a system that is the product of the human mind? Therefore, to approach the reality of nature, we must abandon the idea of systems and observe and experiment. Indeed, in the early stages of research, introducing the concept of systems and establishing boundaries facilitated analysis and made it easier to understand the results.

However, as the research progresses and things that have been excluded in the previous analysis become apparent, the question arises about how well the research reflects nature. That is the time to reconsider the concept of a system. Such a time appears to be coming for the immune system. There is currently no effective methodology to grasp the whole picture of phenomena in living organisms, so the age-old question of how to think about the relationship between the whole and the parts, or which method is better for getting to the whole, remains. Unlike systems in physics, the whole cannot be reached by simply adding up the analysis of the parts in biological systems. The mechanism of emergence, in which new components emerge when the levels that constitute organisms change, has also been advocated. Therefore, the question always arises whether it is possible to understand the whole with the information obtained from the parts.

In this section, I will rethink the immune system concept by examining the relationship between the immune system and other systems that comprise the body. As already noted, there are many reports on the interaction of the various cells and factors that comprise the immune system with the cells and factors of the nervous and endocrine systems (Ader, 1981). However, these themes have not been taken up as a central program in immunology for a long time. One reason is that immunological research has been directed toward the mechanisms for generating diversity; the structure of antigen receptors involved in specific recognition; the identification of regulatory factors such as interleukins, cytokines, and chemokines produced by immune cells and their receptors; and intracellular signal transduction, among others. Another reason may be that the study of intersystemic interactions was considered "soft science" because it was limited to discovering correlations rather than causal relationships. However, since intersystemic interactions have been demonstrated to be based on solid molecular bases and mechanisms, the immune system's role in the overall organism is being seriously reconsidered.

First, I would like to review the history leading up to this point. The trend to view organisms from such a holistic perspective may be traced back to the time of Hippocrates of Kos and Galen of Pergamon (129–c. 216). Hippocrates is considered the first to separate medicine from religion, holding that disease was not caused by a deity or supernatural cause but was induced by natural factors such as environment, diet, and habits. One of the principles of Hippocratic medicine is the theory that the human body has four humors (body fluids): blood, phlegm or mucus, yellow bile, and black bile. When their harmony is maintained (*eucrasia*), the body is healthy; when their harmony is disturbed (*dyscrasia*), the body becomes ill. In other words, he took the view that disease was not localized but a change in the whole. This view may have been influenced by the theory of the four elements advocated by Empedocles (c. 494–c. 434 BC). This theory held that there were four elements (water, air, fire, and earth) as the *arche* (the first principle) of the world, and that their combination and dissociation gave rise to various "things and phenomena" in the world. Hippocrates' humors were also associated with the human personality, with blood being optimistic, vivacious, and sociable; phlegm being calm, reserved, and mild; yellow bile being angry, moody, but decisive; and black bile being gloomy and melancholic.

Another characteristic of Hippocratic medicine is its emphasis on the natural healing power (*vis medicatrix naturae*) that is said to be inherent in our bodies. When an imbalance of the four humors causes disease, this natural healing power restores the body to its original state of equilibrium. Therefore, while it appears passive because it relies on the healing power of nature, Hippocrates' treatment appears based on trust in our bodies. Galen's theory, which holds that humoral imbalance is the cause of all disease and that health can be achieved by restoring the equilibrium of the humors in the body, is essentially a continuation and refinement of Hippocrates' ideas. These holistic views dominated Western medicine for a long time, well into the 18th and 19th centuries.

In the 19th century, a series of theories were proposed that brought attention to the locality. For example, the cell theory of plants by Matthias Jakob Schleiden (1804–1881); the cell theory of plants and animals by Theodor Schwann (1810–1882); the cellular pathology by Rudolf Virchow (1821–1902), who advocated the view, "all cells come from cells" (*omnis cellula e cellula*); and ultimately the germ theory of disease by Louis Pasteur and Robert Koch. These trends led research toward localizing diseases and establishing treatments directed at them, a direction that has flourished to the present day. However, even during the 19th and 20th centuries, when these changes took place, the holistic view remained alive. For example, the ideas and sciences of Claude Bernard's "milieu intérieur" (internal environment) (Bernard, 1878d), Walter Cannon's (1871–1945) "homeostasis" (Cannon, 1926, 1929), or Hans Selye's "stress theory" (Selye, 1956), will be discussed below.

In the early 20th century, Ivan Pavlov, who was also interested in the type of human personality advocated by Hippocrates and Galen, studied conditioned reflexes (Section 2.2, Chapter 2).

As we shall see, his research has inspired researchers in various fields, and its influence has continued to the present day. For example, in 1918, Tohru Ishigami (1857–1919) published a study on tuberculosis patients that suggested a correlation between psychological state and the ability to resist the disease (Ishigami, 1918). Inspired by Pavlov and Cannon, Ishigami conducted a series of studies that revealed a relationship between mental state and immune capacity, disease progression, and prognosis. Specifically, he examined the effects of mental state on glucose and adrenaline levels and of glucose and adrenaline on opsonization (enhancement of bacterial phagocytosis by phagocytes, which he used as an indicator of immune function). He observed that opsonization was lower in patients with advanced tuberculosis than in nonadvanced patients but could be increased by appropriate treatment. Interestingly, patients with decreased opsonization were more likely to receive bad news or to have psychological stresses such as job failure, family problems, or the death of a close relative. He also observed that nervous individuals were more likely to show mental effects on their immunocompetence and have an unfavorable prognosis. In contrast, patients who were optimistic and unperturbed by negative events had relatively high phagocytosis and a good prognosis. While Ishigami's study does not address the mechanism, it is probably the first to show a correlation between psychological state and immunity. It might also be considered the origin of psychoneuroimmunology.

If I may add one more episode about Ishigami, when he was a naval medical captain in his late 30s, he was an assistant to Shibasaburo Kitasato when they sought to identify the pathogen of a plague that had broken out in Hong Kong in 1894. About two weeks after they started their investigation, Ishigami and Tanemichi Aoyama (1859–1917), a professor at Tokyo Imperial University who was also participating in the investigation, developed axillary lymph gland swelling and fever, and were on the verge of death. Fortunately, both survived, but the plague pathogen was first discovered by Alexandre Yersin (1863–1943) of the Pasteur Institute (Yersin, 1894) and named *Yersinia pestis* in his honor.

In 1926, Sergei Métalnikov's group of the Pasteur Institute published a paper in the Bulletin of the Pasteur Institute entitled "The role of conditioned reflexes in immunity" (Métalnikov and Chorine, 1926). They used the classical method established by Ivan Pavlov to perform the following experiment. Filtrates of *Bacillus anthracis* or *Staphylococcus* were injected into the abdominal cavity of guinea pigs as an unconditioned stimulus. At the same time, they were conditioned by scratching the skin or applying local heat as a neutral (conditioned) stimulus. Subsequent experiments showed that neutral stimulation alone without pathogenic stimuli increased the number of cells (polynuclear leukocytes, monocytes, and finally lymphocytes) exudating into the abdominal cavity compared to the group without neutral stimulation. In another series of experiments, they examined the effect of Pavlovian conditioning on antibody production. Rabbits conditioned with heat or a scratch and an emulsion of *Vibrio cholerae* were challenged with the conditioned stimulus alone. Antibody titers consistently increased in rabbits challenged with the conditioned stimulus compared to controls. In other words, their findings indicate that an immune response can be induced by skin stimuli, which normally cannot induce an immune response. The implication of their findings is that mental influences other than the original cause cannot be ignored when considering disease, and this research is thought to have laid the foundation for neuroimmune associative learning.

After studying zoology at St. Petersburg University and working in the Metchnikoff laboratory at the Pasteur Institute, Métalnikov returned once to Russia but came back to the Pasteur Institute in 1919, where he worked mainly on insect immunity until he died in 1946. In Russia, the trend toward neo-Lamarckism persisted, and his work was based on the idea that antibody production and phagocytosis depended on a Pavlovian-style reflex mechanism. Métalnikov believed that "to immunize is mainly to immunize the nervous centers which govern the cells' sensitivity" (Métalnikov, 1934).

In the 1930s, Hans Selye researched the effects of stress on the endocrine and immune systems. Selye was born in Vienna during the Austro-Hungarian Empire, grew up in Hungary, received his medical education in Prague, then went on to Johns Hopkins University in the United States,

McGill University in Canada, and finally founded the Institute of Stress at the University of Montreal where he continued his research. The observations that formed the basis of his research date back to his student days, when he noticed that patients who were ill from different causes shared common symptoms (e.g., fatigue, lack of appetite, and unwillingness to work) and called it the "syndrome of just being sick" (Tan and Yip, 2018). It was during his research at McGill University that he began to consider stress as a cause of these nonspecific symptoms. He made the following observation: When rats were subjected to stress, such as being placed in the cold on the roof of a building or being kept running on a treadmill, they showed adrenal enlargement, atrophy of lymphoid organs (including the thymus), and gastroduodenal ulcers. There, Selye recognized the involvement of Claude Bernard's milieu intérieur and Walter Cannon's homeostasis and linked the organism's response to stress to the hypothalamus–pituitary–adrenal (HPA) axis. The HPA axis comprises the hypothalamus, which comprehensively controls sympathetic, parasympathetic, and endocrine functions; the pituitary gland, which is anatomically located below the hypothalamus; and the adrenal glands, which are small organs located above the kidneys. For example, when stressed, messages are transmitted from the hypothalamus to the pituitary gland and from the pituitary gland to the adrenal glands, which eventually produce cortisol and are ready to respond to stress. The HPA axis also controls immunity, digestion, emotions, and energy balance.

Furthermore, Selye distinguished between acute and chronic stress and named the systemic response to chronically induced stress the "general adaptation syndrome" (Selye, 1936). Selye's central concept is that when subjected to stresses, such as surgery, cold exposure, or sublethal drug administration, the organism responds defensively to the stress regardless of the cause that induced the stress and that the HPA-derived hormones are the essence of this response. The syndrome is divided into three phases. The first phase is the response to the new change that occurs within two days and is called the alarm phase. The second resistance or adaptation phase is the response seen after two days, which is increased resistance to the initial change. The third or exhaustion phase occurs after one to three months of continuous stimulation once the subject can no longer cope with the change and becomes exhausted; its basic condition is the same as in the first phase (Selye, 1936). It is interesting to see how the idea of the "syndrome of just being sick," which occurred to him as a student, matured over time into a new concept of "general adaptation syndrome" by clarifying the changes behind the phenomena and the mechanisms involved.

In 1964, George Solomon (1931–2001) at Stanford University studied the relationship between disease progression and psychological factors such as patient personality in the autoimmune disease rheumatoid arthritis, finding a correlation between them (Moos and Solomon, 1964). He named this area of research on the relationship between stress, emotion, immunity, and disease "psychoimmunology," but it did not gain immediate acceptance at the time. It may be that studies that only revealed correlations were regarded as soft.

In 1975, Robert Ader (1932–2001) and Nicholas Cohen (1938–) of the University of Rochester conducted the following experiment using the Pavlovian system of conditioned reflexes. They studied the effects on antibody production after conditioning rats with an unconditioned stimulus of an immunosuppressant (cyclophosphamide) and a neutral stimulus of saccharin. They showed that only the neutral stimulus of saccharin administration could suppress the immune response (Ader and Cohen, 1975). In a lecture to the American Psychosomatic Society in 1980, Ader named the new field "psychoneuroimmunology," in which biological phenomena are analyzed from the perspective of the interaction between the immune and nervous systems (Ader, 1980). This area is sometimes referred to as "psychoneuroendocrinoimmunology" with the addition of endocrine involvement. The extent of Pavlov's influence on the development of this field can also be seen here.

A book entitled *Psychoneuroimmunology* was published the following year (Ader, 1981). Its basic message was that the immune system alone is insufficient for the organism to protect itself from environmental invaders and stress, so it must interact with other systems (e.g., the nervous and endocrine systems) and their components. In other words, it introduced the viewpoint that these systems function in an integrated manner. This perspective is quite natural considering the often-forgotten nature of the concept of system, as highlighted in Bernard's epigraph in this chapter. Therefore, its analysis requires the participation of diverse fields such as immunology, neuroscience, endocrinology, psychology, and basic sciences such as biochemistry, molecular biology, and physiology. Countless studies suggest that there is interaction between the various systems that are currently divided for convenience. Here, I will provide a glimpse of how intersystemic interactions occur in the body by presenting a few specific examples, focusing mainly on the relationship between the immune and nervous systems.

The nervous system is divided into the somatic and autonomic nervous systems. The somatic nervous system includes afferent or sensory nerves that receive information and transmit it to the central nervous system and efferent or motor nerves that send commands to muscles and other parts of the body. While the somatic nervous system is involved in voluntary processes, the autonomic nervous system constantly controls involuntary processes, such as circulation, respiration, digestion, body temperature, endocrine functions, and metabolism. The autonomic nervous system includes the sympathetic and parasympathetic nervous systems. The sympathetic nervous system is stimulated in crisis, increasing heart rate and blood pressure, mobilizing energy sources, and secreting increased amounts of adrenaline and noradrenaline. This reaction mediates the "fight-or-flight response" (Cannon, 1915). In contrast, the parasympathetic nervous system has sedative effects, such as reducing heart rate and cardiac contraction. Because the primary neurotransmitter involved in this process is acetylcholine, this nerve is also called the cholinergic nerve.

The central nervous system has long been considered an immunologically privileged site, inaccessible to immune cells except for microglia. This separation is accomplished by the blood-brain barrier, which restricts the exchange of substances between the blood and cerebrospinal fluid. Therefore, under physiological conditions, there is no immune response in the central nervous system, and only when there is a lesion does it becomes problematic. However, it has become evident that even under physiological conditions there is a two-way exchange between the nervous and immune systems (McAllister and van de Water, 2009; Kipnis, 2016). This situation reminds us of the two-way communication between mother and child via the placenta, which was thought to provide iron-clad protection (Section 2.3, Chapter 2). These findings seem to indicate that there is no such thing as a perfect barrier in a living organism.

One example of the connection between the nervous and immune systems is a mechanism named the "inflammatory reflex" (Tracey, 2002; Rosas-Ballina and Tracey, 2009). In essence, the autonomic nervous system is responsible for the mechanism by which the nervous system reflexively suppresses inflammation and maintains homeostasis. The autonomic nervous system widely extends nerve fibers to internal organs and exerts its innervation over immune organs, such as bone marrow, thymus, lymph nodes, and spleen, using various neurotransmitters. For example, injection of bovine serum albumin under the rat skin increases the number of nerve endings in nearby lymph nodes (Novotny et al., 1994), and injection of tuberculin into the murine spleen also increases nerve endings (Yang et al., 1998). These findings suggest that the nervous system is not a bystander but is actively and dynamically involved in the local immune response.

When inflammation occurs locally, its four signs—redness (*rubor*), fever (*calor*), pain (*dolor*), and swelling (*tumor*)—observed by Aulus Cornelius Celsus of Ancient Rome (c. 25–c. 50 AD) appear. These changes are thought to be due to the effects of cytokines and other substances produced by immune cells. The inflammatory reflex arc comprises afferent nerves that directly detect substances produced by infection or injury and transmit local information to the central nervous system and efferent nerves that contain cholinergic anti-inflammatory pathways that transmit signals to suppress inflammation. The nerve involved here is the vagus (or the 10th cranial) nerve that ultimately secretes the neurotransmitter acetylcholine, which acts on innate immunity cells with its receptors to inhibit their secretion of proinflammatory cytokines (e.g., tumor necrosis factor, IL-1, and HMGB1). Indeed, direct stimulation of the efferent vagus nerve toward the local area suppresses the production of the aforementioned cytokines (Borovikova et al., 2000; Bernik et al., 2002), whereas suppression of the vagus nerve increases the inflammatory response and makes it uncontrollable (Andersson and Tracey, 2012). Using this mechanism, treating inflammation by electrically stimulating the vagus nerve is currently being tested.

Next, I will examine the relationship between acquired immunity and the nervous system, mainly focusing on the regulation of nervous system functions by T cells. As mentioned in Section 2.1, Chapter 2, it has been reported that T cells that recognize self-antigens (e.g., MBP) are not only involved in the destruction of brain tissue but also play a neuroprotective function (Moalem et al., 1999; Yoles et al., 2001). One mouse model of PTSD is created by having the mice sniff predators to induce stress symptoms. Using this model, Cohen et al. conducted experiments with immunodeficient mice, which lack T and B cells, and nude mice, which lack T cells. Their results showed that both deficient mice had intense PTSD-like symptoms. However, transgenic mice expressing T cells that recognize self-antigens (i.e., MBP) showed improved symptoms (Cohen et al., 2006). It is suggested that peripheral immune cells may regulate psychological processes.

Similarly, the role of T cells in neurogenesis and spatial learning and memory in the hippocampus was examined using immunodeficient mice and transgenic mice with autoreactive T cells. These results showed that both neurogenesis and spatial learning ability were depressed in immunocompromised mice, which was restored in transgenic mice with autoreactive (e.g., MBP-reactive) T cells, but not in mice with T cells recognizing a nonself antigen (e.g., ovalbumin) (Ziv et al., 2006). Therefore, it is not just a matter of having T cells present but of having T cells that recognize some self-antigen, which may not be limited to MBP.

An interesting report was recently published on an experimental system using Pavlov's conditioned reflex (Koren et al., 2021). The researchers found neurons activated during two experimental inflammations (sodium dextran sulfate-induced colitis and zymosan-induced peritonitis) in the insular cortex of the cerebral cortex, and restimulation of these neurons could induce an inflammatory response in the abdomen. The insular cortex is involved in sensing the body's physiological state and integrating bodily sensations, such as pain, hunger, and visceral signals. The results of this experiment indicate that cells in the nervous system store information about immune responses that occur in the periphery and that the stored information can be retrieved by restimulating the neurons. In other words, the nervous system is also involved in forming and extracting immune memory.

A century after Métalnikov's work in the first half of the 20th century, the specific cells and mechanisms involved appear to be coming to light. The same group also used optogenetics to stimulate specific sympathetic nerves in the mouse colon and then studied their effects on colitis induced by dextran sodium sulfate. The sympathetic nervous system is responsible for systemic control by innervating the adrenal glands and regulating adrenaline and noradrenaline, and local control by directly innervating tissues, including immune organs. In this experiment, sympathetic stimulation of the colon caused colitis to abate (Schiller et al., 2021). The mechanism was found to be reduced expression of the molecule (mucosal addressin cell adhesion molecule 1) important for the extravasation of immune cells in vascular endothelial cells, preventing the accumulation of immune cells. While it was already known that many types of inflammation are affected by psychological states, this study has established one mechanism.

If we accept the results of this experiment, specific parts of the brain induce immune responses in the periphery, implying that the nervous and immune systems are anatomically and inseparably linked, and the structure of the nervous and immune connections has been revealed. Kevin Tracey (1957–) has named such neural control of the immune response the "immunological homunculus" (Tracey, 2007), a term introduced by Irun Cohen in Section 2.1.6, Chapter 2. Cohen's idea was to metaphorically superimpose the function of tissue maintenance and homeostatic control by the immune system's baseline recognition of selected self-antigens on Wilder Penfield's brain homunculus, which depicts the neural control of motor and sensory functions dedicated to various parts of the body. However, if the aforementioned analysis continues to progress and the specific neural controls of various immune responses are clarified, it is no longer a metaphor for Penfield's homunculus but a new brain map linking specific nerves to specific immune functions. In this respect, the results are very promising.

3.3 IMMUNITY AS AN INFORMATION SENSING SYSTEM

In the historical background described in the previous section, James Blalock (1949–) published an opinion in *The Journal of Immunology* entitled "The immune system as a sensory organ" in 1984, conceived from the interaction of the immune system with the central nervous and endocrine systems (Blalock, 1984). His points were threefold: first, there are logical biochemical reasons for the interaction of the immune, nervous, and endocrine systems; second, the immune system may function as a sensory organ; and third, the signals and receptors that these three systems use to exchange information may be unable to identify their origin in the future. Indeed, immune cells produce neurotransmitters and neuropeptides that affect the nervous system and have their receptors, allowing immune cells to accept information from the nervous system. In addition, nerves are distributed in the immune organs and tissues, and humoral factors produced by immune cells, such as cytokines, can act directly on nerves. Conversely, it has been shown that mental stresses stimulate the HPA and sympathetic-adrenal medullary systems to produce glucocorticoids and catecholamines, which have inhibitory effects on the immune response. Based on these results, Blalock proposed to view the immune system as a sensory organ that carries a sixth sense, which detects what our bodies' five senses of sight, hearing, smell, taste, and touch cannot detect (Blalock, 1984, 2005).

However, Jonathan Kipnis proposed that the immune system should be considered the seventh sense because some people call the process by which the vagus nerve transmits information from internal organs to the brain (Zagon, 2001) and the deep senses that detect the position and movement of various parts of the body (Smith, 2011) the sixth sense. Kipnis defines the function of the immune system as sensing internal and external information, including pathogens, and transmitting it to the nervous system. In other words, this definition assumes that the immune response is directly linked to the brain, almost wholly overlapping with the idea advocated by Métalnikov that "to immunize is mainly to immunize the nervous centers which govern the cells' sensitivity" (Métalnikov, 1934). This perspective is supported by a growing number of examples, such as IFN-γ derived from immune cells directly acting on neurons to regulate neural circuits involved in social behavior in mice (Filiano et al., 2016) or a major proinflammatory cytokine IL-17 directly acting on nematode neurons to alter their reactivity and influence their behavior (Chen et al., 2017). In any case, the view of the immune system as a systemic sensory organ that perceives internal and external changes has the effect of broadening the conventional perception of immunity as a defense against pathogens as its primary function and restoring a view of the whole organism. This point will be important in approaching the essence of immunity.

Henrique Veiga-Fernandez (1972–) and Antonio Freitas (1947–) have recently made a similar proposal (Veiga-Fernandes and Freitas, 2017). They attempt to consider immune cells and the immune system as involved in maintaining homeostasis, which guarantees the survival of cells and organisms by integrating signals from interactions between and within tissues or from the ecosystem. In other words, the immune system functions like a sensor that receives, integrates, and responds to signals from its surroundings. They call their theory the "s(c)ensory immune system theory." The neuro-immune cell unit proposed by Veiga-Fernandes et al. refers to neurons and immune cells coexisting and functioning at specific anatomical sites (e.g., lymphoid organs, adipose tissue, and mucous membranes that serve as barriers), integrally regulating physiological processes such as hematopoiesis, organogenesis, inflammation, tissue repair, and thermogenesis by brown fat cells (Veiga-Fernandes and Pachnis, 2017; Godinho-Silva et al., 2019). Humoral factors such as neurotransmitters and cytokines mediate the interaction between nerves and immunity; immune cells have receptors that can recognize nerve-derived molecules, and nerve cells have receptors that recognize immune-derived molecules. Therefore, nerve cell disturbances cause abnormal activation of immune cells and autoimmune diseases.

If the specific connections between the immune system and the cells that comprise the nervous system and their products are more extensively confirmed, the network that extends throughout the body may become even more complex. Their progressive confirmation would increasingly reveal a picture in which the immune system cannot be viewed as an isolated system but rather as regulating the homeostasis of the entire organism together with other systems. These perspectives partially resonate with what I am about to reveal in this book. The initial trigger of an immune response may well be local. However, its effects are highly likely to affect the whole body, including the mind, and the holistic view that originated in ancient Greece cannot be ignored. Speaking from personal experience, the body often follows suit when the mind is at peace and the spirit is firmly aware. To paraphrase Métalnikov, I sometimes feel that "mental activity immunizes the immune system." It will be important not only to consider the cooperation between the mind and the body with an emphasis on the mind but also to practice from this perspective.

In Chapter 1, we reviewed research on defense against foreign enemies, which is considered the immune system's primary function. However, it is now evident that the range of roles played by the immune system is broader than previously known, extending throughout the body. Furthermore, a complex picture emerges in which immune cells throughout the body naturally exert local and systemic effects beyond the currently defined system by releasing various humoral factors and receiving various factors from the nervous and endocrine systems, thereby regulating the whole body. The complex nature of the system is expected to be clarified in the future. As Claude Bernard noted, there is no such thing as a system in nature, and if biological functions, including immunity, work as a whole, this is a natural consequence. In his book *Discourse on the Method*, published in 1637, Descartes presents four precepts to arrive at knowledge. One of them is to start with the simplest and easiest-to-know objects and then ascend step by step to the knowledge of the more complex objects (Descartes, 2000). If we assume that this process is a staircase leading from the part to the whole, the research progress to date may have already reached the bottom of the staircase. However, this staircase cannot be ascended by reductionist thinking at the present stage. Therefore, what is required now is philosophical thinking that moves toward synthesis.

3.4   RETHINKING THE MILIEU INTÉRIEUR AND HOMEOSTASIS

Once we realize that the phenomenon of immunity or the immune system is not localized but extends throughout the entire organism and is an important mechanism controlling the organism's fluctuations between normal and pathological states, we find a major stream of thought that has developed a holistic view of disease. In our time, it may be the concept of homeostasis as a mechanism that living organisms actively use to maintain the homeostatic conditions necessary for survival. In 2007, 21 U.S. biology teachers met and chose homeostasis as one of the eight core concepts in biology, along with cell, evolution, and ecosystem (Michael, 2007). However, awareness of homeostasis is low and often ignored (Billman, 2020), and even when this concept is discussed, it varies from person to person (Modell et al., 2015). The original concept of homeostasis goes back to Claude Bernard's milieu intérieur. However, if we look back in human history, the seeds of the idea that the equilibrium of opposing forces is important for the organism's health can be found in ancient Greece.

Alcmaeon, born in Croton in southern Italy, was a man of such ideas (Huffman, 2021). His birth and death dates are unknown, but he was a Greek natural philosopher who is thought to have been active in the first half of the 5th century BC. Due to the scarcity of primary sources, we must rely on third-party testimonies from across the ages for his real image, but based on them, some peculiarities become apparent. For example, he uses political metaphors to define health and pathology. Health is maintained when the opposing forces comprising the body (e.g., wet and dry, cold and warm, sweet and bitter) are in equilibrium (*isonomia*). However, disease develops when any of these forces dominate the monarchy. Sometimes metaphors go in the opposite direction; they are used to explain phenomena in human society by what was revealed in the organism. I will discuss the problems and dangers of this application at the end of this section. This view of interpreting health in terms of the balance of two opposing forces was later carried over to Hippocrates' and then to Galen's medicine and became the central concept of Western medicine for more than 2,000 years.

Alcmaeon also offered some other interesting ideas. He is regarded as the first person to identify the brain as the site of what is called the mind or soul at a time when the heart was thought to be that site. Furthermore, he not only referred to the difference between perceiving and understanding—or primary and secondary consciousness, to use Gerald Edelman's expression (Section 4.5, Chapter 4)—but also advocated the eternity of the soul and is said to have influenced Plato.

Claude Bernard's concept of the milieu intérieur, on which homeostasis is based, is introduced in his works, including *An Introduction to the Study of Experimental Medicine*, originally published in 1865 (Bernard, 1949d). For example, it was explained in detail in the second lecture, "The Three Forms of Life," in his *Lectures on the Phenomena of Life Common to Animals and Plants*, published in the year of his death (Bernard, 1878b). In it, Bernard classified the forms of life into three categories—latent life (unmanifested), oscillating life (fluctuating and dependent on the external environment), and constant life (free and independent of the external environment)—based on the view that life exists as a result of the competition or coordination of two factors. One is the external environmental factor, and the other is the within-organism factor. Bernard often uses the word "cosmique" to describe external factors. I feel the vastness of his vision. He describes the first type of latent life as that which appears to have ceased life activity due to reduced chemical requirements, such as seeds, brewer's yeast (*Saccharomyces cerevisiae*), nematodes, and tardigrades. The second, fluctuating and dependent life, applies to all plants and most animals that live under the direct influence of the external environment. The third, free and independent life, has a milieu intérieur separate from the external environment and can therefore live independently of external influence. This is because in highly evolved organisms, tissues and organs are surrounded and immersed in a milieu intérieur comprising interstitial fluid derived from plasma and lymph fluid and are thus insulated from the effects of the external world. Bernard stated that "the fixity of the milieu intérieur is the condition of free and independent life" (Bernard, 1878a). The British physiologist Denis Noble (1936–) credits Bernard, who also distinguished himself as an excellent experimenter, as the first systems biologist, emphasizing that the milieu intérieur concept suggests a mechanism that controls the entire system (Noble, 2008).

In this lecture, too, Bernard urges caution, pointing out that the vitalistic view that there is some kind of internal principle of life struggling against external physical influences is false, and that the principle of life is actually due to mechanisms brought about by the relationship between the internal and external environment (Bernard, 1878c). Bernard's rather harsh attitude toward vitalism is evident in his *An Introduction to the Study of Experimental Medicine* and other works. The historical situation at the time was as follows: it had long been believed that there were clearly demarcated entities in this world: minerals, plants, and animals. However, in the 18th century, Antoine Lavoisier (1743–1794) revealed that plants and animals share common elements—carbon, hydrogen, nitrogen, and phosphorus—which blurred the boundary between plants and animals. In 1828, Friedrich Wöhler (1800–1882) succeeded in making urea (an organic compound) from ammonium cyanate (an inorganic compound), which blurred the boundary between inorganic and organic substances and opened the possibility that life phenomena could be reduced to physicochemical science.

In Bernard's time, there was a fierce attack from the mechanists and reductionists against vitalists, who considered that life is special and cannot be explained by mechanisms. Bernard appears to have been trying to put an end to vitalism by saying the following:

> These ideas, which were current in other times, are now gradually disappearing; but it is essential to extirpate their very last spawn, because the so-called vitalistic ideas still remaining in certain minds are really an obstacle to the progress of experimental science.
>
> **Bernard (1949c)**

However, we can see that he had a certain sympathy for the vitalists, on the assumption that they recognized the peculiarities of living organisms but did not jump to non-physicochemical arguments using life principles. For example:

I should agree with the vitalists if they would simply recognize that living beings exhibit phenomena unique to themselves and unknown in inorganic nature. I admit, indeed, that manifestations of life cannot be wholly elucidated by the physicochemical phenomena known in inorganic nature.

Bernard (1949b)

The special perception of life that any researcher dealing with life phenomena would experience seems to be manifested here.

Bernard's milieu intérieur concept would be redefined under the name "homeostasis" by the American physiologist Walter Cannon. The following description appears in the "Defense (Function of)" section of Volume IV of the *Dictionary of Physiology*, compiled in 1900 by Charles Richet (1850–1935), who would win the Nobel Prize in Physiology or Medicine in 1913 for his discovery of the anaphylactic reaction:

In short, the living being is stable; and it has to be in order not to be destroyed, dissolved, and decomposed by the colossal and often adverse forces that surround it. But, by a kind of contradiction which is only apparent, it maintains its stability only if it is excitable, capable of modifying itself according to the irritations of the external world and of conforming its response to the irritation so that it is stable only because it is modifiable. Defense is only compatible with a certain degree of instability. This instability must be exercised ceaselessly but within narrow limits, and this moderate instability is the necessary condition for the true stability of being.

Life is a perpetual self-regulation, an adaptation to changing external conditions. The level has to be constantly shifting, but it has to oscillate around an almost invariable average.

So, if I could try to give a formula to this defense of the organism, which, considered in this way, constitutes the entire physiology, I would say of the living being: *It undergoes all impressions and resists them all; it is always renewed and is always the same.*

Richet (1900)

As seen in this description, the paradox that a certain instability or flexibility supports the homeostasis of an organism, and the fact that this is a characteristic of the organism, were recognized as early as 1900. Following this historical trend, Cannon developed the concept of milieu intérieur and defined this characteristic of living organisms as homeostasis (Cannon, 1929). Highly evolved organisms are open systems with many relationships with their environment through the respiratory, digestive, and other organs. Changes in the external environment cause disturbances within the system, but these disturbances are usually automatically adjusted to remain within a narrow range by a feedback mechanism. This state of equilibrium results from the joint action of many organs, including the blood, brain, nerves, heart, lungs, kidneys, and spleen. This physiological response is homeostasis, unique to living organisms, maintaining a steady state by cooperation.

This term combines *homeo* (an abbreviation of *homoios* meaning a certain range of similarity) rather than *homos* (meaning identity) and *stasis* (meaning a state brought about by equilibrium rather than a fixed and immobile stagnation). Cannon acknowledged the existence of a certain threshold in homeostasis but assumed it is not fixed in advance but is maintained by moving up and down. Biological control is sometimes analogized to a thermostat that keeps the temperature of a system constant, but this would not reflect reality. Like Richet, Cannon believed that homeostasis and stability were based on the dynamic instability surrounding both internal and external environments.

However, the term "fixity," which Bernard used to describe the milieu intérieur, might have given the impression of rigid and inflexible control not only to the milieu intérieur but also to the concept of homeostasis. As a result, several alternative concepts emphasizing the aspect of dynamic regulation have been proposed to explain various aspects of physiological regulation that have since been reported. One of the most influential is the concept of "allostasis" (Sterling and Eyer, 1988). The term combines *allos* (meaning "other" or "different") and *stasis*, which differs from homeostasis as follows. First, homeostasis appears to function relatively well when the regulation of isolated organs and tissues is examined in the Bernardian fashion. However, the diurnal fluctuations of blood pressure, for example, which vary with changes in mental states during wakefulness, sleep, or preparation for meetings, make the automatic adjustment to one normal value a fiction. Instead, allostasis emphasizes holistic control involving all body organs. Second, allostasis considers environmental and social influences, referring to a state in which they alter all physiological parameters, not just one parameter, such as blood pressure. Third, allostasis considers how social environmental influences are transmitted to the internal environment, which is explained as being mediated by the brain and defined as "stability through change."

However, not only does this definition appear to be essentially the same as that of the milieu intérieur and homeostasis, but as mentioned earlier, Cannon also points to the coordinated involvement of the brain, nerves, and organs throughout the body, such as the heart, lungs, kidneys, and spleen (Cannon, 1939a). Some believe that allostasis not only encompasses the ability to anticipate and respond to changes in the life cycle and seasonal changes but also contributes to explaining the mechanism of "allostatic overload," a pathological condition that occurs when external influences such as stress exceed the body's processing capacity (McEwen and Wingfield, 2010). However, others have criticized the allostasis concept as merely a paraphrasing of homeostasis that does not improve understanding of physiological control (Carpenter, 2004; Day, 2005; Cabanac, 2006).

As already mentioned, homeostatic control could be considered a consistent theme throughout the history of medicine, beginning with the ancient Greeks. When we turn to modern biology and medicine, it is no exaggeration to say that what is being done is a study of the mechanisms of homeostatic regulation at each level of interest to the researcher: genetic, molecular, cellular, organ, or organism. Immune responses, such as the development of autoimmunity and tumorigenesis, are regulated and determined by the interplay between positive and negative factors, and the analysis of these mechanisms has produced results that have led to therapies. Georges Canguilhem's basic conception of life was not based on an ideal norm fixed from the beginning but on the idea that in times of crisis, a new physiological order, different from the previous one, must be maintained to remain healthy (Canguilhem, 1991). New norms must be created in response to circumstances. It is a view that emphasizes the flexibility and creativity of life, without which it would be impossible to live and survive (Section 5.3, Chapter 5).

The epilogue to Cannon's *The Wisdom of the Body*, originally published in 1932, is entitled "Relations of Biological and Social Homeostasis" (Cannon, 1939b). In it, he attempts to use the homeostasis found in living organisms to explain societal stability. In an article published in *Science* in 1941, he also attempts to compare the state of freedom from internal and external influences in human society by analogy with an organism's physiological state (Cannon, 1941). While it may be tempting to compare organisms and societies, it seems challenging to make a concrete contrast between individual organisms and societies, which are originally entirely different constructs. The human body is a complex structure, but society is even more complex, and, unlike the human body, it appears to have some areas where autonomic control is less likely to work. In *The Wisdom of the Body*, homeostasis in society is described as follows:

> At the outset it is noteworthy that the body politic itself exhibits some indications of crude automatic stabilizing processes. [...] A display of conservatism excites a radical revolt and that in turn is followed by a return to conservatism. Loose government and its consequences bring the reformers into power, but their tight reins soon provoke restiveness and the desire for release. The noble enthusiasms and sacrifices of war are succeeded by moral apathy and orgies of self-indulgence. Hardly any strong tendency in a nation continues to the stage of disaster; before that extreme is reached corrective forces arise which check the tendency and they commonly prevail to such an excessive degree as themselves to cause a reaction.
>
> **Cannon (1939c)**

Even to a non-specialist, this argument gives the impression of being somewhat naïve. This impression is reinforced by the fact that when one looks at the world situation, it is not uncommon to find events that seem to have crossed the threshold beyond which recovery by homeostasis is possible. Rather than going into the specifics of Cannon's argument, I will briefly touch on the problems and dangers associated with uncritically trying to apply phenomena and theories revealed in the biological world to analyze and explain human society without philosophical consideration.

What immediately comes to mind is the example of Herbert Spencer's (1820–1903) theory of social evolution, in which he summarized Darwin's theory in terms of "survival of the fittest" and attempted to apply it to society (Spencer, 1864). This perspective negatively influenced the understanding and solution of social problems, and the idea survives to this day. In 1975, the American naturalist Edward O. Wilson (1929–2021) published *Sociobiology*, which attempted to clarify human social behavior, and thus human nature, by integrating the biological and social sciences: new population genetics, animal behavior, and evolutionary theory (Wilson, 1975). There appears to be an assertion that human social behavior studied in the humanities and social sciences can be explained by biology. The book was heavily criticized by those who saw the dangers of leading to genetic determinism, racism, and even eugenics. According to the author, he was attacked for distorting the facts based on partisan ideology, despite his own reminder that we should not uncritically shift from the fact that "it is so" as revealed in non-human organisms to the ethic that humans "should be so."

Here is another example. The phenomenon of programmed cell death or apoptosis is found in the biological world. This phenomenon, which can be interpreted as a single cell being destined to die for the good of the whole, has been shown to extend not only to multicellular organisms but also to unicellular organisms such as bacteria (Engelberg-Kulka et al., 2006; Lee and Lee, 2019). When one looks back at history, sacrifices were made for the good of the whole. Therefore, there is always a concern that these biological phenomena, which can be seen as altruistic acts, will be used as arguments in debating the place of humans in society. We should always be wary of the dangers of applying phenomena observed in the biological world to human society.

NOTE

1 Bernard, C. (1949). *An Introduction to the Study of Experimental Medicine* (H. C. Greene, Trans.). Henry Schuman. (Originally published 1865) 221.

REFERENCES

Abdul-Careem, M. F., Lee, A. J., Pek, E. A., Gill, N., Gillgrass, A. E., Chew, M. V., Reid, S., & Ashkar, A. A. (2012). Genital HSV-2 infection induces short-term NK cell memory. *Journal of Immunology, 7*, e32821. doi: 10.1371/journal.pone.0032821.

Ader, R. (1980). Psychosomatic and psychoimmunologic research. *Psychosomatic Medicine, 42*, 307–321. doi: 10.1097/00006842-198005000-00001.

Ader, R. (Ed.) (1981). *Psychoneuroimmunology*. Academic Press.

Ader, R., & Cohen, N. (1975). Behaviorally conditioned immunosuppression. *Psychosomatic Medicine, 37*, 333–340. doi: 10.1097/00006842-197507000-00007.

Ahmadzadeh, M., Hussain, S. F., & Farber, D. L. (2001). Heterogeneity of the memory CD4 T cell response: Persisting effectors and resting memory T cells. *Journal of Immunology, 166*, 926–935. doi: 10.4049/jimmunol.166.2.926.

Andersson, U., & Tracey, K. J. (2012). Neural reflexes in inflammation and immunity. *Journal of Experimental Medicine, 209*, 1057–1068. doi: 10.1084/jem.20120571.

Artis, D., & Spits, H. (2015). The biology of innate lymphoid cells. *Nature, 17*, 293–301. doi: 10.1038/nature14189.

Bernard, C. (1878a). *Leçons sur les phénomènes de la vie communs aux animaux et aux végétaux (Lessons on the Phenomena of Life Common to Animals and Plants)*. (H. Yakura, Trans.). J.-B. Baillière. 113.

Bernard, C. (1878b). *Leçons sur les phénomènes de la vie communs aux animaux et aux végétaux (Lessons on the Phenomena of Life Common to Animals and Plants)*. (H. Yakura, Trans.). J.-B. Baillière. 65–124.

Bernard, C. (1878c). *Leçons sur les phénomènes de la vie communs aux animaux et aux végétaux (Lessons on the Phenomena of Life Common to Animals and Plants)*. (H. Yakura, Trans.). J.-B. Baillière. 124.

Bernard, C. (1878d). *Leçons sur les phénomènes de la vie communs aux animaux et aux végétaux (Lessons on the Phenomena of Life Common to Animals and Plants)*. J.-B. Baillière. 1–404.

Bernard, C. (1949a). *An Introduction to the Study of Experimental Medicine*. (H. C. Greene, Trans.). Henry Schuman. (Originally published 1865). 221.

Bernard, C. (1949b). *An Introduction to the Study of Experimental Medicine*. (H. C. Greene, Trans.). Henry Schuman. (Originally published 1865). 69.

Bernard, C. (1949c). *An Introduction to the Study of Experimental Medicine*. (H. C. Greene, Trans.). Henry Schuman. (Originally published 1865). 60.

Bernard, C. (1949d). *An Introduction to the Study of Experimental Medicine*. (H. C. Greene, Trans.). Henry Schuman. (Originally published 1865). 1–314.

Bernik, T. R., Friedman, S. G., Ochani, M., DiRaimo, R., Ulloa, L., Yang, H., Sudan, S,, Czura, C. J., Ivanova, S. M., & Tracey, K. J. (2002). Pharmacological stimulation of the cholinergic antiinflammatory pathway. *Journal of Experimental Medicine, 195*, 781–788. doi: 10.1084/jem.20011714.

Billman, G. E. (2020). Homeostasis: The underappreciated and far too often ignored central organizing principle of physiology. *Frontiers in Physiology, 11*, 200. doi: 10.3389/fphys.2020.00200.

Blalock, J. E. (1984). The immune system as a sensory organ. *Journal of Immunology, 132*, 1067–1070.

Blalock, J. E. (2005). The immune system as the sixth sense. *Journal of Internal Medicine, 257*, 126–138. doi: 10.1111/j.1365-2796.2004.01441.x.

Borovikova, L. V., Ivanova, S., Zhang, M., Yang, H., Botchkina, G. I., Watkins, L. R., Wang, H., Abumrad, N., Eaton, J. W., & Tracey, K. J. (2000). Vagus nerve stimulation attenuates the systemic inflammatory response to endotoxin. *Nature, 405*, 458–462. doi: 10.1038/35013070.

Cabanac, M. (2006). Adjustable set point: To honor Harold T. Hammel. *Journal of Applied Physiology, 100*, 1338–1346. doi: 10.1152/japplphysiol.01021.2005.

Canguilhem, G. (1991). *The Normal and the Pathological*. (C. R. Fawcett & R. S. Cohen, Trans.). Zone Books. 181–201.

Cannon, W. B. (1915). *Bodily Changes in Pain, Hunger, Fear and Rage: An Account of Recent Researches into the Function of Emotional Excitement*. D. Appleton.

Cannon, W. B. (1926). Physiological regulation of normal states: some tentative postulates concerning biological homeostatics. *Charles Richet, Ses Amis, ses collégues, ses Elèves*. Editions Medicales. 91–93.

Cannon, W. B. (1929). Organization for physiological homeostasis. *Physiological Reviews, 9*, 399–431. doi: 10.1152/physrev.1929.9.3.399.

Cannon, W. B. (1939a). *The Wisdom of the Body*. W. W. Norton. 24.

Cannon, W. B. (1939b). *The Wisdom of the Body*. W. W. Norton. 305–324.

Cannon, W. B. (1939c). *The Wisdom of the Body*. W. W. Norton. 311–312.

Cannon, W. B. (1941). The body physiologic and the body politic. *Science, 93*, 1–10. doi: 10.1126/science.93.2401.1.

Carpenter, R. H. S. (2004). Homeostasis: A plea for a unified approach. *Advances in Physiology Education, 28*, 180–187. doi: 10.1152/advan.00012.2004.

Chen, C., Itakura, E., Nelson, G. M., Sheng, M., Laurent, P., Fenk, L. A., Butcher, R. A., Hegde, R. S., & de Bono, M. (2017). IL-17 is a neuromodulator of *Caenorhabditis elegans* sensory responses. *Nature, 542*, 43–48. doi: 10.1038/nature20818.

Cohen, H., Ziv, Y., Cardon, M., Kaplan, Z., Matar, M. A., Gidron, Y., Schwartz, M., & Kipnis, J. (2006). Maladaptation to mental stress mitigated by the adaptive immune system via depletion of naturally occurring regulatory CD4+CD25+cells. *Journal of Neurobiology, 66*, 552–563. doi: 10.1002/neu.20249.

Cooper, M. A., & Yokoyama, W. M. (2010). Memory-like responses of natural killer cells. *Immunological Reviews, 235*, 297–305. doi: 10.1111/j.0105-2896.2010.00891.x.

Cummins, R. (1975). Functional analysis. *Journal of Philosophy, 72*, 741–765. doi: 10.2307/2024640.

Day, T. A. (2005). Defining stress as a prelude to mapping its neurocircuitry: No help from allostasis. *Progress in Neuro-Psychopharmacology and Biological Psychiatry, 29*, 1195–1200. doi: 10.1016/j.pnpbp.2005.08.005.

Descartes, R. (2000). *Discours de la méthode (Discourse on the Method)*. Flammarion. (Originally published 1637). 49–50.

Dogan, I., Bertocci, B., Vilmont, V., Delbos, F., Mégret, J., Storck, S., Reynaud, C. A., & Weill, J. C. (2009). Multiple layers of B cell memory with different effector functions. *Nature Immunology, 10*, 1292–1299. doi: 10.1038/ni.1814.

Eberl, G., Colonna, M., Di Santo, J. P., & McKenzie, A. N. (2015). Innate lymphoid cells: A new paradigm in immunology. *Science, 348*, aaa6566. doi: 10.1126/science.aaa6566.

Engelberg-Kulka, H., Amitai, S., Kolodkin-Gal, I., & Hazan, R. (2006). Bacterial programmed cell death and multicellular behavior in bacteria. *PLoS Genetics, 2*, e135. doi: 10.1371/journal.pgen.0020135.

Farber, D. L., Netea, M. G., Radbruch, A., Rajewsky, K., & Zinkernagel, R. M. (2016). Immunological memory: Lessons from the past and a look to the future. *Nature Reviews Immunology, 16*, 124–128. doi: 10.1038/nri.2016.13.

Filiano, A. J., Xu, Y., Tustison, N. J., Marsh, R. L., Baker, W., Smirnov, I., Overall, C. C., Gadani, S. P., Turner, S. D., Weng, Z., Peerzade, S. N., Chen, H., Lee, K. S., Scott, M. M., Beenhakker, M. P., Litvak, V., & Kipnis, J. (2016). Unexpected role of interferon-γ in regulating neuronal connectivity and social behaviour. *Nature, 535*, 425–429. doi: 10.1038/nature18626.

Gebhardt, T., Wakim, L. M., Eidsmo, L., Reading, P. C., Heath, W. R., & Carbone, F. R. (2009). Memory T cells in nonlymphoid tissue that provide enhanced local immunity during infection with herpes simplex virus. *Nature Immunology, 10*, 524–530.

Giamarellos-Bourboulis, E. J., Tsilika, M., Moorlag, S., Antonakos, N., Kotsaki, A., Domínguez-Andrés, J., Kyriazopoulou, E., Gkavogianni, T., Adami, M. E., Damoraki, G., Koufargyris, P., Karageorgos, A., Bolanou, A., Koenen, H., van Crevel, R., Droggiti, D. I., Renieris, G., Papadopoulos, A., & Netea, M. G. (2020). Activate: Randomized clinical trial of BCG vaccination against infection in the elderly. *Cell, 183*, 315–323. doi: 10.1016/j.cell.2020.08.051.

Gillard, G. O., Bivas-Benita, M., Hovav, A. H., Grandpre, L. E., Panas, M. W., Seaman, M. S., Haynes, B. F., & Letvin, N. L. (2011). Thy1+ NK cells from vaccinia virus-primed mice confer protection against vaccinia virus challenge in the absence of adaptive lymphocytes. *PLoS Pathogens, 7*, e1002141. doi: 10.1371/journal.ppat.1002141.

Godinho-Silva, C., Cardoso, F., & Veiga-Fernandes, H. (2019). Neuro-immune cell units: A new paradigm in physiology. *Annual Review of Immunology, 37*, 19–46. doi: 10.1146/annurev-immunol-042718-041812.

Halliley, J. L., Tipton, C. M., Liesveld, J., Rosenberg, A. F., Darce, J., Gregoretti, I. V., Popova, L., Kaminiski, D., Fucile, C. F., Albizua, I., Kyu, S., Chiang, K. Y., Bradley, K. T., Burack, R., Slifka, M., Hammarlund, E., Wu, H., Zhao, L., Walsh, E. E., Falsey, A. R., et al. (2015). Long-lived plasma cells are contained within the CD19−CD38hiCD138+ subset in human bone marrow. *Immunity, 43*, 132–145. doi: 10.1016/j.immuni.2015.06.016.

Hammer, Q., Rückert, T., Borst, E. M., Dunst, J., Haubner, A., Durek, P., Heinrich, F., Gasparoni, G., Babic, M., Tomic, A., Pietra, G., Nienen, M., Blau, I. W., Hofmann, J., Na, I. K., Prinz, I., Koenecke, C., Hemmati, P., Babel, N., Arnold, R., et al. (2018). Peptide-specific recognition of human cytomegalovirus strains controls adaptive natural killer cells. *Nature Immunology, 19*, 453–463. doi: 10.1038/s41590-018-0082-6.

Herberman, R. B., Nunn, M. E., Holden, H. T., & Lavrin, D. H. (1975a). Natural cytotoxic reactivity of mouse lymphoid cells against syngeneic and allogeneic tumors. II. Characterization of effector cells. *International Journal of Cancer, 16*, 230–239. doi: 10.1002/ijc.2910160205.

Herberman, R. B., Nunn, M. E., & Lavrin, D. H. (1975b). Natural cytotoxic reactivity of mouse lymphoid cells against syngeneic and allogeneic tumors. I. Distribution of reactivity and specificity. *International Journal of Cancer, 16*, 216–229. doi: 10.1002/ijc.2910160204.

Huffman, C. (2021). Alcmaeon. (E. N. Zalta, Ed.). *Stanford Encyclopedia of Philosophy*. https://plato.stanford.edu/archives/sum2021/entries/alcmaeon/.

Ishigami, T. (1918). The influence of psychic acts on the progress of pulmonary tuberculosis. *American Review of Tuberculosis, 2*, 470–484.

Iwasaki, A., & Medzhitov, R. (2015). Control of adaptive immunity by the innate immune system. *Nature Immunology, 16*, 343–353. doi: 10.1038/ni.3123.

Jerne, N. K. (1985). The generative grammar of the immune system. Nobel Lecture, 8 December 1984. *Bioscience Reports, 5*, 439–451. doi: 10.1007/BF01116941.

Kaji, T., Ishige, A., Hikida, M., Taka, J., Hijikata, A., Kubo, M., Nagashima, T., Takahashi, Y., Kurosaki, T., Okada, M., Ohara, O., Rajewsky, K., & Takemori, T. (2012). Distinct cellular pathways select germ-line-encoded and somatically mutated antibodies into immunological memory. *Journal of Experimental Medicine, 209*, 2079–2097. doi: 10.1084/jem.20120127.

Kiessling, R., Klein, E., Pross, H., & Wigzell, H. (1975a). "Natural" killer cells in the mouse. II. Cytotoxic cells with specificity for mouse Moloney leukemia cells. Characteristics of the killer cell. *European Journal of Immunology, 5*, 117–121. doi: 10.1002/eji.1830050209.

Kiessling, R., Klein, E., & Wigzell, H. (1975b). "Natural" killer cells in the mouse. I. Cytotoxic cells with specificity for mouse Moloney leukemia cells. Specificity and distribution according to genotype. *European Journal of Immunology, 5*, 112–117. doi: 10.1002/eji.1830050208.

Kipnis, J. (2016). Multifaceted interactions between adaptive immunity and the central nervous system. *Science, 353*, 766–771. doi: 10.1126/science.aag2638.

Kleinnijenhuis, J., Quintin, J., Preijers, F., Joosten, L. A., Ifrim, D. C., Saeed, S., Jacobs, C., van Loenhout, J., de Jong, D., Stunnenberg, H. G., Xavier, R. J., van der Meer, J. W., van Crevel, R., & Netea, M. G. (2012). Bacille Calmette-Guérin induces NOD2-dependent nonspecific protection from reinfection via epigenetic reprogramming of monocytes. *Proceedings of the National Academy of Sciences of the United States of America, 109*, 17537–17542. doi: 10.1073/pnas.1202870109.

Koren, T., Yifa, R., Amer, M., Krot, M., Boshnak, N., Ben-Shaanan, T. L., Azulay-Debby, H., Zalayat, I., Avishai, E., Hajjo, H., Schiller, M., Haykin, H., Korin, B., Farfara, D., Hakim, F., Kobiler, O., Rosenblum, K., & Rolls, A. (2021). Insular cortex neurons encode and retrieve specific immune responses. *Cell, 184*, 5902–5915. doi: 10.1016/j.cell.2021.10.013.

Kourilsky, P. (2014). *Le Jeu du hasard et de la complexité: La nouvelle science de l'immunologie (The Game of Chance and Complexity: The New Science of Immunology)*. Odile Jacob. 159–160.

Kurosaki, T., Kometani, K., & Ise, W. (2015). Memory B cells. *Nature Reviews Immunology, 15*, 149–159. doi: 10.1038/nri3802.

Lee, H., & Lee, D. G. (2019). Programmed cell death in bacterial community: Mechanisms of action, causes and consequences. *Journal of Microbiology and Biotechnology, 29*, 1014–1021. doi: 10.4014/jmb.1904.04017.

Lee, J., Zhang, T., Hwang, I., Kim, A., Nitschke, L., Kim, M., Scott, J. M., Kamimura, Y., Lanier, L. L., & Kim, S. (2015). Epigenetic modification and antibody-dependent expansion of memory-like NK cells in human cytomegalovirus-infected individuals. *Immunity, 42*, 431–442. doi: 10.1016/j.immuni.2015.02.013.

Métalnikov, S. (1934). *Rôle du système nerveux et des facteurs biologiques et psychiques dans l'immunité (Role of the Nervous System and Biological and Psychological Factors in Immunity)*. Masson.

Métalnikov, S., & Chorine, V. (1926). Rôle des réflexes conditionnels dans l'immunité (The role of conditioned reflexes in immunity). *Annales de l'Institut Pasteur, 40*, 893–900.

Mackaness, G. B. (1964). The immunological basis of acquired cellular resistance. *Journal of Experimental Medicine, 120*, 105–120. doi: 10.1084/jem.120.1.105.

Martinez-Gonzalez, I., Ghaedi, M., Steer, C. A., Mathä, L., Vivier, E., & Takei, F. (2018). ILC2 memory: Recollection of previous activation. *Immunological Reviews, 283*, 41–53. doi: 10.1111/imr.12643.

Masopust, D., & Picker, L. J. (2012). Hidden memories: Frontline memory T cells and early pathogen interception. *Journal of Immunology, 188*, 5811–5817. doi: 10.4049/jimmunol.1102695.

McAllister, A. K., & van de Water, J. (2009). Breaking boundaries in neural-immune interactions. *Neuron, 64*, 9–12. doi: 10.1016/j.neuron.2009.09.038.

McEwen, B. S., & Wingfield, J. C. (2010). What is in a name? Integrating homeostasis, allostasis and stress. *Hormones and Behavior, 57*, 105–111. doi: 10.1016/j.yhbeh.2009.09.011.

Michael, J. (2007). Conceptual assessment in the biological sciences: a National Science Foundation-sponsored workshop. *Advances in Physiology Education, 31*, 389–391. doi: 10.1152/advan.00047.2007.

Moalem, G., Leibowitz-Amit, R., Yoles, E., Mor, F., Cohen, I. R., & Schwartz, M. (1999). Autoimmune T cells protect neurons from secondary degeneration after central nervous system axotomy. *Nature Medicine, 5*, 49–55. doi: 10.1038/4734.

Modell, H., Cliff, W., Michael, J., McFarland, J., Wenderoth, M. P., & Wright, A. (2015). A physiologist's view of homeostasis. *Advances in Physiology Education, 39*, 259–266. doi: 10.1152/advan.00107.2015.

Moos, R. H., & Solomon, G. F. (1964). Personality correlates of the rapidity of progression of rheumatoid arthritis. *Annals of the Rheumatic Diseases, 23*, 145–151. doi: 10.1136/ard.23.2.145.

Netea, M. G., Giamarellos-Bourboulis, E. J., Domínguez-Andrés, J., Curtis, N., van Crevel, R., van de Veerdonk, F. L., & Bonten, M. (2020). Trained immunity: A tool for reducing susceptibility to and the severity of SARS-CoV-2 infection. *Cell, 181*, 969–977. doi: 10.1016/j.cell.2020.04.042.

Netea, M. G., Joosten, L. A. B., Latz, E., Mills, K. H. G., Natoli, G., Stunnenberg, H. G., O'Neill, L. A. J., & Xavier, R. J. (2016). Trained immunity: A program of innate immune memory in health and disease. *Science, 352*, aaf1098. doi: 10.1126/science.aaf1098.

Netea, M. G., Quintin, J., & van Der Meer, J. W. M. (2011). Trained immunity: A memory for innate host defense. *Cell Host & Microbe, 9*, 355–361. doi: 10.1016/j.chom.2011.04.006.

Noble, D. (2008). Claude Bernard, the first systems biologist, and the future of physiology. *Experimental Physiology, 93*, 16–26. doi: 10.1113/expphysiol.2007.038695.

Novotny, G. E., Heuer, T., Schöttelndreier, A., & Fleisgarten, C. (1994). Plasticity of innervation of the medulla of axillary lymph nodes in the rat after antigenic stimulation. *Anatomical Record, 238*, 213–224. doi: 10.1002/ar.1092380208.

O'Leary, J. G., Goodarzi, M., Drayton, D. L., & von Andrian, U. H. (2006). T cell- and B cell-independent adaptive immunity mediated by natural killer cells. *Nature Immunology, 7*, 507–516. doi: 10.1038/ni1332.

O'Neill, L. A. J., & Netea, M. G. (2020). BCG-induced trained immunity: Can it offer protection against COVID-19? *Nature Reviews Immunology, 20*, 335–337. doi: 10.1038/s41577-020-0337-y.

O'Sullivan, T. E., Sun, J. C., & Lanier, L. L. (2015). Natural killer cell memory. *Immunity, 43*, 634–645. doi: 10.1016/j.immuni.2015.09.013.

Pape, K. A., Taylor, J. J., Maul, R. W., Gearhart, P. J., & Jenkins, M. K. (2011). Different B cell populations mediate early and late memory during an endogenous immune response. *Science, 331*, 1203–1207. doi: 10.1126/science.1201730.

Paust, S., & von Andrian, U. H. (2011). Natural killer cell memory. *Nature Immunology, 12*, 500–508. doi: 10.1038/ni.2032.

Quintin, J., Saeed, S., Martens, J. H. A., Giamarellos-Bourboulis, E. J., Ifrim, D. C., Logie, C., Jacobs, L., Jansen, T., Kullberg, B. J., Wijmenga, C., Joosten, L. A. B., Xavier, R. J., van der Meer, J. W. M., Stunnenberg, H. G., & Netea, M. G. (2012). *Candida albicans* infection affords protection against reinfection via functional reprogramming of monocytes. *Cell Host & Microbe, 12*, 223–232. doi: 10.1016/j.chom.2012.06.006.

Reeves, R. K., Li, H., Jost, S., Blass, E., Li, H., Schafer, J. L., Varner, V., Manickam, C., Eslamizar, L., Altfeld, M., von Andrian, U. H., & Barouch, D. H. (2015). Antigen-specific NK cell memory in rhesus macaques. *Nature Immunology, 16*, 927–932. doi: 10.1038/ni.3227.

Richet, C. (1900). Défense (Fonctions de). (Vol. IV) *Dictionnaire de physiologie*. (H. Yakura, Trans.). Félix Alcan. 721.

Rosas-Ballina, M., & Tracey, K. J. (2009). The neurology of the immune system: Neural reflexes regulate immunity. *Neuron, 64*, 28–32. doi: 10.1016/j.neuron.2009.09.039.

Sallusto, F., Lenig, D., Förster, R., Lipp, M., & Lanzavecchia, A. (1999). Two subsets of memory T lymphocytes with distinct homing potentials and effector functions. *Nature, 401*, 708–712. doi: 10.1038/44385.

Schiller, M., Azulay-Debby, H., Boshnak, N., Elyahu, Y., Korin, B., Ben-Shaanan, T. L., Koren, T., Krot, M., Hakim, F., & Rolls, A. (2021). Optogenetic activation of local colonic sympathetic innervations attenuates colitis by limiting immune cell extravasation. *Immunity, 54*, 1022–1036. doi: 10.1016/j.immuni.2021.04.007.

Selye, H. (1936). A syndrome produced by diverse nocuous agents. *Nature, 138*, 32. doi: 10.1038/138032a0.

Selye, H. (1956). *The Stress of Life*. McGraw-Hill.

Slifka, M. K., Antia, R., Whitmire, J. K., & Ahmed, R. (1998). Humoral immunity due to long-lived plasma cells. *Immunity, 8*, 363–372. doi: 10.1016/s1074-7613(00)80541-5.

Smith, R. (2011). "The sixth sense": Towards a history of muscular sensation. *Gesnerus, 68*, 218–271.

Spencer, H. (1864). *Principles of Biology. Vol. I*. Williams and Norgate. 444–445.

Spits, H., Artis, D., Colonna, M., Diefenbach, A., Di Santo, J. P., Eberl, G., Koyasu, S., Locksley, R. M., McKenzie, A. N., Mebius, R. E., Powrie, F., & Vivier, E. (2013). Innate lymphoid cells--a proposal for uniform nomenclature. *Nature Reviews Immunology, 13*, 145–149. doi: 10.1038/nri3365.

Sterling, P., & Eyer, J. (1988). Allostasis: A new paradigm to explain arousal pathology. *Handbook of Life Stress, Cognition and Health*. John Wiley & Sons. 629–649.

Sun, J. C., Beilke, J. N., & Lanier, L. L. (2009). Adaptive immune features of natural killer cells. *Nature, 457*, 557–561. doi: 10.1038/nature07665.

Sun, J. C., Ugolini, S., & Vivier, E. (2014). Immunological memory within the innate immune system. *EMBO Journal, 33*, 1295–1303. doi: 10.1002/embj.201387651.

Tan, S. Y., & Yip, A. (2018). Hans Selye (1907–1982): Founder of the stress theory. *Singapore Medical Journal, 59*, 170–171. doi: 10.11622/smedj.2018043.

Taylor, J. J., Pape, K. A., & Jenkins, M. K. (2012). A germinal center-independent pathway generates unswitched memory B cells early in the primary response. *Journal of Experimental Medicine, 209*, 597–606. doi: 10.1084/jem.20111696.

Teijaro, J. R., Turner, D., Pham, Q., Wherry, E. J., Lefrançois, L., & Farber, D. L. (2011). Cutting edge: Tissue-retentive lung memory CD4 T cells mediate optimal protection to respiratory virus infection. *Journal of Immunology, 187*, 5510–5514. doi: 10.4049/jimmunol.1102243

Tracey, K. J. (2002). The inflammatory reflex. *Nature, 420*, 853–859. doi: 10.1038/nature01321.

Tracey, K. J. (2007). Physiology and immunology of the cholinergic antiinflammatory pathway. *Journal of Clinical Investigation, 117*, 289–296. doi: 10.1172/JCI30555.

Tsuji, R. F., Szczepanik, M., Kawikova, I., Paliwal, V., Campos, R. A., Itakura, A., Akahira-Azuma, M., Baumgarth, N., Herzenberg, L. A., & Askenase, P. W. (2002). B cell-dependent T cell responses: IgM antibodies are required to elicit contact sensitivity. *Journal of Experimental Medicine, 196*, 1277–1290. doi: 10.1084/jem.20020649.

Usherwood, E. J., Hogan, R. J., Crowther, G., Surman, S. L., Hogg, T. L., Altman, J. D., & Woodland, D. L. (1999). Functionally heterogeneous CD8+ T-cell memory is induced by Sendai virus infection of mice. *Journal of Virology, 73*, 7278–7286. doi: 10.1128/JVI.73.9.7278-7286.1999.

van Helden, M. J., de Graaf, N., Boog, C. J., Topham, D. J., Zaiss, D. M., & Sijts, A. J. (2012). The bone marrow functions as the central site of proliferation for long-lived NK cells. *Journal of Immunology, 189*, 2333–2337. doi: 10.4049/jimmunol.1200008.

Veiga-Fernandes, H., & Freitas, A. A. (2017). The s(c)ensory immune system theory. *Trends in Immunology, 38*, 777–788. doi: 10.1016/j.it.2017.02.007.

Veiga-Fernandes, H., & Pachnis, V. (2017). Neuroimmune regulation during intestinal development and homeostasis. *Nature Immunology, 18*, 116–122. doi: 10.1038/ni.3634.

Vivier, E., Raulet, D. H., Moretta, A., Caligiuri, M. A., Zitvogel, L., Lanier, L. L., Yokoyama, W. M., & Ugolini, S. (2011). Innate or adaptive immunity? The example of natural killer cells. *Science, 331*, 44–49. doi: 10.1126/science.1198687.

Wang, N. S., McHeyzer-Williams, L. J., Okitsu, S. L., Burris, T. P., Reiner, S. L., & McHeyzer-Williams, M. G. (2012). Divergent transcriptional programming of class-specific B cell memory by T-bet and RORα. *Nature Immunology, 13*, 604–611. doi: 10.1038/ni.2294.

Wang, X., Peng, H., Cong, J., Wang, X., Lian, Z., Wei, H., Sun, R., & Tian, Z. (2018). Memory formation and long-term maintenance of IL-7Rα+ ILC1s via a lymph node-liver axis. *Nature Communications, 9*, 4854. doi: 10.1038/s41467-018-07405-5.

Wilson, E. O. (1975). *Sociobiology: The New Synthesis.* Harvard University Press.

Wright, L. (1973). Functions. *Philosophical Review, 82*, 139–168. doi: 10.2307/2183766.

Yang, H., Wang, L., Huang, C. S., & Ju, G. (1998). Plasticity of GAP-43 innervation of the spleen during immune response in the mouse. Evidence for axonal sprouting and redistribution of the nerve fibers. *Neuroimmunomodulation, 5*, 53–60. doi: 10.1159/000026326.

Yersin, A. (1894). La peste bubonique à Hong-Kong (The bubonic plague in Hong Kong). *Annales de l'Institut Pasteur, 8*, 662–667.

Yoles, E., Hauben, E., Palgi, O., Agranov, E., Gothilf, A., Cohen, A., Kuchroo, V., Cohen, I. R., Weiner, H., & Schwartz, M. (2001). Protective autoimmunity is a physiological response to CNS trauma. *Journal of Neuroscience, 21*, 3740–3748. doi: 10.1523/jneurosci.21-11-03740.2001.

Zagon, A. (2001). Does the vagus nerve mediate the sixth sense? *Trends in Neurosciences, 24*, 671–673. doi: 10.1016/s0166-2236(00)01929-9.

Zinkernagel, R. M. (2000). On immunological memory. *Philosophical Transactions of the Royal Society of London. Series B: Biological Sciences, 355*, 369–371. doi: 10.1098/rstb.2000.0576.

Zinkernagel, R. M. (2002). On differences between immunity and immunological memory. *Current Opinion in Immunology, 14*, 523–536. doi: 10.1016/s0952-7915(02)00367-9.

Zinkernagel, R. M. (2012). Immunological memory ≠ protective immunity. *Cellular and Molecular Life Sciences, 69*, 1635–1640. doi: 10.1007/s00018-012-0972-y.

Zinkernagel, R. M. (2018). What if protective immunity is antigen-driven and not due to so-called "memory" B and T cells? *Immunological Reviews, 283*, 238–246. doi: 10.1111/imr.12648.

Ziv, Y., Ron, N., Butovsky, O., Landa, G., Sudai, E., Greenberg, N., Cohen, H., Kipnis, J., & Schwartz, M. (2006). Immune cells contribute to the maintenance of neurogenesis and spatial learning abilities in adulthood. *Nature Neuroscience, 9*, 268–275. doi: 10.1038/nn1629.

4 The Immune System Omnipresent in the Biological World

'Life' is the success phase of an immune system.[1]

Peter Sloterdijk

The existence of the immune system in the classical sense has long been examined from an anthropocentric perspective. Specifically, the key molecules that comprise the immune system in humans and mice (e.g., antibodies, antigen receptors on T and B cells, and major histocompatibility complex (MHC)) or the characteristic mechanisms found therein (e.g., the genetic mechanisms by which antigen receptors are generated and the enzymes involved) were used as indicators in the search for species possessing an immune system. Similarly, neuron-like morphology or the electrophysiological phenomena exhibited by neurons has been considered an indicator in the search for the nervous system, another complex system, in other species. This could be considered an approach that looks down from the top of the phylogenetic tree, in which humans are considered the most evolved species. This approach remains prevalent, and it is not uncommon to find people who do not consider any system other than the human-like system to be an immune system. In Chapter 4, I abandon this view and instead adopt a more open-minded approach, first examining the defense systems of organisms living in nature and then discussing the systems revealed in this study.

As previously mentioned, there are two types of immunity in humans and mice: innate and acquired. Acquired immunity is controlled by B and T cells, which can recognize a nearly infinite number of antigens and also possess immunological memory. These cells have specificity and can react with greater speed and strength when they encounter the same antigen again. In contrast, innate immunity is primarily regulated by antigen-presenting cell (APCs), which are believed to lack specificity and immunological memory. From an evolutionary perspective, acquired immunity emerged approximately 500 million years ago among the jawed vertebrates (Gnathostomata). However, 95% of the organisms on Earth do not have acquired immunity in the classical sense; yet, they live without significant problems. Does this indicate that acquired immunity is not necessary for the survival of most organisms, or is it possible that systems and functions corresponding to acquired immunity exist in these organisms but have not been identified?

Since the discovery of Toll's role in *Drosophila* infection defense (Lemaitre et al., 1996), the role of innate immunity has been extensively studied and has become increasingly important (Section 1.6, Chapter 1). These studies have revealed the following: First, innate immunity and acquired immunity must function harmoniously to effectively respond to pathogens. Second, TLRs are found in vertebrates, invertebrates (including everything down to sponges), and even plants. Third, innate immunity has immunological memory as well. Fourth, bacteria and archaea have systems that correspond not only to innate immunity but also to acquired immunity with their own memory function.

As discussed in Chapter 3, it has also become clear that, even within the system of a single species, cells that were thought to belong to the innate immune system possess specificity and memory. These recent findings force us to reconsider the fundamental nature of the immune system and the ontological meaning of immunity. In Chapter 4, I have decided to extract the minimal conditions that constitute immunity by tracing the evolutionary phylogenetic tree from bacteria and examining each immune system. The reason for this is that I believe the minimal requirements for immunity can only be clarified through such comparative studies. Furthermore, the framework that supports immunity may be easier to grasp in organisms in the early stages of evolution than in highly differentiated organisms whose components are intricately intertwined.

4.1 BACTERIAL IMMUNE SYSTEM

In eukaryotes, genetic information is transmitted vertically from parents to offspring. The genetic recombination that occurs during sexual reproduction introduces genetic mutations, which subsequently become the target of natural selection during evolution. However, this engenders the question of how genetic diversity emerges in bacteria and archaea that reproduce asexually. The earliest organisms on Earth used mutation and horizontal gene transfer as the primary mechanisms of genetic variation, and the resulting changes underwent natural selection. In horizontal gene transfer, genes from one independent organism are passed on to other organisms, resulting in the creation of organisms with new characteristics. A famous example is methicillin-resistant *Staphylococcus aureus*, which emerged due to the acquisition of a gene encoding a peptidoglycan synthase enzyme that prevents the binding of previously effective β-lactam antibiotics, such as penicillin, methicillin, and cephalosporins, making effective treatment difficult. This is a major problem due to nosocomial infections and other complications. Horizontal gene transfer is also involved in the process of creating new pathogens by spreading genes encoding the virulence factors of the pathogen to other bacteria. Although this is advantageous to bacteria, only a small fraction of the transmitted genes function immediately to their advantage. Thus, bacteria are constantly exposed to the invasion of foreign genes from the external environment and must have strategies in place to avoid horizontal gene transfer.

This engenders the question of how bacteria avoid this danger and maintain their integrity. First, I discuss the three types of horizontal gene transfer that exist in bacteria: conjugation, in which DNA is directly transmitted through physical contact between two cells; transformation, in which DNA is introduced from outside the cell; and transduction, in which DNA is transported to another cell by a virus or a bacteriophage (phage). Following this, I analyze the structure and function of the two systems considered to be the bacterial immune system—namely, the restriction modification system and clustered regularly interspaced short palindromic repeats (CRISPR)–CRISPR-associated protein (Cas) system—and consider their implications.

4.1.1 Horizontal Gene Transfer in Bacteria

Bacteria and archaea have the ability to incorporate heterogeneous genetic information from the external world and acquire new traits, such as antibiotic resistance, toxin production, and virulence factors. Three mechanisms are involved in this process: conjugation, transformation, and transduction. Conjugation is the transfer of DNA via direct contact between two cells, a donor and a recipient. This phenomenon was discovered in 1946 by Joshua Lederberg and Edward Tatum (1909–1975; Nobel Prize in Physiology or Medicine 1958). They used two mutant *E. coli* strains: One was *E. coli* that grows only when biotin, phenylalanine, and cystine are added to a minimal medium containing only the minimum nutrients necessary for cell growth (strain Y-24), and the other was *E. coli* that grows only when threonine, leucine, and thiamine are added (strain Y-10). Both strains have a mutation that prevents them from synthesizing the components necessary for cell growth; therefore, they cannot grow in a minimal medium. However, when the two strains were mixed for several hours and subsequently transferred to a minimal medium, colonies appeared. Lederberg and Tatum reported that these colonies exhibited behaviors that were consistent with being derived from a single cell that had exchanged genetic information between the two strains and was able to synthesize the nutrients necessary for growth. They viewed this process as the equivalent of sexual reproduction (Lederberg and Tatum, 1946). However, these experiments did not clarify whether direct cell-to-cell contact was necessary. In 1950, Bernard Davis (1916–1996), using a U-shaped tube containing a filter through which liquid could pass but bacteria could not, showed physical contact between donor and recipient cells to be essential for the gene transfer shown by Lederberg and Tatum (Davis, 1950). In 1952, it was also found that horizontal gene transfer in *E. coli* is not bidirectional, with one cell functioning as a donor and the other as a recipient (Hayes, 1952).

In transformation, a plasmid or naked DNA fragment released into the environment from the donor bacterium is taken up directly through the cell membrane of the recipient bacterium and incorporated into the host genome through homologous recombination. This phenomenon was discovered by the British bacteriologist Frederick Griffith (1877–1941) in 1928 through experiments using two types of *Streptococcus pneumoniae*—the S (smooth) and R (rough) types (Griffith, 1928). The S-type bacteria are capsular, form smooth colonies, and are pathogenic; in contrast, the R-type bacteria lack capsules, form rough surface colonies, and are not pathogenic. The study showed that, when either R-type or heat-killed S-type bacteria alone were administered to mice, they were not pathogenic, but when the two bacteria were mixed and injected, the mice died of pneumonia and bacteremia. In essence, the nonpathogenic *S. pneumoniae* strain became pathogenic when exposed to the heat-killed pathogenic strain. Based on these results, Griffith hypothesized that some factor derived from the strain that lost virulence was responsible for the transformation of the nonpathogenic strain into the pathogenic strain. This transforming factor was thought to be DNA, not protein, according to the experiments conducted by Oswald Avery (1877–1955), Colin MacLeod (1909–1972), and Maclyn McCarty (1911–2005) in 1944 (Avery et al., 1944). However, this was not widely accepted. The experiments of Alfred Hershey (1908–1997; Nobel Prize in Physiology or Medicine 1969) and Martha Chase (1927–2003) in 1952, which used a phage composed of protein capsule and DNA, confirmed that the genetic material was DNA and not protein (Hershey and Chase, 1952).

In transduction, genes from one bacterium are transferred to other bacteria by phage viruses that specifically infect bacteria. For example, when a phage with bacteriolytic activity infects a bacterium, it hijacks the host's replication, transcription, and translation machinery and replicates the phage's genes. In this process, virions (infectious viral particles) containing the bacterial DNA are released with the lysis of the bacterium to infect another bacterium. The process of transduction was first demonstrated by Norton Zinder (1928–2002) and Joshua Lederberg in 1952 using *Salmonella* bacteria (Zinder and Lerderberg, 1952).

4.1.2 Defense Mechanisms in Bacteria

Bacteria, due to being exposed to the danger of invasion by phage-derived heterologous DNA, have had to devise complex and diverse defense mechanisms. To maintain their integrity and stability, they must distinguish between their own DNA and the invading heterologous DNA. One strategy for this is the restriction modification system, which uses restriction enzymes to only cleave the foreign DNA. The other strategy is the CRISPR–Cas system. Some scientists consider the restriction modification system to be the innate immunity and CRISPR–Cas to be the acquired immunity of bacteria; however, those familiar with the mammalian immune system were skeptical that an organism in the early stages of evolution, without T cells, B cells, or antibodies, could have an immune system. The structural and mechanistic differences between the two were too great. Below, I examine the restriction modification system and the CRISPR–Cas system in more detail to clarify their functioning.

4.1.2.1 Restriction Modification System

The restriction modification system involves a strategy through which bacteria and archaea restrict the entry of foreign DNA from the external world. It consists of two enzymes: restriction enzymes and DNA methyltransferases. Restriction enzymes specifically recognize and cleave DNA sequences of four to ten bases, thereby destroying the invading DNA. However, the sequences recognized by the restriction enzymes are short, and the corresponding sequences are also found in self-DNA.

Methyltransferase prevents the cleavage of self-DNA by modifying (methylating) the recognition site of the restriction enzyme, thus preventing the cleavage of self-DNA by the restriction enzyme. In essence, the restriction modification system provides bacteria and archaea with a mechanism to discriminate between self-DNA and invading nonself-DNA.

It has been shown that at least one restriction modification system is found in 90% of the bacterial genomes examined; furthermore, several possess multiple systems. One reason this system is called the bacterial immune system is that it can discriminate between self and nonself. Moreover, this is classified as innate immunity because it has no clear specificity for invading DNA and cannot remember its encounters with DNA. This may be because of the classical view that discrimination between self and nonself is the primary criterion for being an immune system and that the memory of encounters with nonself is a requirement for acquired immunity. Nevertheless, the restriction modification system contributes to the process of defending bacteria against phages. However, phages have evolved to counteract bacteria through strategies such as the methylation of their own DNA and the production of proteins that resist restriction enzymes. As discussed below, this is an aspect of what has been called the evolutionary arms race in the biological world. From the bacteria's perspective, completely eliminating horizontal gene transfer would deprive them of the opportunity to expand their genetic diversity, and they would not have access to new genes from the environment that their progeny would need to survive in a constantly changing and thus challenging world. Furthermore, evolution based on natural selection is less likely to occur. Conversely, the unrestricted incorporation of DNA from the external world into the bacterium engenders a significant risk of lethal infection by phages. If bacteria cannot eliminate all invading genes, the invasion of DNA from the environment must be balanced, and they need a mechanism to facilitate this.

Among highly evolved organisms such as mice and humans, discrimination between self and nonself is achieved by altering the composition of the repertoire of antigen-recognizing cells. In the case of B cells, self-reactive cells are physically eliminated or functionally suppressed in the bone marrow. In T cells, cells with antigen receptors that recognize self but not too strongly are selected in the thymus to exit to the periphery. Essentially, the side that recognizes the antigen is altered. In contrast, in the bacterial restriction modification system, the self-component is altered to escape attack by restriction enzymes. Interestingly, in addition to immune functions, the restriction modification system is involved in other functions including the regulation of gene expression via epigenetic changes (Vasu and Nagaraja, 2013).

4.1.2.2 CRISPR–Cas System

Recently, a genetic mechanism called the CRISPR–Cas system was shown to function as a defense mechanism against phages and plasmid invasion in bacteria and archaea (Bolotin et al., 2005; Brouns et al., 2008; Marraffini and Sontheimer, 2008; Sorek et al., 2008; Karginov and Hannon, 2010; Marraffini and Sontheimer, 2010a). This system is expressed in approximately 45% of bacteria and 85% of archaea (Grissa et al., 2007). In 1987, while analyzing the intestinal alkaline phosphatase gene of *E. coli*, Yoshizumi Ishino (1957–) and colleagues discovered a region in which highly homologous and closely repeated sequences alternate with sequences unrelated to them (Ishino et al., 1987). Similar reports followed this discovery. In 2002, these sequences were named CRISPR (Jansen et al., 2002); however, their function has not been clarified.

The CRISPR locus is composed of alternating repeats and spacer sequences, each consisting of several dozen bases. The repeats are the same length and sequence, but the spacer sequences vary from bacterium to bacterium, with the number of spacer sequences sometimes exceeding 500. In many cases, the spacer sequences match those of phages and plasmids (Bolotin et al., 2005; Mojica et al., 2005; Pourcel et al., 2005). Located in close proximity to the CRISPR locus is the *cas* locus, which encodes Cas and other proteins with endonuclease activity. The CRISPR–Cas system is divided into 2 classes, 6 types, and 33 subtypes (Makarova et al., 2020). Recent studies in comparative sequence analysis suggest that all CRISPR–Cas systems employ the same structural and functional principles and share a common ancestry (Makarova et al., 2013).

Notably, it was found that bacteria with a spacer sequence in common with a particular phage are resistant to that phage; otherwise, the phage is infectious. Therefore, bacteria have an immunological memory at the genetic level that guarantees the elimination of foreign DNA. These facts suggest that the CRISPR–Cas system is responsible for acquired immunity in bacteria and archaea. Furthermore, the CRISPR–Cas system may be an example of Lamarckian inheritance, as environmental factors (viral DNA) are incorporated into the host genome and transmitted to daughter cells (Koonin and Wolf, 2009). For more information on the ideas proposed by Lamarck, please refer to Section 2.5, Chapter 2.

The action of CRISPR–Cas can be divided into three functional stages: adaptation, expression, and interference. The adaptation stage is the acquisition of spacers, in which the Cas protein cleaves the invading phage or plasmid DNA into fragments of approximately 30 bases, called protospacers, which are incorporated into the CRISPR sequence as new spacers. This process constitutes the formation of an immune memory. In this stage, a few nucleotides neighboring the protospacer, called the protospacer-adjacent motif (PAM), are required. In the expression stage, the CRISPR gene region consisting of the spacers and repeats is transcribed to generate a long pre-CRISPR RNA (pre-crRNA), which is further cleaved by the Cas protein to form a short crRNA. This is a fragment of memory that has been encountered in the past and incorporated into the bacterium. In the interference stage, this crRNA forms a complex with trans-activating crRNA (tracrRNA), which guides the nuclease-active Cas protein to the sequence corresponding to the invading DNA (protospacer). There, the Cas protein specifically cleaves the strand complementary to the crRNA and its opposite strand, inhibiting the growth of the foreign gene. Thus, CRISPR–Cas, unlike restriction modification systems, achieves memory-based specific immunity to foreign phages and plasmids. Therefore, it is considered bacterial acquired immunity.

It is noteworthy that there are several functional similarities between bacterial and mammalian immunity. First, the adaptation stage corresponds to antigen recognition and memory of the event. Interestingly, if the same phage is not encountered thereafter, the incorporated spacer degenerates. This indicates that bacterial memory lasts only for a brief period, suggesting that the maintenance of memory requires successive encounters with foreign DNA (Makarova et al., 2006; Andersson and Banfield, 2008). There has been controversy regarding the requirements for T cells to maintain memory. In the past, memory T cells were assumed to have a lower antigen requirement than naïve T cells because they proliferate at lower concentrations of antigen. However, it was recently reported that memory T cells have a higher antigen requirement than naïve T cells (Mehlhop-Williams and Bevan, 2014). This finding, if accepted, suggests the existence of similarities in the mechanisms of immune memory in bacteria and highly evolved species. Second, the expression and interference stages are similar to the mammalian immune response to the same antigen after immunization or vaccination. Furthermore, it is clear that even phages that cannot replicate can induce spacer acquisition, and commonalities with human vaccination involving inactivated pathogens can be observed (Hynes et al., 2014). Third, bacteria have two systems to inactivate phages, namely the restriction modification system and the CRISPR–Cas system, and the cooperative action of these systems can enhance defense (Dupuis et al., 2013). If it is assumed that the restriction modification system is the bacterial innate immune system and CRISPR–Cas is the acquired immune system, there is a resemblance to the interaction between innate immunity and acquired immunity in mammals. While the immune systems present in bacteria and humans, which are at the extremes of evolution, are not similar from a structural standpoint, their functional elements are remarkably similar.

As mentioned above, the CRISPR–Cas system adapts to and eliminates causative pathogens by physically incorporating elements from the environment (phage and plasmid DNA) into the host genome and transmitting the incorporated DNA to the next generation. This mode of inheritance appears to correspond to the inheritance of acquired traits, which Lamarck described as "everything that has been acquired, traced or changed in the organization of individuals during the course of their lives is preserved by generation, and transmitted to the new individuals" (Lamarck, 1815). Moreover, this system recognizes invading DNA in a sequence-specific manner and has a diverse repertoire of recognition. Its specificity and diversity in preparing to adapt to environmental factors are shared with the human immune system and are reminiscent of Darwin's mechanism of natural selection.

In 2010, Jennifer Doudna (1964–; Nobel Prize in Chemistry 2020), Emmanuelle Charpentier (1968–; Nobel Prize in Chemistry 2020), and colleagues showed that CRISPR and an endonuclease called Cas9 can be used to cut DNA in a sequence-specific manner (Jinek et al., 2012). DNA strands that are complementary and noncomplementary to the introduced crRNA are cleaved by separate regions of Cas9. This demonstrated that this technology could be easily applied to genome editing. In a sense, they took advantage of the technology possessed by the bacterial immune system. Since then, this technology has been applied to a wide range of fields, to the point that there is virtually no laboratory that does not use it; thus, it has transformed the life sciences.

However, because this technology can easily alter the human genome, ethical issues may arise. For instance, in 2018, this technique was applied to confer resistance to the human immunode-ficiency virus on twin babies. However, immediately afterward, it was severely criticized by the scientific community as premature and potentially dangerous. Another problem is the use of CRISPR–Cas9 and other technologies to induce a phenomenon known as gene drive. In sexually reproducing species, there are pairs of alleles that offspring inherit from parents with a probability of 50%. Gene drive is the process of stimulating the biased inheritance of specific genes. To arti-ficially induce this, the expected gene is modified to be transmitted to offspring with a probability of nearly 100% by introducing the expected gene into the DNA double-strand, thereby increasing the frequency of the expected trait over time in the population. For example, this is used to combat pathogen-transmitting insects (e.g., mosquitoes that transmit malaria, Zika fever, and dengue fever) or exotic species. In this case, the possibility of unwanted traits spreading due to mutations or gene drives spreading beyond the targeted species is assumed. Therefore, ethical issues such as the impact on humans and ecosystems have been discussed (Gurwitz, 2014; Oye et al., 2014; Champer et al., 2016).

4.1.3 Autoimmunity in Bacteria

If CRISPR–Cas is a true immune system, there must be a mechanism to discriminate between self and nonself. As in the case of organisms in the later stages of evolution (Section 2.1, Chapter 2), without such a mechanism, there is a risk of misidentifying self as nonself and attacking it. This engenders the question of how self and nonself are distinguished during the adaptation (acquisition of DNA) and interference (destruction of DNA) stages that occur when DNA invades from the out-side. When self-DNA is targeted, chromosome breaks result in defects. This phenomenon is called bacterial autoimmunity.

Research has yielded some interesting results regarding this. An analysis of the CRISPR loci of 330 bacterial species revealed that one in 250 spacers (0.4% of all spacers) is a "self-targeting spacer," and of the 330 bacterial species with CRISPR, 59 (18%) have at least one self-targeting spacer (Stern et al., 2010). Although the numbers differ, subsequent studies have also confirmed the presence of self-targeting spacers. If these results are assumed to be accurate, the CRISPR–Cas system has autoimmunity (or self-recognition) embedded in it. Thus, the following questions must be considered: Why does autoimmunity exist in bacteria, and what exactly does it do? Are self-targeting spacers involved in autoimmunity? If they are, how is the process leading to host death circumvented (a question asked of human autoimmunity as well)? Or does the presence of self-targeting spacers serve a different function?

In this regard, the hypothesis that CRISPR–Cas functions as a DNA repair system in thermo-philes was proposed; however, it was never proven (Makarova et al., 2002). Instead, a new hypoth-esis was proposed that the immunity encoded by the CRISPR gene is mediated by a mechanism similar to RNA interference (RNAi) or RNA silencing in eukaryotic cells (Makarova et al., 2006). In RNAi, RNA is involved in the sequence-specific regulation of gene expression triggered by double-stranded RNA, through translational or transcriptional repression. Andrew Fire (1959–; Nobel Prize in Physiology or Medicine 2006) and Craig Mello (1960–; Nobel Prize in Physiology or Medicine 2006) discovered it in the nematodes *Caenorhabditis elegans* (Fire et al., 1998). If the self-targeting spacer of the CRISPR system is involved in gene repression that is useful to bacteria, it can be assumed that it would be selected for and conserved during evolution; however, this has not been the case (Stern et al., 2010). Conversely, it has often been observed that the presence of self-targeting spacers can degenerate the CRISPR system and reduce its activity. Taking this information into account, it is reasonable to speculate that self-targeting spacers are accidentally incorporated into the CRISPR–Cas locus and become deleterious to the bacteria, as opposed to being present to participate in specific gene regulation. This may also explain why this system is present in only approximately half of bacteria. It is also interesting whether the incorporation of self-DNA is completely coincidental or the result of recognizing sequences identical to self-DNA present in viruses and plasmids as foreign.

According to one study, mismatches between the target DNA and the crRNA at a specific position outside the spacer guarantee DNA interference, and prolonged pair formation between the crRNA and the CRISPR locus (self-DNA) inhibits autoimmunity (Marraffini and Sontheimer, 2010b). In essence, the complementarity of the sequence outside the spacer determines the discrimination between self and nonself; furthermore, the absence of pair formation in that part results in interference or autoimmunity, while prolonged pair formation suppresses the destruction of self-DNA. Another study revealed that 37% of the self-targeting spacers are located on the leader sequence end of the CRISPR locus, suggesting that they were incorporated early (Stern et al., 2010). If that is the case, it can be assumed that the memory acquisition function of CRISPR is maintained even after the self-targeting spacer is incorporated and that a mechanism to avoid the deleterious effects of autoimmunity exists. For example, mutations or deletions in genes such as *cas* comprising the CRISPR system could prevent the host from suffering destructive effects. The significance of autoimmunity in bacteria requires further study.

4.1.4 NONIMMUNOLOGICAL FUNCTIONS OF THE CRISPR–CAS SYSTEM

Recent studies have shown that not all CRISPR–Cas systems are involved in acquired immunity and that some have completely lost their immune function; furthermore, some systems are responsible for functions beyond immunity. The most prominent nonimmune function is the regulation of transcription (Westra et al., 2014; Barrangou, 2015). Genes regulated by CRISPR–Cas include those that control pathogenicity and bacterial population behavior (Bille et al., 2005; Gunderson and Cianciotto, 2013; Sampson et al., 2013).

First, I consider this problem in terms of the control of virulence. In the Gram-negative bacterium *Francisella novicida*, Cas9 of the CRISPR–Cas system has been shown to repress the expression of a bacterial lipoprotein associated with pathogenicity. This lipoprotein is a MAMP and is recognized by the human PRR (TLR2), inducing an inflammatory immune response. Therefore, the suppression of bacterial lipoprotein expression attenuates the human immune response, thereby enhancing virulence. The mechanism of lipoprotein suppression is understood as follows: The complex formed by the factors comprising CRISPR–Cas binds to the transcripts of bacterial lipoprotein genes, causing them to lose stability (Sampson et al., 2013). Thus, CRISPR–Cas is essential for *F. novicida* to be pathogenic. Similar roles have been identified in other bacteria. For *Legionella pneumophila*, the causative agent of Legionnaires' disease, to grow within amoebae, Cas2 is required (Gunderson and Cianciotto, 2013). These results indicate that CRISPR–Cas is not only involved in bacterial defense against foreign DNA but also required for bacterial intracellular infection of the host cells.

Furthermore, the *cas* gene has been shown to be involved in the social behavior and developmental processes of *Myxococcus xanthus* (Thöny-Meyer and Kaiser, 1993; Boysen et al., 2002). *Myxococci*—Gram-negative, spore-forming, and obligate aerobes—are abundant in cultivated soils and glide across the surface of soil particles, feeding on other bacterial colonies. Each *Myxococcus* surrounding a colony secretes an extracellular enzyme to digest its prey and share its products with the other bacteria. However, as nutrients in the soil become depleted, tens of thousands of bacteria stop multiplying and form aggregates to ensure their survival and spread. Aggregates of cells adopt a hill-like shape and subsequently form fruiting bodies, which contain spherical spores that are resistant to environmental conditions such as desiccation and high temperatures. Although the formation of aggregates was once thought to be due to chemotaxis, which acts in response to a concentration gradient of chemicals around the cell, direct cell-to-cell interactions appear to be essential to this process. Mutation experiments on genes involved in the program that causes these changes in *Myxococci* have revealed that the *cas* gene is involved in the developmental processes, including the formation of aggregates, fruiting bodies, and spores (Thöny-Meyer and Kaiser, 1993; Boysen et al., 2002).

It is believed that the developmental processes in *M. xanthus* and the virulence of *F. novicida* were selected for during evolution. The involvement of bacterial CRISPR–Cas—the prototype of the immune system—in a wide range of functions, such as the modulation of bacterial behavior induced by signals from the external world, and its ability to adapt to the original environmental cues are suggestive of the fundamental nature of the immune system. This mechanism is reminiscent of not only the mammalian immune response but also the function of the central nervous system in humans. This point will be elaborated in Sections 4.4–4.6, Chapter 4, and Chapter 5 from a broader perspective.

4.1.5 VIEWS FROM AN EVOLUTIONARY PERSPECTIVE

As already explained, the bacterial immune system faces a dilemma; To maintain genome stability and integrity, it is essential to contain invading mobile genetic elements using CRISPR–Cas. However, too much restriction of foreign gene entry also prevents the uptake of foreign genes that would be useful for bacteria, such as antibiotic resistance and virulence factors, resulting in the loss of strategies for adapting to the environment. The exact frequency at which new spacers are incorporated is unknown, but it is assumed to be higher than the mutation rate of the genome. Therefore, the function of CRISPR–Cas in bringing genetic variation to bacteria is critical for better facilitating their adaptation to the external world. In essence, for bacteria and archaea to survive, a balance must be maintained between defending against invading DNA and ensuring genome variability.

Similar to other predator–prey relationships, the following is an interesting aspect of the evolutionary arms race between bacteria and phages; The ever-present risk of predation by phages forces bacteria to counter with new immune mechanisms; this, in turn, leads to the evolution of phage strategies for evading bacterial immunity. To counteract bacterial restriction modification systems, phages have acquired several mechanisms (Samson et al., 2013). For example, some phages may have few restriction sites, or the phage genome may be modified by a host methyltransferase and escape cleavage when infected by bacteria. Alternatively, the phage genome may encode a methyltransferase. Furthermore, phages utilize various strategies to counter bacterial defense strategies, including the production of over 20 CRISPR–Cas-opposing proteins (Samson et al., 2013). A recent report has stated that, to counteract bacterial genomic islands (genetic regions acquired through horizontal gene transfer) that act in a repressive manner against phages, phages prepare their own CRISPR–Cas to attack bacterial genes that repress phages (Seed et al., 2013). This warrants further investigation of the battle being waged for survival among the smallest beings in the biological world.

4.2 PLANT IMMUNE SYSTEM

The immune systems of organisms belonging to Gnathostomata, such as humans and mice, are equipped with T cells, B cells, and antibodies that circulate throughout the body to prepare for invasion by any pathogens. Plants do not have such cells, molecules, or mechanisms, but they still survive harsh environments. Notably, plants can also specifically recognize pathogens, eliminate them based on the information acquired, and remember the experience. Moreover, plant immune memory sometimes transcends generations. Such functions overlap with the four functional steps of the immune response observed in CRISPR–Cas. This is only a functional component, as opposed to a structural condition. Both bacteria and plants perform the function of immunity in their own way. This engenders the question of how they recognize and memorize a vast number of pathogens. Below, I examine the specific mechanisms related to this.

4.2.1 STRUCTURE OF INNATE IMMUNITY IN PLANTS

Microorganisms, such as viruses, bacteria, fungi, and oomycetes, must penetrate the plant to be pathogenic. Specifically, these microorganisms must penetrate the leaf and root surfaces; alternatively, they can enter through wounds or physiologically present pores and drainage tissues. The cell wall, the first line of defense against pathogens, functions as a physical barrier and dynamically regulates host defenses as well. For example, they prevent pathogens from entering by producing and accumulating polysaccharides called callose at the site of pathogen invasion. Although these are not antigen-specific responses, two receptors are responsible for defense against pathogens. One is a transmembrane PRR on the cell surface, which corresponds to the animal TLR (Janeway and Medzhitov, 2002; Jones and Dangl, 2006). It recognizes MAMPs that have been conserved over the course of evolution. MAPMs include lipopolysaccharide (LPS; a major component of the outer membrane of Gram-negative bacteria), two peptides derived from flagellar proteins (flg22), peptidoglycan (a polymeric compound composed of peptides and sugars that constitute the bacterial cell wall), and chitin (a mucopolysaccharide that is a major component of fungal cell walls and other components) (Newman et al., 2013).

MAMPs are typically not present in the host and are recognized by the host as foreign. Plants may use lytic enzymes to release MAMPs from bacteria. Some PRRs have intracellular phosphotransferase serine/threonine kinase activity; this, after binding to MAMPs, transmits the information to the cell and inhibits pathogen growth (Zipfel, 2014). This process is called pattern-triggered immunity (PTI). While most plants are able to defend against infection at this stage, adapted pathogens deliver diverse effector proteins (virulence factors) into the host in various ways, suppressing PTI and activating genes that promote microbial growth and facilitating infection (Dangl and Jones, 2001; Jones and Dangl, 2006).

The second step is effector-triggered immunity (ETI), which intracellularly responds to a variety of effectors, conferring resistance to bacteria, viruses, fungi, oomycetes, nematodes, insects, and other organisms. The intracellular receptor for this is the nucleic acid-binding–leucine-rich repeat (NB–LRR)-type receptor (NLR), which is also present in animals. This receptor has been shown to be the product of a resistance gene (R protein), which has been studied as a molecule that confers resistance to pathogens (Bent, 1996; Ellis et al., 2000; Dangl and Jones, 2001); this is addressed in the next section. The changes induced by ETIs are known as hypersensitivity reactions, which is programmed cell death (apoptosis) of infected cells. This appears to prevent the spread of the pathogen to other parts of the plant. This local response induces a plant-wide immune response known as systemic acquired resistance.

The sequencing of PTI and ETI from the perspective of host–microbe coevolution has been proposed (Chisholm et al., 2006). According to this report, there is an evolutionary trend in which, after PTI is effective, the pathogen injects more effective effector proteins into the plant cells; this, in turn, causes the plant to produce more effective R proteins. This is an evolutionary arms race scenario that can be seen throughout the biological world. The following sections focus on specific recognition in plants, local and systemic responses, immune memory, autoimmunity, and antiviral immunity.

4.2.2 MECHANISMS OF SPECIFIC RECOGNITION

The first report that disease resistance in plants is inherited according to Mendelian laws was made in 1907 (Biffen, 1907). In the mid-20th century, Harold Henry Flor (1900–1991) studied the genetics of resistance to the pathogen (*Melampsora lini*) that causes flax rust and proposed the "gene-for-gene hypothesis" (Flor, 1956, 1971). According to this hypothesis, resistance to disease is regulated by the compatibility of the resistance (*R*) gene present in the plant with the avirulence (*avr*) gene derived from the pathogen. More specifically, R proteins, which function as receptors, bind to the Avr protein of the pathogen that serves as the ligand, thereby rendering the plant resistant to the pathogen. Furthermore, the plant genome was estimated to contain *R* genes corresponding to many pathogens. Subsequent studies revealed that the majority of what were believed to be R proteins were NLRs, as described in the previous section. Furthermore, it found that the direct binding of R proteins to Avr proteins was not always observed; in addition, the number of *R* genes was also insufficient for dealing with many pathogens: approximately 150, 235, 400, and 1,500 for *Arabidopsis*, *Populus*, rice, and wheat, respectively (Hammond-Kosack and Kanyuka, 2007). Therefore, the gene-for-gene hypothesis, in which the direct binding of pathogen proteins to their receptors is responsible for dealing with diverse pathogens, is either false or inadequate for explaining all phenomena.

Thus, the question of how plants deal with numerous pathogens with a limited number of NLR proteins remains. Several mechanisms have been identified (Kourelis and van der Hoorn, 2018). One of them is the guard hypothesis, which assumes that NLR proteins do not bind directly to pathogen proteins but recognize host proteins that have been modified by pathogen effectors (Chisholm et al., 2006; Jones and Dangl, 2006). Specifically, effectors as virulence factors have targets on the host and contribute to virulence by modifying their host targets. The target is assumed to become the modified self by the pathogen and activates a defense response via the corresponding NLR protein. For example, in *Arabidopsis*, a target protein called resistance to *Pseudomonas syringae* pv. maculicola 1 (RPM1)-interacting protein 4 (RIN4), which does not bind to NLR proteins in the absence of infection, is recognized by NLR proteins only after it becomes the modified self through threonine phosphorylation upon infection with *P. syringae*. In essence, NLR proteins do not directly recognize the nonself (pathogen); rather, they indirectly sense the traces of physicochemical effects left on the self-protein by the effectors of the pathogen. Moreover, multiple mutually distinct effectors may affect the same target. This may prompt the evolution of new NLR proteins to recognize the differentially modified self on a single target. Such a strategy would allow NLR proteins to transcend a one-to-one correspondence to deal with pathogens.

The aforementioned mechanism is reminiscent of the danger theory proposed by Polly Matzinger in the 1990s to explain the human immune response (Section 1.6.6, Chapter 1). According to this theory, the PRRs on APCs do not directly recognize pathogens or nonself; rather, they recognize infection- or damage-induced molecular patterns in host cells and tissues. Based on this, Matzinger argued that the immune response does not begin with the discrimination between self and nonself but is determined by whether it is detrimental to the host. In the guard hypothesis, the target is the self as modified by the pathogen, and in the danger theory, the trigger is not limited to the pathogen; despite this difference, conceptually, the two overlap completely. This mode of recognition, namely reacting to one's own tissues, is somewhat reminiscent of the self-referentiality inherent in the immune system.

4.2.3 LOCAL HYPERSENSITIVITY REACTIONS AND SYSTEMIC ACQUIRED RESISTANCE

As noted above, plants have neither mobile immune cells nor antibodies. Naturally, this raises the question of how the overall defense is executed under such conditions. Before addressing this question, I examine the local response. First, ETI is induced through direct or indirect interactions between NLR proteins and pathogen effectors. This is a hypersensitivity reaction that induces apoptosis in infected cells. After this reaction occurs locally, resistance is seen systemically. This phenomenon had been reported since the 1930s (Chester, 1933) and was named systemic acquired resistance by Frank Ross (1911–1989) in 1961 (Ross, 1961). He infected local areas of tobacco (*Nicotiana tabacum*) leaves with the tobacco mosaic virus and observed that the opposite leaves were also resistant to this virus.

Plants do not have a circulatory system like animals, but they do have a tissue involved in transport; it is called the phloem. Through this tissue, immune signals important for systemic acquired resistance are transported to the entire plant. The major immune signals are assumed to be salicylic acids, and methylsalicylic acid, jasmonic acid, and azelaic acid are also included. It is believed that the crosstalk of these signals contributes to effective systemic defense by transmitting local information to uninfected distant sites. Plants have mechanisms that compensate for the absence of mobile cells and antibodies (Shah and Zeier, 2013).

4.2.4　Immunological Memory in Plants

Another important aspect of Ross's finding is that the second infection resulted in resistance not only to the tobacco mosaic virus but also to other viruses. The resistance to a wide range of pathogens exhibited by systemic acquired resistance is indicative of the nature of plant immune memory; furthermore, it is considered to be due to an overall nonspecific increase in the level of immunity upon contact with the first pathogen. This is labeled immune priming or innate immune memory, and its importance became evident in the COVID-19 pandemic; however, it was first proposed in relation to plants (Chester, 1933). Immune memory in bacteria is supported by a Lamarckian mode of inheritance transmitted to the next generation at the gene level via the CRISPR–Cas system (Section 4.1, Chapter 4). Thus, the following question emerges: What mechanisms operate in plants?

When a pathogen infects a plant, various changes occur in the plant that enhance the subsequent defense response. I will elucidate the molecular basis underlying this priming or immune memory. For example, it has been reported that mRNA and protein levels of systemic mitogen-activated protein kinases (MPK3 and MPK6) are elevated by local infection in *Arabidopsis thaliana*; furthermore, suppressing the function of these two kinases also attenuates the priming effect (Beckers et al., 2009). A few scholars have also suggested that a transcriptional regulatory cofactor called non-expressor of pathogenesis-related genes 1 (NPR1), which plays a role in the activation of genes related to immunity, is involved in priming (Cao et al., 1994; Dong, 2004). More interestingly, the memory of systemic acquired resistance that occurs when *Arabidopsis* is infected with *P. syringae* not only showed resistance to pathogens other than *P. syringae* but was also transmitted across generations (Luna et al., 2012). The mechanism involved here is assumed to be epigenetic changes involving the methylation and acetylation of histones around the genes related to systemic acquired resistance and the *NPR1* gene.

4.2.5　Autoimmunity in Plants

Speciation has been a major theme in biology since Darwin. While reproduction is possible between conspecifics, different species are unable to produce viable offspring. Therefore, reproductive isolation occurs. The mechanisms of reproductive isolation are classified into prezygotic mechanisms, which act before fertilization, and postzygotic mechanisms, which act after it. Hybrid necrosis, the reproductive isolation seen in plants, is considered to be due to a postzygotic mechanism. In this phenomenon, yellowing, wilting, dwarfing, cell death and tissue necrosis are seen in hybrids originating from normal parents (Bomblies and Weigel, 2007). One explanation for hybrid incompatibility is the famous Bateson–Dobzhansky–Muller model (Orr, 1996). When two populations derived from the same ancestor are isolated and each accumulates gene mutations independently, hybridization between them may fail because of incompatibility between the mutated genes. A genetic analysis of two strains causing hybrid necrosis in *Arabidopsis* identified *Dangerous Mix 1* (*DM1*) and *Dangerous Mix 2d* (*DM2d*) as the respective responsible gene regions (Bomblies et al., 2007). Interestingly, both regions contain NLR genes encoding receptors that recognize self-proteins modified with pathogen effectors.

As previously mentioned, NLRs initiate an immune response and produce cell death; this is the hypersensitivity reaction. On examining hybrid necrosis in lettuce (*Lactuca sativa*), the molecule incompatible with NLR was found to be homologous to RIN4, which is a target of pathogen effectors in *Arabidopsis* (Jeuken et al., 2009). Furthermore, increased levels of NLRs resulted in hybrid necrosis, but when NLR expression was suppressed, hybrid necrosis was absent (Kim et al., 2010; Li et al., 2010; Cheng et al., 2011). In essence, it was revealed that hybrid necrosis involves the recognition of self-components by NLRs. Furthermore, when *Arabidopsis* was examined extensively, 2% showed similar hybrid necrosis symptoms. As NLR is expressed in all cells of the plant, although there are no mobile immune cells, all cells play the role of immunocompetent cells. Therefore, NLRs must be strictly controlled to prevent them from activating and attacking their own components when there is no infection. However, there can be no perfect control in an organism, and autoimmunity cannot be eliminated. From a different perspective, autoimmunity can be considered to be embedded in the system in plants, as in the case of mammals and bacteria.

4.2.6 RNA-Based Antiviral Immunity

This section explores the plant response to a virus. This process involves RNA silencing, which relies on small RNA molecules. There are two major strategies for gene silencing: One is to act on the process of transcription to prevent the production of messenger RNA, and the other is to act on the messenger RNA after transcription to degrade it. RNA silencing was first discovered in the plant genus *Petunia*. In 1990, an attempt was made to obtain genetically modified dark purple *petunias* by introducing an enzyme gene that promoted pigmentation; however, *petunias* with no pigmentation appeared instead (Napoli et al., 1990; van der Krol et al., 1990). The mechanism of this phenomenon was elucidated in research using *C. elegans* in 1998 (Fire et al., 1998), as described in Section 4.1, Chapter 4. Small RNAs can be divided into three types: small interfering RNAs (siRNAs) involved in the sequence-specific degradation of RNAs introduced from the outside, microRNAs (miRNAs) involved in regulating the expression of other genes in the genome, and Piwi protein-binding RNAs (piRNAs) involved in monitoring transposons and ensuring genome stability and fertility in the animal germline. These are noncoding RNAs that are not translated into proteins.

As in the case of bacteria, the immune function of plants against viral infection involves a process comprising target recognition, degradation, and memory. Viruses that enter the cell are recognized and degraded in a sequence-specific manner. From the resulting single-stranded RNA, double-stranded RNA is synthesized and stored (memorized) as the genetic information of the invading virus. Simultaneously, this information is transmitted throughout the plant as small RNA molecules to prepare for the degradation of newly invading viruses. Following this, during the process in which the immune system works to degrade the invading virus (effector phase), small RNA molecules degrade the viral genome in a sequence-specific manner to protect the plant from infection.

Thus, the plant defense system has several important features. First, it possesses adaptability and specificity with regard to any virus. These depend on the invading viral genome, opposed to the host genome preparing the specificity as in mammals. Second, RNA silencing is not localized; rather, it propagates sequence-specific recognition molecules to distant locations, allowing for systemic defense. Third, RNA is synthesized and stored in memory based on information from the invading virus. Owing to the specificity, adaptability, systemic defense, and memory of the plant defense system, it is appropriate to call it an immune system; and some scientists have called it the acquired immunity of plants. If plants have a defensive response, it is a rule of the biological world that viruses will engage in an evolutionary arms race to generate strategies to counter it. Viruses produce molecules called RNA silencing suppressors that inhibit various processes of RNA silencing to counter the immune response of plants (Ding and Voinnet, 2007). Similar to other predator–prey relationships, plants and viruses are likely to continue to coevolve.

4.3   THE IMMUNE SYSTEMS OF INVERTEBRATES AND JAWLESS FISHES

In the classical view of the immune system, acquired immunity and innate immunity were clearly distinguished, and invertebrates, such as insects, were thought to possess only innate immunity. However, this distinction has gradually deteriorated, and there have been several reports that invertebrates also show immune memory and specificity, which have been considered characteristics of acquired immunity. In this section, I consider several invertebrates as examples and examine the mechanisms through which they deal with pathogens in the external world, in addition to comparing them with other organisms.

4.3.1   SPONGES

Sponges are mostly found attached to rocks in seawater and have no distinct organs such as muscles or nervous systems. They have a water flow system as an important structure, which allows them to filter and feed on large amounts of seawater. Specifically, they take in nutrients and oxygen through small pores on their surfaces; their collar cells ingest microorganisms and organic matter as nutrients; and their flagella generate water currents that expel waste products and carbon dioxide through their large pores. Sponges and *Ctenophora* (derived from the Greek words *kteis*, meaning "comb," and *pherō*, meaning "carry") were both considered likely to be candidates as the earliest multicellular animals to emerge in evolution; although *Ctenophora* were favored for a time, sponges are now considered the oldest multicellular animals (Feuda et al., 2017). This seems reasonable; sponges do not have organs, whereas *Ctenophora* have muscles, a gut, and a nervous system, which complicates the evolutionary explanation of the origin of multicellular animals. As a natural consequence of their mode of life, sponges are forced to come into contact with microorganisms, including pathogens. The symbiosis with microorganisms was discussed in Section 2.2, Chapter 2, and sponges are no exception, enjoying essential functions for survival via symbiosis with microorganisms that account for approximately 40% of their own volume (Thomas et al., 2016). However, they are exposed to large numbers of pathogens, making defense mechanisms essential.

At the end of the 19th century, Metchnikoff pointed out the existence of innate immunity in sponges on the basis of phagocytosis (Metchnikoff, 1892). Recent studies have shown that there are PRRs involved in the recognition of MAMPs and molecules involved in signal transduction from these receptors to NF-κB (a transcription factor involved in the immune response to infection) (Wiens et al., 2007; Brennan and Gilmore, 2018). The recognition of MAMPs by PRRs, a mechanism characteristic of innate immunity, is commonly observed in the animals examined below. Furthermore, a study that stimulated two types of sponges with a mixture of LPS and peptidoglycan, which constitute MAMPs, and examined their gene expression showed that the expression of *NLR* gene for cytoplasmic PRR was increased in one, whereas the expression of another gene for G protein-coupled receptors was induced in the other (Pita et al., 2018). This result may indicate the existence of a species-specific immune response in sponges.

The transition from unicellular to multicellular organisms was a decisive moment in evolution. At the beginning of the 20th century, Henry Van Peters Wilson (1863–1939) conducted the following experiment with sponges (Wilson, 1907). The sponges were broken apart through a sieve, and when those cells were put back together, they again formed aggregates and eventually became sponges. However, when the same experiment was performed between sponges of different species, no cellular cohesion was observed. It is highly likely that such a phenomenon occurred when multicellular organisms emerged. This is a type of transplantation experiment, and the results indicate that the recognition of self and nonself (allorecognition) occurs in sponges.

Approximately 40 years ago, the existence of histocompatibility in sponges was pointed out by William Hildemann (1927–1983) and colleagues (Hildemann et al., 1979; Hildemann et al., 1980). In an allorecognition system, it was reported that a second transplant performed up to 2–3 weeks after the first transplant resulted in faster rejection compared to the first transplant (Bigger et al., 1982).

In essence, it was shown that the immune memory indexed to the transplantation is retained for 2–3 weeks. The fact that a sponge that emerged approximately 600 million years ago (Li et al., 1998) was at the source of present-day sponges and all other animals, and shared mechanisms that lead to our immune system, further stimulates our imagination regarding the evolutionary process.

4.3.2 CNIDARIANS

Cnidarians, a type of animal that appeared approximately 500 million years ago (Technau and Steele, 2011), include jellyfish, sea anemones, and corals. There are two types of cnidarians: adherent polypoidal and jellyfish-like floating forms. The cnidae that characterize these animals are organelles on the surface of their bodies that, when stimulated, eject a harpoon-like structure that can sting or wrap around their prey. Thus, they function as a defense against predators. Some of these animals can survive for hundreds of years. The relevant question here concerns how they deal with pathogens in the absence of specifically functioning immune cells.

Cells constitute a physicochemical barrier against invaders through phagocytosis and mucus secretion. Regarding the selective recognition of pathogens, cnidarians have innate immunity in the form of PRRs that recognize MAMPs and DAMPs in the host (Shinzato et al., 2011). When cnidarians' cells combine between incompatible individuals of the same species, rejection occurs and adhesion is not observed with the release of cnidae. Histocompatibility is necessary to maintain tissue integrity, and there is an allorecognition mechanism that discriminates between self and nonself (Hildemann et al., 1977). It has been confirmed that cnidarians have histocompatibility genes for this purpose (Karadge et al., 2015).

Furthermore, cnidarians live in symbiosis with a wide variety of microorganisms (Thompson et al., 2015). In addition to eliminating pathogens, the cnidarian immune system identifies microorganisms that are beneficial to its own survival. This activity provides an idea of the holobiont involved in the regulation of cnidarians' metabolism, development, and behavior. Furthermore, given the characteristics of the immune system, a phenomenon that corresponds to an autoimmune disease that destroys its own tissues has been observed during the reproductive process of *Hydractinia echinata*, an animal belonging to the Hydrozoa (Buss et al., 1985). Another important question is whether immune memory exists in cnidarians; regarding this, interesting results have recently been reported by research involving anemones (Brown and Rodriguez-Lanetty, 2015). According to this study, when anemones were primed with a sublethal dose of a pathogen and given a lethal dose of the pathogen 2, 4, and 6 weeks later, survival was significantly increased compared to the unprimed group after 2–4 weeks; however, there was no difference between the two groups after 6 weeks. This indicates that immune memory as a priming effect persisted for 4 weeks. Immune memory being observed, albeit for a short period, in invertebrate sponges and cnidarians is yet another indication that this function is essential for the survival of an organism.

4.3.3 INSECTS

Analysis of the genes encoding the major insect proteins and fossil analysis revealed that insects appeared on Earth approximately 480 million years ago (Misof et al., 2014). Since then, insects have continued to survive, accounting for nearly 90% of all arthropods. This suggests that insects can adapt to any environment and that they are equipped with an excellent immune system. The immune function of insects is further explored below.

As in other organisms, there is a physical barrier between an insect and the external world. One is an outer skin composed of one layer of epithelial cells and covered with a cuticle, and the other is an enclosing membrane composed of chitin and other materials that covers the inside of the digestive tract. When pathogens pass through this barrier, the host's humoral immunity and cellular immunity are triggered. In insect humoral immunity, the production of antimicrobial peptides, melanin reaction via the activation of phenoloxidase precursors, and the production of reactive oxygen species occur. Antimicrobial peptides are produced after infection mainly by the fat body, which corresponds to the human liver and adipose tissue. The first insect antimicrobial peptide discovered was lysozyme, which degrades the plasma membrane peptidoglycan of Gram-positive bacteria. Others include defensins, which act on Gram-positive bacteria and fungi; cecropin, drosocin, attacin, and diptericin, which act on Gram-negative bacteria; and drosomycin and metchnikowin from *Drosophila melanogaster*, which act on fungi.

Cellular immunity includes phagocytosis, nodule formation (nodulation), in which hemocytes that have phagocytosed pathogens assemble, and encapsulation, in which multiple blood cells encircle and sequester foreign substances. Insects have an open vascular system, and hemolymph—arthropods' fluid analog of blood—fills the body cavity. Nutrients, hormones, and mobile blood cells are transported throughout the body via the hemolymph. Phagocytosis is mediated by plasmatocytes in *Drosophila* and granulocytes and plasmacytes in Lepidoptera (butterflies and moths); nodulation is mediated by granulocytes and plasmatocytes in Lepidoptera; and encapsulation is mediated by granulocytes and plasmatocytes in Lepidoptera and plasmatocytes and lamellocytes in *Drosophila* (Eleftherianos et al., 2021). After infection, the elimination of the pathogen by blood cells occurs first, followed by humoral immunity involving antimicrobial peptides and other substances. However, humoral and cellular immunity do not function independently, instead cooperating with each other. For example, plasmatocytes in *Drosophila* act on the fat body to stimulate the production of antimicrobial peptides.

Immune priming, which exhibits specificity and immune memory, is also observed in the following insects: for example, the fruit fly (*Drosophila melanogaster*) (Pham et al., 2007), the red flour beetle (*Tribolium castaneum*) (Sadd and Schmid-Hempel, 2006; Roth et al., 2009), the Indian meal moth (*Plodia interpunctella*) (Tidbury et al., 2011), and the *Anopheles* mosquito (*Anopheles gambiae*) (Rodrigues et al., 2010). It is also found in social insects, such as the buff-tailed bumblebee (*Bombus terrestris*) (Sadd and Schmid-Hempel, 2006) and the European honey bee (*Apis mellifera*) (Hernández López et al., 2014). When these insects were primed by sublethal doses of bacteria, viruses, or protozoa, they acquired resistance to subsequent lethal doses of infection, and in some cases the resistance was observed beyond their generation. The mechanism of the specific recognition is unknown in insects. However, homologues of the human Down syndrome cell adhesion molecule (Dscam) expressed in insects and crustaceans have been considered candidates (Kurtz and Armitage, 2006). It is assumed that the *Dscam* gene in *Drosophila* consists of four exons and that the combination of the possible types of each exon yields over 18,000 isoforms, accommodating diverse pathogens and supporting specificity (Watson et al., 2005). This molecule is said to be involved in axon guidance because of its remarkable diversity (Schmucker et al., 2000). However, it remains controversial whether this corresponds to acquired immunity in vertebrates (Armitage et al., 2017). The reasons are threefold: First, the diversity of Dscam is due to alternative splicing rather than gene rearrangement like antigen receptors. Second, the diversity arising from it is not as large as that of T cells and B cells. Third, it is unclear whether this molecule is involved in memory formation. Therefore, while it is possible that it is involved in some immune processes, there exists no evidence that it is responsible for specific recognition.

4.3.4 Urochordates

The golden star tunicate (*Botryllus schlosseri*), a colonial ascidian tunicate, forms colonies that are interconnected by a vascular system and is covered by a gelatinous capsule. When the blood vessels of two colonies come into contact with each other, either the two systems fuse to form a new colony with a different genetic makeup, or an inflammatory reaction destroys the contacting vessels, resulting in scar formation. This phenomenon can be said to embody acceptance and rejection by allorecognition. At Stanford University, Irving Weissman (1939–) and colleagues conducted research on this and, in 1982, revealed that a gene similar to the human MHC is responsible for determining whether colonies fuse or reject (Scofield et al., 1982). Furthermore, in 2005, the locus involved in fusion (fusibility/histocompatibility [FuHC]) was identified, showing that fusion occurs when two colonies share at least one allele of *FuHC* (e.g., AA and AB) and rejection occurs when they share none of *FuHC* (in the case of AA and BB) (De Tomaso et al., 2005). Since MHC has only been identified in highly evolved Gnathostomata, this study demonstrates that MHC-like molecules are present and involved in allorecognition in invertebrates.

However, it was not clear whether *FuHC* is the gene that determines allorecognition in *Botryllus schlosseri*, or whether it is only in close proximity to the original responsible gene. In 2013, the *Botryllus* histocompatibility factor (BHF) was reported to be as the responsible factor (Voskoboynik et al., 2013). BHF is frequently expressed in the vascular system, suggesting that it is involved in allorecognition. However, the structure of *BHF* was not found to be related to the histocompatibility genes of cnidarians or the *MHC* of Gnathostomata. While the function of allorecognition has been observed since early animal evolution, it is possible that the recognition mechanism in ascidians is different from that observed in other organisms.

Furthermore, there are other molecules that generate unique diversity. For example, the snail (*Biomphalaria glabrata*), which belongs to the mollusk family, has a molecule called fibrinogen-related protein (FREP). This molecule is upregulated during infection and can bind to pathogens or their products. The structure consists of an amino-terminal Ig superfamily region and a carboxy-terminal fibrinogen region, and alternative splicing and point mutations produce various molecules (Loker et al., 2004; Litman et al., 2005). Variable region-containing chitin-binding proteins (VCBPs) are also present in the Florida lancelet (*Branchiostoma floridae*) (Cannon et al., 2002). Its structure is highly diverse with two Ig-like variable regions and a chitin-binding region. In the vase tunicate (*Ciona intestinalis*), VCBP is secreted into the gut and has the ability to bind to bacteria (Dishaw et al., 2011). The presence of Ig-like variable region genes in these animals and their involvement in bacterial recognition is an important finding regarding the origin of genes involved in antigen recognition in Gnathostomata.

4.3.5 AGNATHA

The lamprey and the hagfish, which belong to the same jawless vertebrate family, have immune systems that are most similar to those of Gnathostomata (to which humans belong). In Gnathostomata, antibodies (immunoglobulins and B cell receptors) are prepared to recognize a myriad of antigens through their *V(D)J* gene combinations, and the basic mechanism is similar for T cell receptors. However, no enzymes (RAGs) that cause the *V(D)J* gene rearrangement of antigen receptors have been found in jawless animals, and the mechanism of immune response in these animals remained unknown for a period.

To solve this problem, Max Cooper and colleagues examined gene expression after lamprey larvae were immunized with a mixture of bacteria and mitogenic factors. However, they did not find B cell receptors, T cell receptors or MHC, which are important in acquired immunity. Instead, they found a gene that generates high diversity. This gene is incomplete in the germ line and cannot code for a protein; however, when it differentiates into lymphocyte-like cells, it encodes a protein with high diversity. As this gene is reminiscent of the genetic rearrangement in antibodies, they assumed that it might be an antigen receptor in this animal and named it variable lymphocyte receptor (VLR) (Pancer et al., 2004). A module encoding a highly diverse LRR exists in the vicinity of this gene, which generates diversity via sequential incorporation into the *VLR* gene during differentiation. Although this is different from the mechanism of antibody gene rearrangement, it has been postulated that VLRs' level of diversity is comparable to that of antibodies (Alder et al., 2005).

To date, VLRs corresponding to T cell and B cell receptors have been identified (Guo et al., 2009). VLRB+ cells proliferate and differentiate into antibody-producing cells upon antigen stimulation, suggesting that they are expressed on cells corresponding to B cells. In contrast, VLRA+ cells are thought to be expressed on cells corresponding to T cells, as T cell mitogenic factors induce cell proliferation and increase the production of proinflammatory cytokines.

Furthermore, VLRC, which is expressed on T cell-like cells, has been identified (Kasamatsu et al., 2010). The gene expression suggests the following: While VLRA⁺ cells correspond to αβ T cells (with α and β chains as antigen receptors), which constitute the majority of T cells, VLRC⁺ cells correspond to γδ T cells (with γ and δ chains as antigen receptors), which are a minority and are distributed mostly in the intestinal mucosa (Hirano et al., 2013). This indicates that the prototype cells for B cells and two series of T cells are prepared at the jawless stage. However, further studies on immunological memory in lampreys and hagfish are needed (Sharrock and Sun, 2020).

4.4 MINIMAL FUNCTIONAL UNITS THAT CONSTITUTE THE IMMUNE SYSTEM

It has been established that bacterial immunity is considerably different from both plant and animal immunity. Considering appearances alone, it is natural to question whether the bacterial system can even be considered an immune system. Moreover, the immune systems of plants and invertebrates are markedly different from that of human beings, although not as different as that of bacteria. However, in vertebrate Agnathans, the major cells that constitute the immune system are basically similar, although the mechanisms by which they are generated are different. In this section, I discuss some of the features of the immune system that have become clear from the analyses at the organismal level in Chapter 3 and from the phylogenetic perspective in Chapter 4.

First, a version of the immune system exists in all living organisms, from bacteria to humans, although the structure and mechanisms differ considerably. This indicates that the immune system has the same extent as life and overlaps with the existence of life. As defects in the components of the immune system threaten the survival of organisms and may lead to death, it is clear that immunity is essential for organisms to live and survive.

Second, although there are many interpretations of immunity, a self- and nonself-distinguishing mechanism lies at the core of immune function. However, the mechanism that produces tolerance to self is not always perfect, and the possibility of autoreactivity escalating into autoimmune disease is always present. Autoimmunity has been reported since the beginning of the 20th century, when the history of modern immunology began. Further studies have demonstrated that autoimmunity is present in all organisms with immune systems.

Third, tolerance to nonself has also been observed, as in the case of symbiosis with microorganisms. As these phenomena seemingly contradict the Burnetian framework, some scientists have argued for a new paradigm in which the existence of autoimmunity is the norm.

Fourth, all organisms' immune systems have a memory function, although the mechanisms differ. This is surprising as the classical view of immunity posits that immunological memory is a feature of adaptive acquired immunity, which is limited to organisms with T cells and B cells. As noted above, given that the immune system has the same extent as life itself, immunological memory is an indispensable component of life.

Fifth, in highly evolved organisms, the immune system does not function alone; rather it interacts in complex ways with other systems, especially the nervous, endocrine, and metabolic systems. The interactions among these systems are multidirectional, and the immune system exists and functions in such a way that it is almost integrated into the entire organism. In essence, immunity should not be viewed as a local phenomenon at the site of antigen entry but as a phenomenon that involves other systems and ultimately affects the entire organism. Therefore, to examine immune phenomena, the discussion must be extended beyond the so-called immune system.

This holistic view is also reminiscent of Jerne's idiotypic network theory. As shown in Section 1.7.1, Chapter 1, this theory postulates that a network formed by the interaction of antibodies via idiotypes, which are characteristic structures of each antibody, regulates immune responses and immunosuppression. Despite approximately 15 years of extensive search, it disappeared from the center stage of immunology without scientific confirmation. However, the view that immune function is controlled by a currently unidentified network that covers the entire organism could be partially true. If any local event can affect the activity of the entire organism, it will be essential to move away from the traditional intra-systemic logic and apply more flexible holistic thinking.

Similar developments can be seen within research on the immune system. Early analyses focused on local phenomena in which antigen–antibody reactions occur, but it soon became clear that humoral factors and many other cell types are involved. Insights into the relationship between innate immunity and acquired immunity, which have been studied separately, are also undergoing significant changes. The two types of immunity must cooperate for effective defense against pathogens. Furthermore, the boundary between innate immunity and acquired immunity is eroding as it becomes increasingly clear that cells that were thought to belong to innate immunity, or organisms from earlier stages of evolution, possess antigen specificity and immune memory, which were considered characteristics of acquired immunity. These findings cast doubt on the nature and very existence of the immune system.

Sixth, the functional elements common to the immune systems of all living organisms can be summarized as four functions: (1) detecting signals in the internal and external environment, (2) integrating the information received, (3) responding effectively to the initial signal based on that information, and (4) storing that experience as a memory for future use. In essence, information reception, integration, appropriate response, and memory are the basic functions of immunity. If this assumption is accepted, there is a perfect overlap between the basic functional elements of immunity and the functional properties of the nervous system. The functional similarities between the two systems in humans and mice have been noted in previous research (Cohen, 1992a; Hershberg and Efroni, 2001; Habibi et al., 2009; Kioussis and Pachnis, 2009; Nataf, 2014). These functional features having been preserved in the organism during evolution warrants a reconsideration of the relationship between the immune system and the nervous system from a different perspective.

The idea that bacteria and archaea, which are considered the most primitive organisms, have immune systems was initially unimaginable. The strong influence of the anthropocentric worldview means that the immune systems of humans and mice are what people reflexively think of when immunity is considered. Other species are not afforded much attention. Therefore, when I first read the report that bacteria have an immune system, I was not sure whether the term "immune system" was being used metaphorically or if it was referring to the actual immune system. The supposed immune system in bacteria is far removed from the human immune system. What I found interesting was that the CRISPR–Cas system, which seemed strange at first, was critical for understanding the fundamental nature of immunity.

Strict use of language is conducive to scientific progress, but at the same time, inclusive use of language can also promote scientific development. The immune system may be an example of this. The first question is why the scientific community, including the editors of the relevant journals, immediately used the term "immune system" to describe the CRISPR–Cas system. The most likely explanation is that they were already thinking of a particular definition of the immune system and that the CRISPR–Cas system fits that definition. As discussed in Chapter 1, there are different views on the immune system. The most persistent view is that it is a defense system centered on the discrimination of self and nonself, but there are other views as well; for example, Irun Cohen proposed considering it a sensing or homeostatic system (Cohen and Young, 1991; Cohen, 1992a, 1992b, 2000), and Anne-Marie Moulin saw the cognitive paradigm in immunity, in addition to defense and selection paradigms (Moulin, 1995).

Recent findings on CRISPR–Cas reinforce the classical view of the immune system as a defense system. Because of its simple structure and function, CRISPR–Cas provides a clear visualization of the basic minimal units of the immune system. There are three stages and four functional elements. The first adaptive stage involves a step in which the Cas protein recognizes and cleaves the viral DNA that has entered the bacterium, and the resulting short DNA fragment is incorporated into the CRISPR locus as a corresponding memory to counter for later invasion by the same virus. Comparing this to the human immune response, the first step corresponds to antigen recognition and the second step to the memory of the encounter with the antigen. In the second stage, namely expression, the information stored in the genome is processed to prepare for the next stage. In the third stage, namely interference, the stored information is used to effectively eliminate the invading foreign DNA.

These analyses make it clear that any mechanism involved in the defense of an organism against external invaders can be called an immune system. Thus, when we look at what is considered an immune system, the details of the anatomical structure and mechanisms of the system do not constitute a condition for calling it an immune system; rather, only the system's function is relevant. The smallest units of immune system function present in bacteria and archaea are also found in the immune systems of plants, insects, and even humans and mice. Nevertheless, there are many newly emerging and complex regulatory mechanisms in highly evolved organisms that play an important role in immune function and its maintenance in those organisms. Therefore, if we observe only highly evolved organisms, it is difficult to see the minimal conditions that constitute immunity. For an organism's defense mechanism to be called an immune system, it would only have to fulfill the four functional conditions involved in defense against invaders.

However, the situation is not so simple. The immune system, especially in highly evolved organisms such as humans and mice, is not limited in its function; it is also closely related to the nervous and endocrine systems. It is surprising, however, that this trend is also observed in bacteria and archaea. As already explained, the CRISPR–Cas system is involved not only in bacterial immunity but also in the regulation of genes that define virulence and control the behavior of bacterial populations (Bille et al., 2005; Sampson and Weiss, 2013; Westra et al., 2014; Barrangou, 2015) and the *cas* gene is involved in the social behavior and developmental processes of myxobacteria (Thöny-Meyer and Kaiser, 1993; Boysen et al., 2002). This is important for understanding the fundamental nature of the immune system.

These results suggest that, since the appearance of life on Earth, the immune system has played a role, beyond immunity in the classical sense, in maintaining biological functions. The CRISPR–Cas system also regulates the social behavior of bacteria by receiving information from the external world, integrating it, and responding appropriately to the original signal. The manner in which the bacterial immune system regulates the behavioral responses induced by environmental signals is reminiscent of the action of the human central nervous system, and it is tempting to consider the functions executed by the bacterial immune system as "proto-neural." At present, no nervous system has been identified in bacteria. Regardless of whether an organism possesses a brain, nervous system-like activity must be essential for its survival. If this is the case, it is possible to infer that the immune system is responsible for the proto-neuronal function in bacteria.

Bacteria have other systems that receive information from the outside and control their behavior. One example is chemotaxis, a phenomenon in which bacteria behave in response to a concentration gradient of a particular chemical in the external environment. Signaling occurs from receptors, and ultimately, flagellar rotation controls the movement of the bacteria, which move away from potentially harmful substances and toward favorable ones. In this case, the bacteria measure the concentration of the substance that causes chemotaxis over time, and it is believed that they remember past data. This entails a chemical reaction called methylation, which is said to last from 1 to 10 seconds (Koshland, 1974). Whether the state of methylation is considered memory may be a point of contention, but if this is considered memory, the phosphorylation and dephosphorylation reactions and conformational changes in protein structure that are widely carried out would also be included in the category of memory, and the discussion may extend beyond reasonable bounds. This is a definitional issue, but at this stage, I shall refrain from adopting this perspective.

A fundamental characteristic of the CRISPR–Cas system is that it senses signals in the environment in a broad sense, integrates them in a meaningful way, and responds appropriately. At the same time, this system serves multiple functions, including those not directly related to immunity. The immune system in highly evolved organisms is also involved in diverse functions. Perhaps a new name is needed to describe these multifunctional systems. In any case, the inclusive view adopted here with regard to the immune system provides important insights and flexibility when considering the anatomy and physiology of various systems in other organisms.

An issue that has emerged from the examination of the immune systems of other species is auto-immunity. This phenomenon has evidently been an inherent part of the immune system since the appearance of life on Earth. In bacteria, 0.4% of all spacers are directed to self-genes, and approximately 18% of bacteria with the CRISPR–Cas system have at least one spacer corresponding to self (Stern et al., 2010). Bacteria with this inherent potential for autoimmunity already possess strategies to avoid it. This may be natural in the logic of life, but it is surprising nevertheless.

4.5 THE MINIMAL COGNITION PROBLEM

When I came to the conclusion that the bacterial immune system is equipped with the smallest unit of cognitive function, I realized that the minimal cognition problem is being debated (Beer, 2003; Keijzer, 2003; Barandiaran and Moreno, 2006; van Duijn et al., 2006; Lyon, 2015; Godfrey-Smith, 2016): What is the minimum requirement for cognition? A wide range of ideas have emerged regarding this issue. At one extreme is brain-centrism or neurocentrism. This view, which is still influential, posits that the existence of a brain or brain-related structures (e.g., neurons) and functions (e.g., electrophysiological activity) is the minimum requirement for cognitive ability. Thus, an organism without a brain or neurons is said to be cognitively inept. Recent events have shown that this view continues to exert significant influence on the field of biology, remaining one of its central concepts. The emerging field of "plant neurobiology" has been harshly criticized for its unscientific use of the term "neuro" to describe plants without neurons. Consequently, the name of a journal focusing on this field had to be changed from *Plant Neurobiology* to *Plant Signaling & Behavior* (Alpi et al., 2007; Struik et al., 2008).

However, at the opposite end of the spectrum is the view that the minimum requirement for cognition is the demonstration of a sensorimotor response initiated by the reception of an external signal (van Duijn et al., 2006; Lyon, 2015). According to this criterion, it is essential that an element of motility be present in the output, a typical example of which is found in bacterial chemotaxis. Therefore, processes such as the lactose (*lac*) operon of *E. coli*, for example, cannot be considered cognition (van Duijn et al., 2006). This definition implies that the presence of a nervous system is not necessary for cognition and is based on the position that functional and physiological criteria are important, as opposed to structural and anatomical organization. According to a more inclusive view that has recently been proposed, information processing and decision-making occur in organisms and biological systems, and when information is acquired, stored, processed, and used at any level of organization in an organism, it is considered cognition (Lyon, 2015; Baluška and Levin, 2016).

Furthermore, some scientists have argued for "embodied cognition" that goes beyond the brain (Lakoff and Johnson, 1980; Varela et al., 1991; Clark, 1998) and "extended cognition" that goes beyond the body, involving the environment that surrounds the organism (Clark and Chalmers, 1998; Wilson, 2004; Menary, 2010). Although such diverse views have been proposed, within each criterion, cases of cognitive capacity and cases of non-cognitive capacity are relatively well discriminated. Therefore, the question of which criterion is best to use arises, but a clear consensus has yet to be reached. An important aspect regarding this issue is which criterion has the broadest explanatory power when cognition is viewed from various perspectives—structural, functional, and evolutionary. Furthermore, it will be essential to be clearly aware of the importance of memory in cognition.

In immunology, there has been a similar debate about what constitutes the immune system. The classical view, as in neurocentrism in the definition of cognition, has made the presence of structural elements such as T cells, B cells, antibodies, and MHC found in humans and mice or the presence of highly diverse and specific recognition mechanisms a necessary condition for the immune system.

Based on this criterion, the immune system would exist only in Gnathostomata or, at best, in jawless organisms such as lampreys and hagfish.

However, as already addressed, there is a growing view that what is considered the immune system exists in almost all organisms that do not have lymphocytes or antibodies, including bacteria and archaea (Rimer et al., 2014). This has valuable implications for the criteria of cognition. Perhaps the most important of these is the need to distance oneself from anthropocentric or neurocentric thinking by focusing on function. Furthermore, when answering the question of where to look for the most basic components of cognition, it is important to consider which criteria have the broadest explanatory power in light of the framework of modern biology.

Functions involving subjectivity, such as cognition and consciousness, are difficult to define and often ambiguous. In general, there are at least two levels of consciousness: One involves being aware of one's surroundings, and the other involves being aware of what one perceives there. If the former is thinking, the latter is reflecting on one's thoughts. Ned Block (1942–) of New York University divided consciousness into two levels: phenomenal consciousness and access consciousness (Block, 1995). Phenomenal consciousness involves qualitative content, such as subjective experiences and sensations, and corresponds to what is called qualia. Access consciousness is a state of being able to access information once it has been accepted through language, reasoning, and action, and it is responsible for higher-order functions.

Later, Gerald Edelman classified consciousness into primary consciousness (sensory consciousness) and secondary consciousness (higher consciousness) (Edelman, 2004). The former involves the present and the immediate past in which we perceive the world, and it is present not only in humans but also in certain animals. The latter is the consciousness of being aware, and it involves abstract thought, will, or self-reflective awareness involving the past, the present, and the future. Edelman stated that, in both cases, memory is essential to the integration of the events around the subject. Thomas Nagel (1937–) of New York University labeled the former as simply consciousness and the latter as cognition to mean higher mental functions such as thinking, reasoning, and judgment (Nagel, 2012). Regardless the terms used, it is believed that there are at least two levels of mental activity in humans.

The term "cognition" used in the discussion of minimal cognition does not refer to higher consciousness in the typical sense but to a much broader concept that includes primary consciousness; this calls into question the very definition of cognition. The existence of subjectivity can only be confirmed by the organisms that actually experience the world. It is inherently difficult to determine the state of consciousness of other organisms and, moreover, whether they are conscious in the first place. Even if other species have their own subjective worlds, the manifestation of subjectivity is likely to differ from species to species. One lesson I have learned from my study of the immune system through phylogeny is that the anthropocentric perspective must be abandoned. The immune systems of many organisms take forms that are unimaginable from the viewpoint of evolved organisms. To call it an immune system requires a free mind—one that is free from the habitual ways of looking at it.

As pointed out by Theodosius Dobzhansky (1900–1975), "Nothing in biology makes sense except in the light of evolution" (Dobzhansky, 1973). The strongest constraint on modern biology would be neo-Darwinism, which integrates Darwin's theory of evolution and Mendelian genetics. Whether consciously or not, this principle has been espoused by nearly all modern biologists and constitutes the foundation of modern biology's orthodoxy, so to speak. Those who do not adhere to it have come to be severely criticized as unscientific. However, it is also true that this view has been criticized from several perspectives, including those of religious ideologies (Waddington, 1953; Vaz and Varela, 1978; Behe, 1996; Dembski, 1998; Ramos et al., 2006; Hoffmeyer, 2011; Nagel, 2012).

One such criticism is that of Thomas Nagel, who considers himself an atheist. Since the 17th century, science has certainly made tremendous progress, but in the process, it has excluded mental phenomena such as consciousness, meaning, intention, and purpose from its analysis. In his recent book, *Mind and Cosmos* (Nagel, 2012)—provocatively subtitled *Why the Materialist*

Neo-Darwinian Conception of Nature Is Almost Certainly False—he argues that there are aspects of the universe and life that cannot be explained by a neo-Darwinism based on purposeless mutation and natural selection and that these aspects can be better understood by other means. The book challenges the orthodoxy of modern biology. However, it has been criticized by evolutionary biologists and philosophers for bringing teleology into science, favoring intelligent design, and not containing enough substance to reject neo-Darwinism (Sober, 2012; Alwan, 2013). Keeping these in mind, I examine his argument below.

Nagel begins his argument with the mind–body problem. In his view, this problem is not a local problem of analyzing the relationship between the mind, the body, and behavior but a larger problem that concerns the universe and its history. If the scientific method applied to the mind–body problem is not valid in principle, applying this approach to the larger problem becomes questionable. He draws a clear distinction between the incompleteness of the knowledge that has been obtained by modern science and the incompleteness of the capabilities inherent in science as a method for understanding nature. At present, this method is based on physicochemical reductionism. According to Nagel, if this principle has inherent limitations, a new framework for understanding nature must be developed.

In *Mind and Cosmos*, the explanatory power of reductionist neo-Darwinism regarding the origin and evolution of life is called into question. Nagel presents the following points: First, the probability that self-replicating forms of life could have appeared on primitive Earth by random physicochemical processes alone is low. Second, even if life did emerge, would there have been enough time for the organisms we see on Earth today to take their present form through genetic mutation and natural selection? Third, the universe has existed for 13.8 billion years, but the emergence of the mind is a recent event. Even if the seemingly mindless universe is comprehensible through physics, is it possible to understand the subjective world of the mind through physics and chemistry? Fourth, how do life and the mind emerge from inorganic matter? If natural selection was not involved in the origin of life, other factors that modify genetic variation would have been necessary. If these two problems cannot be solved by current theories and methods, current methodologies must be discarded even though alternatives for these are not available at present. Nagel believes that neo-Darwinism cannot provide satisfactory answers to the origin and evolution of life or even the mind–body problem. He predicts that, if a theory that can answer these questions emerges, it will be comparable to relativity theory or the introduction of electromagnetic fields into physics.

Interestingly, Nagel presents four conditions for the conscious mind to fit into the neo-Darwinism's physicalist framework. The first condition is that consciousness plays an essential role in the survival and reproduction of organisms, at least in the later stages of evolution. The second condition is that the characteristics of consciousness must be transmitted genetically in some form. The third condition is that genetic variation, which provides candidates for natural selection, is both a mental change and a physical change, at least at some point. The fourth condition, which Nagel considers the most important, is that these mechanisms must inevitably have been anticipated by organisms that emerged earlier in evolution to create that possibility.

If the neural-like cognitive functions of CRISPR–Cas—recognition, information processing, adaptive response, and memory—correspond to what Nagel calls consciousness, Nagel's four conditions would be satisfied. From this perspective, each condition is examined below.

The first condition is that consciousness must play a fundamental role in survival and reproduction, at least in the later stages of evolution. This is easily met if the immune system has been responsible for neural-like cognitive functions since the beginning of evolution. Immunity is directly related to survival, which favors reproduction in turn. As for the second condition, the immune system is mediated and transmitted by genetic mechanisms. The third condition has two parts: The first is that genetic variation must provide a candidate for natural selection, which would not be problematic. The second is that genetic variation must be both mental and physical; this is slightly more complicated, since it depends on how one defines the mental dimension, and the subjective world is ultimately unknowable to a third party. However, if the mental dimension is interpreted in a broader sense that includes adaptive capacity to the external world and the decision-making process, this condition is also satisfied. The fourth condition is that consciousness should be preceded by organisms at an earlier stage of evolution. This condition would also be satisfied if the immune systems in bacteria and archaea are recognized as the primordial consciousness. In any case, the possibility that the immune system is responsible for neural-like cognitive functions in bacteria suggests that the immune system may be reconsidered as a universal cognitive system. Therefore, the status of the immune system in the organism should be upgraded.

It is unlikely that the mind–body problem will be solved by physicochemical reductionism, as Nagel himself claims. It would also be rather difficult to solve the problem of consciousness. As discussed in more detail in Section 5.4, Chapter 5, subjective experience is difficult without being able to feel "what is it like to be …?" (Nagel, 1974). In other words, the subjective aspect of a cognitive process is only real for the organism actually experiencing it. This engenders the question of whether current science, which excludes subjectivity from its activities, can handle this problem.

If dealing with the subjective aspect of cognition is difficult, shouldn't science consider rethinking cognition to fit within a biological definition? As mentioned above, if cognitive processes can be defined, for example, as the ability to adapt to the environment or the existence of a decision-making process, then it will be possible to deal with the problem of consciousness within the framework of neo-Darwinism and withstand criticisms such as Nagel's. This will not solve the problem of cognition in humans and other organisms, but it will facilitate a discussion of the activities of organisms within a broader framework. In essence, it is only when the most inclusive genetic and biochemical criteria are applied as a definition of minimal cognition that the four conditions raised by Nagel are met and broad explanatory power is guaranteed.

4.6 IMMUNITY AS THE MOST ANCIENT COGNITIVE SYSTEM

There is no living organism that does not have memory. All organisms have at least immunological memory, although the mechanisms differ. This is the conclusion of the analysis thus far. The phenomenon of immunity was described by Thucydides in the 5th century BC, characterized by memory and specificity. As it has been confirmed that immune memory is ubiquitous in the living world, it is impossible for any living organism to be without immune memory. Thus, the principle should apply to the discovery of what appears to be extraterrestrial life, and novel questions regarding what new mechanisms for immunity or immunological memory may be at work there will be of interest.

In *Mind-Energy*, Bergson offers the following reflections: Mind is consciousness, and consciousness is first and foremost memory and a bridge between the past and the future. All consciousness is an anticipation of the future. To know with scientific certainty that a particular being is conscious, one must enter into it, coincide with it, and be it. Consciousness does not depend on the existence of a brain and, in principle, is coextensive with life. The role of an organism is to create, and it must prepare something now to create the future. The only way to prepare for the future is to refer to what has happened before. In other words, memory, which preserves the past, is essential. This is how a world in which the past, the present, and the future are formed as a continuum without division emerges (Bergson, 1920).

To continue surviving, organisms must be aware of their internal and external environments and respond effectively to these; for this purpose, it is essential to store the information obtained in the past. Thus, an organism must have cognitive capabilities. Furthermore, cognitive functions are not necessarily monopolized by the nervous system, and a major question concerns what is responsible for cognitive functions in each organism. In Chapter 4, I have reasoned that bacteria and plants, which do not have a nervous system, survive in harsh conditions and that the immune system may be responsible for their cognitive function and may support their survival. There seems to be very little contradiction in such a hypothesis. If this conclusion is accepted, the immune system constitutes the oldest cognitive system.

NOTE

1 Sloterdijk, P. (2013). *You Must Change Your Life* (W. Hoban, Trans.). Polity Press. (Originally published 2009). 449.

REFERENCES

Alder, M. N., Rogozin, I. B., Iyer, L. M., Glazko, G. V., Cooper, M. D., & Pancer, Z. (2005). Diversity and function of adaptive immune receptors in a jawless vertebrate. *Science, 310*, 1970–1973. doi: 10.1126/science.1119420.

Alpi, A., Amrhein, N., Bertl, A., Blatt, M. R., Blumwald, E., Cervone, F., Dainty, J., De Michelis, M. I., Epstein, E., Galston, A. W., Goldsmith, M. H., Hawes, C., Hell, R., Hetherington, A., Hofte, H., Juergens, G., Leaver, C. J., Moroni, A., Murphy, A., Oparka, K., et al. (2007). Plant neurobiology: no brain, no gain? *Trends in Plant Science, 12*, 135–136. doi: 10.1016/j.tplants.2007.03.002.

Alwan, W. (2013). Evolution is rigged! A review of Thomas Nagel's "Mind and Cosmos". https://partiallyexaminedlife.com/2013/02/07/evolution-is-rigged-a-review-of-thomas-nagels-mind-and-cosmos/.

Andersson, A. F., & Banfield, J. F. (2008). Virus population dynamics and acquired virus resistance in natural microbial communities. *Science, 320*, 1047–1050. doi: 10.1126/science.1157358.

Armitage, S. A. O., Kurtz, J., Brites, D., Dong, Y., Du Pasquier, L., & Wang, H. C. (2017). *Dscam1* in Pancrustacean immunity: Current status and a look to the future. *Frontiers in Immunology, 8*, 662. doi: 10.3389/fimmu.2017.00662.

Avery, O. T., MacLeod, C. M., & McCarty, M. (1944). Studies on the chemical nature of the substance inducing transformation of pneumococcal types: Induction of transformation by a desoxyribonucleic acid fraction isolated from pneumococcus type III. *Journal of Experimental Medicine, 79*, 137–158. doi: 10.1084/jem.79.2.137.

Baluška, F., & Levin, M. (2016). On having no head: Cognition throughout biological systems. *Frontiers in Psychology, 7*, 902. doi: 10.3389/fpsyg.2016.00902.

Barandiaran, X., & Moreno, A. (2006). On what makes certain dynamical systems cognitive: A minimally cognitive organization program. *Adaptive Behavior, 14*, 171–185. doi: 10.1177/1059712306014002008.

Barrangou, R. (2015). The roles of CRISPR-Cas systems in adaptive immunity and beyond. *Current Opinion in Immunology, 32*, 36–41. doi: 10.1016/j.coi.2014.12.008.

Beckers, G. J. M., Jaskiewicz, M., Liu, Y., Underwood, W. R., He, S. Y., Zhang, S., & Conrath, U. (2009). Mitogen-activated protein kinases 3 and 6 are required for full priming of stress responses in *Arabidopsis thaliana*. *Plant Cell, 21*, 944–953. doi: 10.1105/tpc.108.062158.

Beer, R. D. (2003). The dynamics of active categorical perception in an evolved model agent. *Adaptive Behavior, 11*, 209–243. doi: 10.1177/1059712303114001.

Behe, M. J. (1996). *Darwin's Black Box: The Biochemical Challenge to Evolution*. Free Press.

Bent, A. F. (1996). Plant disease resistance genes: Function meets structure. *Plant Cell, 8*, 1757–1771. doi: 10.1105/tpc.8.10.1757.

Bergson, H. (1920). *Mind-Energy: Lectures and Essays*. (H. W. Carr, Trans.). Henry Holt and Company. (Originally published 1919). 3–36.

Biffen, R. H. (1907). Studies on the inheritance of disease resistance. *Journal of Agricultural Science, 2*, 109–128. doi: 10.1017/S0021859600001234.

Bigger, C. H., Jokiel, P. L., Hildemann, W. H., & Johnston, I. S. (1982). Characterization of alloimmune memory in a sponge. *Journal of Immunology, 129*, 1570–1572. doi: 10.4049/jimmunol.129.4.1570.

Bille, E., Zahar, J.-R., Perrin, A., Morelle, S., Kriz, P., Jolley, K. A., Maiden, M. C. J., Dervin, C., Nassif, X., & Tinsley, C. R. (2005). A chromosomally integrated bacteriophage in invasive meningococci. *Journal of Experimental Medicine, 201*, 1905–1913. doi: 10.1084/jem.20050112.

Block, N. (1995). On a confusion about a function of consciousness. *Behavioral and Brain Sciences, 18*, 227–247. doi: 10.1017/S0140525X00038188.

Bolotin, A., Quinquis, B., Sorokin, A., & Ehrlich, S. D. (2005). Clustered regularly interspaced short palindrome repeats (CRISPRs) have spacers of extrachromosomal origin. *Microbiology, 151*, 2551–2561. doi: 10.1099/mic.0.28048-0.

Bomblies, K., Lempe, J., Epple, P., Warthmann, N., Lanz, C., Dangl, J. L., & Weigel, D. (2007). Autoimmune response as a mechanism for a Dobzhansky-Muller-type incompatibility syndrome in plants. *PLoS Biology, 5*, e236. doi: 10.1371/journal.pbio.0050236.

Bomblies, K., & Weigel, D. (2007). Hybrid necrosis: Autoimmunity as a potential gene-flow barrier in plant species. *Nature Reviews Genetics, 8*, 382–393. doi: 10.1038/nrg2082.

Boysen, A., Ellehauge, E., Julien, B., & Søgaard-Andersen, L. (2002). The DevT protein stimulates synthesis of FruA, a signal transduction protein required for fruiting body morphogenesis in *Myxococcus xanthus*. *Journal of Bacteriology, 184*, 1540–1546. doi: 10.1128/JB.184.6.1540-1546.2002.

Brennan, J. J., & Gilmore, T. D. (2018). Evolutionary origins of Toll-like receptor signaling. *Molecular Biology and Evolution, 35*, 1576–1587. doi: 10.1093/molbev/msy050.

Brouns, S. J., Jore, M. M., Lundgren, M., Westra, E. R., Slijkhuis, R. J. H., Snijders, A. P. L., Dickman, M. J., Makarova, L. S., Koonin, E. V., & van der Oost, J. (2008). Small CRISPR RNAs guide antiviral defense in prokaryotes. *Science, 321*, 960–964. doi: 10.1126/science.1159689.

Brown, T., & Rodriguez-Lanetty, M. (2015). Defending against pathogens - immunological priming and its molecular basis in a sea anemone, cnidarian. *Scientific Reports, 5*, 17425. doi: 10.1038/srep17425.

Buss, L. W., Moore, J. L., & Green, D. R. (1985). Autoreactivity and self-tolerance in an invertebrate. *Nature, 313*, 400–402. doi: 10.1038/313400a0.

Cannon, J. P., Haire, R. N., & Litman, G. W. (2002). Identification of diversified genes that contain immunoglobulin-like variable regions in a protochordate. *Nature Immunology, 3*, 1200–1207. doi: 10.1038/ni849.

Cao, H., Bowling, S. A., Gordon, S., & Dong, X. (1994). Characterization of an Arabidopsis mutant that is nonresponsive to inducers of systemic acquired resistance. *Plant Cell, 6*, 1583–1592. doi: 10.1105/tpc.6.11.1583.

Champer, J., Buchman, A., & Akbari, O. S. (2016). Cheating evolution: Engineering gene drives to manipulate the fate of wild populations. *Nature Reviews Genetics, 17*, 146–159. doi: 10.1038/nrg.2015.34.

Cheng, Y. T., Li, Y., Huang, S., Huang, Y., Dong, X., Zhang, Y., & Li, X. (2011). Stability of plant immune-receptor resistance proteins is controlled by SKP1-CULLIN1-F-box (SCF)-mediated protein degradation. *Proceedings of the National Academy of Sciences of the United States of America, 108*, 14694–14699. doi: 10.1073/pnas.1105685108.

Chester, K. S. (1933). The problem of acquired physiological immunity in plants. *Quarterly Review of Biology, 8*, 275–324. doi: 10.1086/394440.

Chisholm, S. T., Coaker, G., Day, B., & Staskawicz, B. J. (2006). Host-microbe interactions: Shaping the evolution of the plant immune response. *Cell, 124*, 803–814. doi: 10.1016/j.cell.2006.02.008.

Clark, A. (1998). *Being There: Putting Brain, Body, and World Together Again*. MIT Press.

Clark, A., & Chalmers, D. (1998). The extended mind. *Analysis, 58*, 7–19. doi: 10.1093/analys/58.1.7.

Cohen, I. R. (1992a). The cognitive paradigm and the immunological homunculus. *Immunology Today, 13*, 490–494. doi: 10.1016/0167-5699(92)90024-2.

Cohen, I. R. (1992b). The cognitive principal challenges clonal selection. *Immunology Today, 13*, 441–444. doi: 10.1016/0167-5699(92)90071-E.

Cohen, I. R. (2000). *Tending Adam's Garden: Evolving the Cognitive Immune Self*. Academic Press.

Cohen, I. R., & Young, D. B. (1991). Autoimmunity, microbial immunity and the immunological homunculus. *Immunology Today, 12*, 105–110. doi: 10.1016/0167-5699(91)90093-9.

Dangl, J. L., & Jones, J. D. G. (2001). Plant pathogens and integrated defence responses to infection. *Nature, 411*, 826–833. doi: 10.1038/35081161.

Davis, B. D. (1950). Nonfiltrability of the agents of genetic recombination in *Escherichia coli*. *Journal of Bacteriology, 60*, 507–508. doi: 10.1128/jb.60.4.507-508.1950.

De Tomaso, A. W., Nyholm, S. V., Palmeri, K. J., Ishizuka, K. J., Ludington, W. B., Mitchel, K., & Weissman, I. L. (2005). Isolation and characterization of a protochordate histocompatibility locus. *Nature, 438*, 454–459. doi: 10.1038/nature04150.

Dembski, W. A. (1998). *The Design Inference: Eliminating Chance through Small Probabilities*. Cambridge University Press.

Ding, S. W., & Voinnet, O. (2007). Antiviral immunity directed by small RNAs. *Cell, 130*, 413–426. doi: 10.1016/j.cell.2007.07.039.

Dishaw, L. J., Giacomelli, S., Melillo, D., Zucchetti, I., Haire, R. N., Natale, L., Russo, N. A., De Santis, R., Litman, G. W., & Pinto, M. R. (2011). A role for variable region-containing chitin-binding proteins (VCBPs) in host gut-bacteria interactions. *Proceedings of the National Academy of Sciences of the United States of America, 108*, 16747–16752. doi: 10.1073/pnas.1109687108.

Dobzhansky, T. (1973). Nothing in biology makes sense except in the light of evolution. *The American Biology Teacher, 35*, 125–129. doi: 10.2307/4444260.

Dong, X. (2004). NPR1, all things considered. *Current Opinion in Plant Biology, 7*, 547–552. doi: 10.1016/j.pbi.2004.07.005.

Dupuis, M.-E., Villion, M., Magadán, A. H., & Moineau, S. (2013). CRISPR-Cas and restriction-modification systems are compatible and increase phage resistance. *Nature Communications, 4*, 2087. doi: 10.1038/ncomms3087.

Edelman, G. M. (2004). *Wider Than the Sky: The Phenomenal Gift of Consciousness*. Yale University Press.

Eleftherianos, I., Heryanto, C., Bassal, T., Zhang, W., Tettamanti, G., & Mohamed, A. (2021). Haemocyte-mediated immunity in insects: Cells, processes and associated components in the fight against pathogens and parasites. *Immunology, 164*, 401–432. doi: 10.1111/imm.13390.

Ellis, J., Dodds, P., & Pryor, T. (2000). Structure, function and evolution of plant disease resistance genes. *Current Opinion in Plant Biology, 3*, 278–284. doi: 10.1016/s1369-5266(00)00080-7.

Feuda, R., Dohrmann, M., Pett, W., Philippe, H., Rota-Stabelli, O., Lartillot, N., Wörheide, G., & Pisani, D. (2017). Improved modeling of compositional heterogeneity supports sponges as sister to all other animals. *Current Biology, 27*, 3864–3870. doi: 10.1016/j.cub.2017.11.008.

Fire, A., Xu, S., Montgomery, M. K., Kostas, S. A., Driver, S. E., & Mello, C. C. (1998). Potent and specific genetic interference by double-stranded RNA in *Caenorhabditis elegans*. *Nature, 391*, 806–811. doi: 10.1038/35888.

Flor, H. H. (1956). The complementary genic systems in flax and flax rust. *Advances in Genetics, 8*, 29–54. doi: 10.1016/S0065-2660(08)60498-8.

Flor, H. H. (1971). Current status of the gene-for-gene concept. *Annual Review of Phytopathology, 9*, 275–296. doi: 10.1146/annurev.py.09.090171.001423.

Godfrey-Smith, P. (2016). Individuality, subjectivity, and minimal cognition. *Biology and Philosophy, 31*, 775–796. doi: 10.1007/s10539-016-9543-1.

Griffith, F. (1928). The significance of pneumococcal types. *Journal of Hygiene, 27*, 113–159. doi: 10.1017/s0022172400031879.

Grissa, I., Vergnaud, G., & Pourcel, C. (2007). The CRISPRdb database and tools to display CRISPRs and to generated dictionaries of spacers and repeats. *BMC Bioinformatics, 8*, 172. doi: 10.1186/1471-2105-8-172.

Gunderson, F. F., & Cianciotto, N. P. (2013). The CRISPR-associated gene *cas2* of *Legionella pneumophila* is required for intracellular infection of ameobae. *mBio, 4*, e00074–00013. doi: 10.1128/mBio.00074-13.

Guo, P., Hirano, M., Herrin, B. R., Li, J., Yu, C., Sadlonova, A., & Cooper, M. D. (2009). Dual nature of the adaptive immune system in lampreys. *Nature, 459*, 796–801. doi: 10.1038/nature08068.

Gurwitz, D. (2014). Gene drives raise dual-use concerns. *Science, 345*, 1010. doi: 10.1126/science.345.6200.1010-b.

Habibi, L., Ebtekar, M., & Jameie, S. B. (2009). Immune and nervous systems share molecular and functional similarities: Memory storage mechanism. *Scandinavian Journal of Immunology, 69*, 291–301. doi: 10.1111/j.1365-3083.2008.02215.x.

Hammond-Kosack, K. E., & Kanyuka, K. (2007). Resistance genes (R genes) in plants. *Encyclopedia of Life Sciences*. John Wiley & Sons. 1–21. Doi: 10.1002/9780470015902.a0020119

Hayes, W. (1952). Recombination in *Bact. coli K* 12: Unidirectional transfer of genetic material. *Nature, 169*, 118–119. doi: 10.1038/169118b0.

Hernández López, J., Schuehly, W., Crailsheim, K., & Riessberger-Gallé, U. (2014). Trans-generational immune priming in honeybees. *Proceedings of the Royal Society B: Biological Sciences, 281*, 20140454. doi: 10.1098/rspb.2014.0454.

Hershberg, U., & Efroni, S. (2001). The immune system and other cognitive systems. *Complexity, 6*, 19–26. doi: 10.1002/cplx.1046.

Hershey, A. D., & Chase, M. (1952). Independent functions of viral protein and nucleic acid in growth of bacteriophage. *Journal of General Physiology, 36*, 39–56. doi: 10.1085/jgp.36.1.39.

Hildemann, W. H., Bigger, C. H., Johnston, I. S., & Jokiel, P. L. (1980). Characteristics of transplantation immunity in the sponge, *Callyspongia diffusa*. *Transplantation, 30*, 362–367. doi: 10.1097/00007890-198011000-00011.

Hildemann, W. H., Johnson, I. S., & Jokiel, P. L. (1979). Immunocompetence in the lowest metazoan phylum: Transplantation immunity in sponges. *Science, 204*, 420–422. doi: 10.1126/science.441730.

Hildemann, W. H., Raison, R. L., Cheung, G., Hull, C. J., Akaka, L., & Okamoto, J. (1977). Immunological specificity and memory in a scleractinian coral. *Nature, 270*, 219–223. doi: 10.1038/270219a0.

Hirano, M., Guo, P., McCurley, N., Schorpp, M., Das, S., Boehm, T., & Cooper, M. D. (2013). Evolutionary implications of a third lymphocyte lineage in lampreys. *Nature, 501*, 435–438. doi: 10.1038/nature12467.

Hoffmeyer, J. (2011). Biology is immature biosemiotics. (C. Emmeche, & K. Kull, Eds.) *Towards a Semiotic Biology: Life Is the Action of Signs*. Imperial College Press. 43–65.

Hynes, A. P., Villion, M., & Moineau, S. (2014). Adaptation in bacterial CRISPR-Cas immunity can be driven by defective phages. *Nature Communications, 5*, 4399. doi: 10.1038/ncomms5399.

Ishino, Y., Shinagawa, H., Makino, K., Amemura, M., & Nakata, A. (1987). Nucleotide sequence of the *iap* gene, responsible for alkaline phosphatase isozyme conversion in *Escherichia coli*, and identification of the gene product. *Journal of Bacteriology, 169*, 5429–5433. doi: 10.1128/jb.169.12.5429-5433.1987.

Janeway, C. A., Jr., & Medzhitov, R. (2002). Innate immune recognition. *Annual Review of Immunology, 20*, 197–216. doi: 10.1146/annurev.immunol.20.083001.084359.

Jansen, R., Embden, J. D., Gaastra, W., & Schouls, L. M. (2002). Identification of genes that are associated with DNA repeats in prokaryotes. *Molecular Microbiology, 43*, 1565–1575. doi: 10.1046/j.1365-2958. 2002.02839.x.

Jeuken, M. J., Zhang, N. W., McHale, L. K., Pelgrom, K., den Boer, E., Lindhout, P., Michelmore, R. W., Visser, R. G., & Niks, R. E. (2009). *Rin4* causes hybrid necrosis and race-specific resistance in an interspecific lettuce hybrid. *Plant Cell, 21*, 3368–3378. doi: 10.1105/tpc.109.070334.

Jinek, M., Chylinski, K., Fonfara, I., Hauer, M., Doudna, J. A., & Charpentier, E. (2012). A programmable dual-RNA-guided DNA endonuclease in adaptive bacterial immunity. *Science, 337*, 816–821. doi: 10.1126/science.1225829.

Jones, J. D. G., & Dangl, J. L. (2006). The plant immune system. *Nature, 444*, 323–329. doi: 10.1038/ nature05286.

Karadge, U. B., Gosto, M., & Nicotra, M. L. (2015). Allorecognition proteins in an invertebrate exhibit homophilic interactions. *Current Biology, 25*, 2845–2850. doi: 10.1016/j.cub.2015.09.030.

Karginov, F. V., & Hannon, G. J. (2010). The CRISPR system: Small RNA-guided defense in bacteria and archaea. *Molecular Cell, 37*, 7–19. doi: 10.1016/j.molcel.2009.12.033.

Kasamatsu, J., Sutoh, Y., Fugo, K., Otsuka, N., Iwabuchi, K., & Kasahara, M. (2010). Identification of a third variable lymphocyte receptor in the lamprey. *Proceedings of the National Academy of Sciences of the United States of America, 107*, 14304–14308. doi: 10.1073/pnas.1001910107.

Keijzer, F. (2003). Making decisions does not suffice for minimal cognition. *Adaptive Behavior, 11*, 266–269. doi: 10.1177/1059712303114006.

Kim, S. H., Gao, F., Bhattacharjee, S., Adiasor, J. A., Nam, J. C., & Gassmann, W. (2010). The Arabidopsis resistance-like gene *SNC1* is activated by mutations in *SRFR1* and contributes to resistance to the bacterial effector AvrRps4. *PLoS Pathogens, 6*, e1001172. doi: 10.1371/journal.ppat.1001172.

Kioussis, D., & Pachnis, V. (2009). Immune and nervous systems: More than just a superficial similarity? *Immunity, 31*, 705–710. doi: 10.1016/j.immuni.2009.09.009.

Koonin, E. V., & Wolf, Y. I. (2009). Is evolution Darwinian or/and Lamarckian? *Biology Direct, 4*, 42. doi: 10.1186/1745-6150-4-42.

Koshland, D. E., Jr. (1974). Chemotaxis as a model for sensory systems. *FEBS Letters, 40*, S3–S9. doi: 10.1016/0014-5793(74)80683-6.

Kourelis, J., & van der Hoorn, R. A. L. (2018). Defended to the nines: 25 years of resistance gene cloning identifies nine mechanisms for R protein function. *Plant Cell, 30*, 285–299. doi: 10.1105/tpc.17.00579.

Kurtz, J., & Armitage, S. A. (2006). Alternative adaptive immunity in invertebrates. *Trends in Immunology, 27*, 493–496. doi: 10.1016/j.it.2006.09.001.

Lakoff, G., & Johnson, M. (1980). *Metaphors We Live By*. University of Chicago Press.

Lamarck, J. B. (1815). *Histoire naturelle des animaux sans vertèbres, Tome 1 (Natural History of the Invertebrate Animals, Volume 1)*. Abel Lanoë. 181–182.

Lederberg, J., & Tatum, E. L. (1946). Gene recombination in *Escherichia coli*. *Nature, 158*, 558. doi: 10.1038/158558a0.

Lemaitre, B., Nicolas, E., Michaut, L., Reichart, J. M., & Hoffmann, J. A. (1996). The dorsoventral regulatory gene cassette *spätzle/Toll/cactus* controls the potent antifungal response in Drosophila adults. *Cell, 86*, 973–983. doi: 10.1016/s0092-8674(00)80172-5.

Li, C. W., Chen, J. Y., & Hua, T. E. (1998). Precambrian sponges with cellular structures. *Science, 279*, 879–882. doi: 10.1126/science.279.5352.879.

Li, Y., Li, S., Bi, D., Cheng, Y. T., Li, X., & Zhang, Y. (2010). SRFR1 negatively regulates plant NB-LRR resistance protein accumulation to prevent autoimmunity. *PLoS Pathogens, 6*, e1001111. doi: 10.1371/ journal.ppat.1001111.

Litman, G. W., Cannon, J. P., & Dishaw, L. J. (2005). Reconstruction immune phylogeny: New perspective. *Nature Reviews Immunology, 5*, 866–879. doi: 10.1038/nri1712.

Loker, E. S., Adema, C. M., Zhang, S. M., & Kepler, T. B. (2004). Invertebrate immune systems - not homogeneous, not simple, not well understood. *Immunological Reviews, 198*, 10–24. doi: 10.1111/j.0105-28 96.2004.0117.x.

Luna, E., Bruce, T. J. A., Roberts, M. R., Flors, V., & Ton, J. (2012). Next-generation systemic acquired resistance. *Plant Physiology, 158*, 844–853. doi: 10.1104/pp.111.187468.

Lyon, P. (2015). The cognitive cell: Bacterial behavior reconsidered. *Frontiers in Microbiology, 6*, 264. doi: 10.3389/fmicb.2015.00264.

Makarova, K. S., Aravind, L., Grishin, N. V., Rogozin, I. B., & Koonin, E. V. (2002). A DNA repair system specific for thermophilic Archaea and bacteria predicted by genomic context analysis. *Nucleic Acids Research, 30*, 482–496. doi: 10.1093/nar/30.2.482.

Makarova, K. S., Grishin, N. V., Shabalina, S. A., Wolf, Y. I., & Koonin, E. V. (2006). A putative RNA-interference-based immune system in prokaryotes: Computational analysis of the predicted enzymatic machinery, functional analogies with eukaryotic RNAi, and hypothetical mechanisms of action. *Biology Direct, 1*, 7. doi: 10.1186/1745-6150-1-7.

Makarova, K. S., Wolf, Y. I., Iranzo, J., Shmakov, S. A., Alkhnbashi, O. S., Brouns, S. J., Charpentier, E., Cheng, D., Haft, D. H., Horvath, P., Moineau, S., Mojica, F. J. M., Scott, D., Shah, S. A., Siksnys, V., Terns, M. P., Venclovas, Č., White, M. F., Yakunin, A. F., Yan, W., et al. (2020). Evolutionary classification of CRISPR-Cas systems: A burst of class 2 and derived variants. *Nature Reviews Microbiology, 18*, 67–83. doi: 10.1038/s41579-019-0299-x.

Makarova, K. S., Wolf, Y. I., & Koonin, E. V. (2013). The basic building blocks and evolution of CRISPR-Cas systems. *Biochemical Society Transactions, 41*, 1392–1400. doi: 10.1042/BST20130038.

Marraffini, L. A., & Sontheimer, E. J. (2008). CRISPR interference limits horizontal gene transfer in straphylococci by targeting DNA. *Science, 322*, 1843–1845. doi: 10.1126/science.1165771.

Marraffini, L. A., & Sontheimer, E. J. (2010a). CRISPR interference: RNA-directed adaptive immunity in bacteria and archaea. *Nature Reviews Genetics, 11*, 181–190. doi: 10.1038/nrg2749.

Marraffini, L. A., & Sontheimer, E. J. (2010b). Self versus non-self discrimination during CRISPR RNA-directed immunity. *Nature, 463*, 568–571. doi: 10.1038/nature08703.

Mehlhop-Williams, E. R., & Bevan, M. J. (2014). Memory CD8+ T cells exhibit increased antigen threshold requirements for recall proliferation. *Journal of Experimental Medicine, 211*, 345–356. doi: 10.1084/jem.20131271.

Menary, R. (Ed.) (2010). *The Extended Mind*. MIT Press.

Metchnikoff, E. (1892). *Leçons sur la pathologie comparée de l'inflammation (Lectures on the Comparative Pathology of Inflammation)*. G. Mason. 51–66.

Misof, B., Liu, S., Meusemann, K., Peters, R. S., Donath, A., Mayer, C., Frandsen, P. B., Ware, J., Flouri, T., Beutel, R. G., Niehuis, O., Petersen, M., Izquierdo-Carrasco, F., Wappler, T., Rust, J., Aberer, A. J., Aspock, U., Aspock, H., Bartel, D., Blanke, A. B., S., et al. (2014). Phylogenomics resolves the timing and pattern of insect evolution. *Science, 346*, 763–767. doi: 10.1126/science.1257570.

Mojica, F. J., Diez-Villasenor, C., Garcia-Martinez, J., & Soria, E. (2005). Intervening sequences of regularly spaced prokaryotic repeats derive from foreign genetic elements. *Journal of Molecular Evolution, 60*, 174–182. doi: 10.1007/s00239-004-0046-3.

Moulin, A. M. (1995). Clés pour l'histoire de l'immunologie (Keys for the history of immunology) (M. Daëron, Ed.). *Le Système immunitaire ou l'immunité cent ans après Pasteur (The Immune System or Immunity a 100 years after Pasteur)*. Nathan. 122–131.

Nagel, T. (1974). What is it like to be a bat? *Philosophical Review, 83*, 435–450. doi: 10.2307/2183914.

Nagel, T. (2012). *Mind and Cosmos: Why the Materialist Neo-Darwinian Conception of Nature Is Almost Certainly False*. Oxford University Press.

Napoli, C., Lemieux, C., & Jorgensen, R. (1990). Introduction of a chimeric chalcone synthase gene into petunia results in reversible co-suppression of homologous genes in trans. *Plant Cell, 2*, 279–289. doi: 10.1105/tpc.2.4.279.

Nataf, S. (2014). The sensory immune system: A neural twist to the antigenic discontinuity theory. *Nature Reviews Immunology, 14*, 280. doi: 10.1038/nri3521-c1.

Newman, M. A., Sundelin, T., Nielsenand, J. T., & Erbs, G. (2013). MAMP (microbe-associated molecular pattern) triggered immunity in plants. *Frontiers in Plant Science, 4*, 139. doi: 10.3389/fpls.2013.00139.

Orr, H. A. (1996). Dobzhansky, Bateson, and the genetics of speciation. *Genetics, 144*, 1331–1335. doi: 10.1093/genetics/144.4.1331.

Oye, K. A., Esvelt, K., Appleton, E., Catteruccia, F., Church, G., Kuiken, T., Lightfoot, S. B., McNamara, J., Smidler, A., & Collins, J. P. (2014). Biotechnology. Regulating gene drives. *Science, 345*, 626–628. doi: 10.1126/science.1254287.

Pancer, Z., Amemiya, C. T., Ehrhardt, G. R. A., Ceitlin, J., Gartland, G. L., & Cooper, M. D. (2004). Somatic diversification of variable lymphocyte receptors in the agnathan sea lamprey. *Nature, 430*, 174–180. doi: 10.1038/nature02740.

Pham, L. N., Dionne, M. S., Shirasu-Hiza, M., & Schneider, D. S. (2007). A specific primed immune response in *Drosophila* is dependent on phagocytes. *PLoS Pathogens, 3*, e26. doi: 10.1371/journal.ppat.0030026.

Pita, L., Hoeppner, M. P., Ribes, M., & Hentschel, U. (2018). Differential expression of immune receptors in two marine sponges upon exposure to microbial-associated molecular patterns. *Scientific Reports, 8,* 16081. doi: 10.1038/s41598-018-34330-w.

Pourcel, C., Salvignol, G., & Vergnaud, G. (2005). CRISPR elements in *Yersinia pestis* acquire new repeats by preferential uptake of bacteriophage DNA and provide additional tools for evolutionary studies. *Microbiology, 151,* 653–663. doi: 10.1099/mic.0.27437-0.

Ramos, G. C., Vaz, N. M., & Saalfeld, K. (2006). Wings for flying, lymphocytes for defense: Spandrels, exaptation and specific immunity. *Complexus, 3,* 211–216. doi: 10.1159/000095881.

Rimer, J., Cohen, I. R., & Friedman, N. (2014). Do all creatures possess an acquired immune system of some sort? *Bioessays, 36,* 273–281. doi: 10.1002/bies.201300124.

Rodrigues, J., Brayner, F. A., Alves, L. C., Dixit, R., & Barillas-Mury, C. (2010). Hemocyte differentiation mediates innate immune memory in *Anopheles gambiae* mosquitoes. *Science, 329,* 1353–1355. doi: 10.1126/science.1190689.

Ross, A. F. (1961). Systemic acquired resistance induced by localized virus infections in plants. *Virology, 14,* 340–358. doi: 10.1016/0042-6822(61)90319-1.

Roth, O., Sadd, B. M., Schmid-Hempel, P., & Kurtz, J. (2009). Strain-specific priming of resistance in the red flour beetle, *Tribolium castaneum. Proceedings of the Royal Society B: Biological Sciences, 276,* 145–151. doi: 10.1098/rspb.2008.1157.

Sadd, B. M., & Schmid-Hempel, P. (2006). Insect immunity shows specificity in protection upon secondary pathogen exposure. *Current Biology, 16,* 1206–1210. doi: 10.1016/j.cub.2006.04.047.

Sampson, T. R., Saroj, S. D., Llewellyn, A. C., Tzeng, Y. L., & Weiss, D. S. (2013). A CRISPR/Cas system mediates bacterial innate immune evasion and virulence. *Nature, 497,* 254–257. doi: 10.1038/nature12048.

Sampson, T. R., & Weiss, D. S. (2013). Alternative roles for CRISPR/Cas systems in bacterial pathogenesis. *PLoS Pathogens, 9,* e1003621. doi: 10.1371/journal.ppat.1003621.

Samson, J. E., Magadán, A. H., Sabri, M., & Moineau, S. (2013). Revenge of the phages: Defeating bacterial defences. *Nature Reviews Microbiology, 11,* 675–687. doi: 10.1038/nrmicro3096.

Schmucker, D., Clemens, J. C., Shu, H., Worby, C. A., Xiao, J., Muda, M., Dixon, J. E., & Zipursky, S. L. (2000). *Drosophila* Dscam is an axon guidance receptor exhibiting extraordinary molecular diversity. *Cell, 101,* 671–684. doi: 10.1016/s0092-8674(00)80878-8.

Scofield, V. L., Schlumpberger, J. M., West, L. A., & Weissman, I. L. (1982). Protochordate allorecognition is controlled by a MHC-like gene system. *Nature, 295,* 499–502. doi: 10.1038/295499a0.

Seed, K. D., Lazinski, D. W., Calderwood, S. B., & Camilli, A. (2013). A bacteriophage encodes its own CRISPR/Cas adaptive response to evade host innate immunity. *Nature, 494,* 489–491. doi: 10.1038/nature11927.

Shah, J., & Zeier, J. (2013). Long-distance communication and signal amplification in systemic acquired resistance. *Frontiers in Plant Science, 4,* 30. doi: 10.3389/fpls.2013.00030.

Sharrock, J., & Sun, J. C. (2020). Innate immunological memory: From plants to animals. *Current Opinion in Immunology, 62,* 69–78. doi: 10.1016/j.coi.2019.12.001.

Shinzato, C., Shoguchi, E., Kawashima, T., Hamada, M., Hisata, K., Tanaka, M., Fujie, M., Fujiwara, M., Koyanagi, R., Ikuta, T., Fujiyama, A., Miller, D. J., & Satoh, N. (2011). Using the *Acropora digitifera* genome to understand coral responses to environmental change. *Nature, 476,* 320–323. doi: 10.1038/nature10249.

Sober, E. (2012). Remarkable facts. Ending science as we know it. *Boston Review.* https://www.bostonreview.net/archives/BR37.6/elliott_sober_thomas_nagel_mind_cosmos.php.

Sorek, R., Koonin, V., & Hugenholtz, P. (2008). CRISPR--a widespread system that provides acquired resistance against phages in bacteria and archaea. *Nature Reviews Microbiology, 6,* 181–186. doi: 10.1038/nrmicro1793.

Stern, A., Keren, L., Wurtzel, O., Amitai, G., & Sorek, R. (2010). Self-targeting by CRISPR: Gene regulation or autoimmunity? *Trends in Genetics, 26,* 335–340. doi: 10.1016/j.tig.2010.05.008.

Struik, P. C., Yin, X., & Meinke, H. (2008). Plant neurobiology and green plant intelligence: Science, metaphors and nonsense. *Journal of the Science of Food and Agriculture, 88,* 363–370. doi: 10.1002/jsfa.3131.

Technau, U., & Steele, R. E. (2011). Evolutionary crossroads in developmental biology: Cnidaria. *Development, 138,* 1447–1458. doi: 10.1242/dev.048959.

Thöny-Meyer, L., & Kaiser, D. (1993). *devRS,* an autoregulated and essential genetic locus for fruiting body development in *Myxococcus xanthus. Journal of Bacteriology, 175,* 7450–7462. doi: 10.1128/jb.175.22.7450-7462.1993.

Thomas, T., Moitinho-Silva, L., Lurgi, M., Björk, J. R., Easson, C., Astudillo-García, C., Olson, J. B., Erwin, P. M., López-Legentil, S., Luter, H., Chaves-Fonnegra, A., Costa, R., Schupp, P. J., Steindler, L., Erpenbeck, D., Gilbert, J., Knight, R., Ackermann, G., Lopez, J. V., Taylor, M. W., et al. (2016). Diversity, structure and convergent evolution of the global sponge microbiome. *Nature Communications, 7*, 11870. doi: 10.1038/ncomms11870.

Thompson, J. R., Rivera, H. E., Closek, C. J., & Medina, M. (2015). Microbes in the coral holobiont: Partners through evolution, development, and ecological interactions. *Frontiers in Cellular and Infection Microbiology, 4*, 176. doi: 10.3389/fcimb.2014.00176.

Tidbury, H. J., Pedersen, A. B., & Boots, M. (2011). Within and transgenerational immune priming in an insect to a DNA virus. *Proceedings of the Royal Society B: Biological Sciences, 278*, 871–876. doi: 10.1098/rspb.2010.1517.

van der Krol, A. R., Mur, L. A., Beld, M., Mol, J. N., & Stuitje, A. R. (1990). Flavonoid genes in petunia: Addition of a limited number of gene copies may lead to a suppression of gene expression. *Plant Cell, 2*, 291–299. doi: 10.1105/tpc.2.4.291.

van Duijn, M., Keijzer, F., & Franken, D. (2006). Principles of minimal cognition: Casting cognition as senso-rimotor coordination. *Adaptive Behavior, 14*, 157–170. doi: 10.1177/1059712306014400207.

Varela, F. J., Thompson, E., & Rosch, E. (1991). *The Embodied Mind: Cognitive Science and Human Experience*. MIT Press.

Vasu, K., & Nagaraja, V. (2013). Diverse functions of restriction-modification systems in addition to cellular defense. *Microbiology and Molecular Biology Reviews, 77*, 53–72. doi: 10.1128/MMBR.00044-12.

Vaz, N. M., & Varela, F. J. (1978). Self and non-sense: An organism-centered approach to immunology. *Medical Hypotheses, 4*, 231–267. doi: 10.1016/0306-9877(78)90005-1.

Voskoboynik, A., Newman, A. M., Corey, D. M., Sahoo, D., Pushkarev, D., Neff, N. F., Passarelli, B., Koh, W., Ishizuka, K. J., Palmeri, K. J., Dimov, I. K., Keasar, C., Fan, H. C., Mantalas, G. L., Sinha, R., Penland, L., Quake, S. R., & Weissman, I. L. (2013). Identification of a colonial chordate histocompatibility gene. *Science, 341*, 384–387. doi: 10.1126/science.1238036.

Waddington, C. H. (1953). Epigenetics and evolution. *Symposia of the Society for Experimental Biology, 7*, 186–199.

Watson, F. L., Püttmann-Holgado, R., Thomas, F., Lamar, D. L., Hughes, M., Kondo, M., Rebel, V. I., & Schmucker, D. (2005). Extensive diversity of Ig-superfamily proteins in the immune system of insects. *Science, 309*, 1874–1878. doi: 10.1126/science.1116887.

Westra, E. R., Buckling, A., & Fineran, P. C. (2014). CRISPR-Cas systems: Beyond adaptive immunity. *Nature Reviews Microbiology, 12*, 317–326. doi: 10.1038/nrmicro3241.

Wiens, M., Korzhev, M., Perovic-Ottstadt, S., Luthringer, B., Brandt, D., Klein, S., & Müller, W. E. (2007). Toll-like receptors are part of the innate immune defense system of sponges (demospongiae: Porifera). *Molecular Biology and Evolution, 24*, 792–804. doi: 10.1093/molbev/msl208.

Wilson, H. V. (1907). On some phenomena of coalescence and regeneration in sponges. *Journal of Experimental Zoology, 5*, 245–258. doi: 10.1002/jez.1400050204.

Wilson, R. A. (2004). *Boundaries of the Mind: The Individual in the Fragile Sciences - Cognition*. Cambridge University Press.

Zinder, N. D., & Lerderberg, J. (1952). Genetic exchange in Salmonella. *Journal of Bacteriology, 64*, 679–699. doi: 10.1128/jb.64.5.679-699.1952.

Zipfel, C. (2014). Plant pattern-recognition receptors. *Trends in Immunology, 35*, 345–351. doi: 10.1016/j.it.2014.05.004.

5 Metaphysics of Immunity

The guiding motto in the life of every natural philosopher should be, Seek simplicity and distrust it.[1]

Alfred North Whitehead

It is difficult to define science that is universally accepted. Rather than seeking to define it here, I will characterize science today by reflecting on what is done in the biological sciences in particular. In order to understand a life phenomenon, scientists formulate a hypothesis, conduct observations and experiments using various methods, deduce the success or failure of the hypothesis, and collect and construct universal facts. If laws are revealed in the process, it becomes possible to predict what may happen in the future. Originally, the word "science" (*scientia*) meant the sum of knowledge. However, what does "the sum" mean?

In 1872, the German physiologist Emile du Bois-Raymond (1818–1896) remarked at the congress of the Society of German Natural Scientists and Physicians in Leipzig, "*Ignoramus et ignorabimus*" (We do not know and will never know) (du Bois-Reymond, 1874). Will something remain unknowable, no matter how science develops? Conversely, as the German mathematician David Hilbert (1862–1943) stated at the 1930 congress of the Society of German Association of Natural Scientists and Physicians in Königsberg, "We must know, we will know" (Smith, 2014), will the development of science eventually go so far as to reveal the totality of all things?

While debates about this issue will undoubtedly continue, I have personally come to believe that not all facts about nature can be illuminated by the light of science. Just looking back at the history of immunology's development, there continues to be a marked fragmentation of the field, with no sign of a move toward integration. As soon as one mystery is resolved, a new one succeeds it, and each opened door reveals an entirely new world to explore. If this is the true structure of reality, we seem hardly different from Sisyphus, who rolls his boulder uphill, knowing that his work has no end. Even if science is omnipotent and capable of revealing everything, it is unlikely to do so in the near future.

5.1 A METHOD CALLED "METAPHYSICALIZATION OF SCIENCE" (MOS)

In this section, I attempt to introduce the process of MOS for a richer understanding of nature (Yakura, 2020c, 2022, 2023). As I mentioned in the Introduction, this idea came to me when I read Auguste Comte's Law of Three Stages (Comte, 1893). Looking back through history, as science progresses and reveals hidden aspects of nature that were previously the domain of philosophy, old philosophical concepts are replaced by newly established scientific concepts. This process has been repeated as various fields of science have developed. Why, then, should we bring back philosophical elements that were excluded from science more than a century ago and discuss scientifically explainable phenomena? Why do we need the power of philosophy to understand scientific problems more profoundly and to reveal the essence of nature?

One reason for adopting this approach is my intuition that current science is insufficient to capture the essence of nature. Because modern science, including immunology, has taken the approach of segmenting nature and revealing the mechanisms of its parts, the whole is often forgotten, and no attempt is made to reach the essence that pervades the whole. Of course, science desires to gain a perspective that leads to the whole, but it does not have the methodology to do so at present. Moreover, due to the inherent nature of science, this possibility may not be guaranteed in the future. If this is the case, one possibility for getting to the core of natural phenomena is to mobilize a metaphysics that stands on the foundations of science but moves away from them to rethink scientific

DOI: 10.1201/9781003486800-5

findings from a broader perspective. This effort is expected to link nature and culture, the past and the present, and fuse them into an understanding of nature as a whole. We believe that the process, called MOS, will be a pivotal way to reach a fundamental and richer understanding in all areas of science.

Another reason is whether the essence of immunity can be clarified by analyzing only organisms on Earth. The same can be said about the definition of life. Unlike the days when the possibility of life in the universe was considered almost nil, this question cannot be ignored today. To answer it, it may help to have a properly abstracted definition ready in addition to the conclusions that emerge from a purely scientific analysis because it may provide an inclusive view of immunity in its diverse ways of being, as we saw in Chapter 4. When we recognize the current situation in this way, it will be essential to have philosophical and metaphysical reflections based on the findings of science on Earth to reach a deeper and more universal understanding of immunity. If the mission of metaphysics is to provide a rational explanation of nature at the broadest and most inclusive level, it may be possible to derive a view that applies to the universe beyond the Earth.

The MOS comprises three steps. The first step is "scientific extraction," which involves collecting as wide a range of scientific results on the subject phenomenon as possible and identifying the fundamental characteristics or minimal elements that characterize the subject from them. The second step is "philosophical reflection," in which the fundamental characteristics and minimal elements identified in the first step are repeatedly reflected upon while introducing philosophical and metaphysical concepts and arguments in an attempt to approach the essence of the subject while maintaining logical consistency. By going back and forth between the physical and the metaphysical, a world that could not be reached by scientific thinking alone may be opened up. This attempt may not directly contribute to solving concrete problems in the daily life of science. However, it may have an invisible but profound effect on scientists' thinking and imagination.

The MOS position holds the science supposedly conducted independently of metaphysics in high regard. It includes the proposal that science be redefined as an activity that includes a metaphysical reflection on its results. In other words, I hope that many scientists will recognize that science is complete only after philosophical reflection, in which scientific discoveries are discussed and their significance is considered. If you feel uncomfortable with the word "complete" used here, you may call it the "ethic of knowledge" because it refers to the desirable way of knowing in the future. It is based on intellectual activity that combines scientific thinking and metaphysical reflection. I believe this method of cognition is valid beyond science to politics, economics, culture, and even everyday events. Therefore, as a third step, the process of practicing the MOS that transcends the individual and opens up to society is conceived (Yakura, 2020c, 2022, 2023).

After studying mathematics, logic, physics, and philosophy of science in England, Alfred North Whitehead (1861–1947) was invited to teach philosophy at Harvard University at the age of 63, where he developed his own metaphysics until his death at 86. His metaphysics was the original philosophy that the substance of the world is not material but processes and is revealed through interaction with other processes. He brought it to fruition as *Process and Reality* (Whitehead, 1929). As this chapter's epigraph states, Whitehead appealed to all who philosophize about nature to "seek simplicity and distrust it" (Whitehead, 2006). He intended to call attention to the fact that because science aims to segment, analyze, simplify, and explain the complex nature, we are prone to perceive the simple conclusions of science about nature as final. If we were to extend our thinking from these words, we would first use science to simplify nature, but that is only the first step. To attain a deeper understanding of complex nature, we must use thought and philosophy to challenge what science has revealed.

In 1930, Martin Heidegger discussed the problem of essence in a lecture entitled "The Essence of Human Freedom: An Introduction to Philosophy" (Heidegger, 1987). According to Heidegger, to shed light on the essence of a thing is not merely to describe its existence in a measurable form but to talk about it in such a way as to shed light on the foundation of its inner potentiality. In other words, Heidegger believed that to discuss the essence of a thing or a phenomenon is not merely to describe it quantitatively and mathematically, as science does today, but to go beyond that point to explore its hidden potential. This view implies that merely summarizing the results of scientific research does not reach the essence of a thing being dealt with in that research. Furthermore, Heidegger cautions that the essence that results from the quest is far from being ultimately established and is constantly transforming. This view encourages us to repeat again and again the process of further contemplation and fundamental awareness of the scientific findings extracted from the immune phenomenon. In Chapter 5, I aim to shed light on what possibilities lie within immunity, what philosophical themes exist therein, and to understand immunity on a level that has never been reached before. If this leads to clarifying the essence of immunity—that is, a new horizon of the possibilities inherent in immunity—then the attempt by MOS will be meaningful.

The results of the studies on immunity that have been reviewed so far can be summarized as follows. First, regardless of the mechanisms or the structures that support it, the function of immunity exists across species, from bacteria to humans, and is essential for survival in a harsh environment where pathogens exist. This conclusion suggests that immunity is universally recognized throughout the living world and is a fundamental requirement for life.

Second, the basic immune function comprises four elements: receiving stimuli from the external world, integrating that information, responding appropriately to the stimuli based on the integrated information, and remembering the experience. These four functional elements are not only conserved in the immune system of all organisms but also overlap with the functional elements of the nervous system. In other words, the possibility emerges that immunity is essentially a neural-like function of cognition and that the function of defense exists under this principle.

Third, from bacteria to humans, the immune system contains mechanisms for self-recognition and its avoidance, and autoimmune diseases develop when the balance between them is disturbed. Here, the question arises whether autoimmunity is merely a phenomenon caused by a system's functional abnormality or whether self-recognition is a physiological necessity for living organisms.

Fourth, in multicellular organisms, the immune function has been assumed to be performed by the part that has been called the immune system, which not only forms a network often referred to as "psycho-neuro-endocrino-immune" but is also involved in the basic function of metabolism. In other words, immunity is supported by the entire organism and can be seen as an expression of its functions as a whole. This situation raises the question of how to define immunity as a system. If the immune system's boundaries overlap with those of the organism, any attempt to explore the nature of immunity will ultimately be concerned with the question of life or its control in general.

In reflecting on this search for the essence of immunity, I was reminded of Spinoza's *conatus*—"effort" or "striving" of a thing to continue to exist—as one of the philosophical themes that immunity encompasses. This concept also has the moral implication that it is good to maintain an equilibrium that leads toward existence and bad to disturb it. I will now reflect on immunity from the two perspectives of *conatus* and the normativity of life to get at its essence.

5.2   IMMUNITY IN LIGHT OF SPINOZA'S PHILOSOPHY

First, let us consider how *conatus*, a principal theme of Spinoza's philosophy, relates to immunity, referring to his main work *The Ethics*, published posthumously in 1677 (Spinoza, 2009). Spinoza's philosophy has an important formula, *Deus sive Natura* (God, or Nature), which is his answer to the mind-body problem that began with Descartes and remains unresolved to this day, as well as to his view of nature. *The Ethics* begins with a discussion of God, but Spinoza's God is not the biblical God. According to his definition, God is "a being absolutely infinite—that is, a substance consisting in infinite attributes, of which each expresses eternal and infinite essentiality" (*The Ethics*, Part I, Definition VI) and is "the indwelling and not the transient cause of all things" (Part I, Proposition XVIII). Here, an attribute is "that which the intellect perceives as constituting the essence of substance" (Part I, Definition IV), and substance is "that which is in itself, and is conceived through itself: in other words, that of which a conception can be formed independently of any other conception" (Part I, Definition III). Spinoza's substance is unique in that it does not result from other causes. It is self-sufficient and generated by its own cause (*sui generis*). Furthermore, there is only one substance, called God, and no other substances (Part I, Propositions VI–VIII and XI). Taking all of this into consideration, God shares boundaries with nature or the totality of what exists within this world.

It has been pointed out that a similar panpsychism appears to be embedded in Tendai Hongaku Buddhist Thought as the core idea of Japanese culture (Umehara, 2013). There are phrases that eloquently illustrate it, such as « 草木国土悉皆成仏 » (*somoku kokudo shikkai jobutsu*), literally meaning "The grasses, trees, and land, all without exception attain Buddhahood" or « 山川草木悉皆成仏 » (*sansen somoku shikkai jobutsu*), meaning "The mountains, rivers, grasses, and trees, all have the Buddha nature." The meaning of these phrases is that not only animate but inanimate things are conscious beings who come to be Buddha (Umehara, 2013; Yakura, 2015). In this light, the findings of immunology to date, that immunity as a cognitive system exists in all organisms, resonate with the deep roots of Japanese culture.

Descartes advocated substance dualism that claims that this world consists of two entities: non-extended thought entities (*res cogitans*) and extended physical entities (*res extensa*). In contrast, Spinoza, who was influenced by Descartes, used Descartes' concept to advance his argument, but his conclusions were quite different. He argued for the monism that entities have both physical and mental aspects that cannot be separated and are connected, constituting an integrated whole. In Descartes' case, the question arises about how two entities that are in different dimensions and do not overlap can interact. Descartes answered this question by positing that when we desire to do something, for example, the thinking entity acts on the brain's pineal gland and drives the muscles to produce the effect that the mind desires. He held that the mental could affect the physical in this way. However, the problem is that because Descartes separated the physical from the mental, his explanation contradicts the principle of physical causal closure (i.e., physical phenomena can be explained only by the laws of physics). The dilemma posed by substance dualism remains unresolved, and one would imagine that only a minority of scientists accept this theory today.

Thus far, I have shown that the boundaries of the immune system extend to those of the entire organism. Furthermore, when we consider that immunity exists in all living organisms and is essential for their life support and that it is involved not only in defense against external microorganisms but also in neural, mental, psychological, endocrine, metabolic, and other functions, an image emerges in which immunity is integrated within the living organisms and functions throughout the body. This image overlaps remarkably with Spinoza's key concept *conatus*. The word derives from Latin, meaning "effort," "attempt," or "tendency," but it has been defined by many philosophers in various ways. Spinoza understood that all things have an important inner tendency to try to sustain their existence. To describe this disposition, Spinoza used the term *conatus*. Of course, Spinoza did not see immunity in *conatus*. However, I saw a similarity between immunity and *conatus* in that it is essential for the existence and survival of all beings. Let us now look back at Spinoza's definition of *conatus* in a little more detail.

In Part III of *The Ethics*, "On the Origin and Nature of the Emotions," Spinoza defines *conatus* as "everything, in so far as it is in itself, endeavours to persist in its own being" (Proposition VI). This definition is well understood when one considers that living organisms strive to maintain the identity and unity of their own structure and function when faced with a life crisis. More importantly, Proposition VII states that "the endeavour, wherewith everything endeavours to persist in its own being, is nothing else but the actual essence of the thing in question." In other words, every being has *conatus*, a force that strives to maintain its existence, but this force is not accidental; it is inherent in the essence of the being. The essence of existence is found in the *conatus*. Proposition VIII further states that the *conatus* "involves no finite time, but an indefinite time." The effort inherent in nature to maintain existence continues while that existence persists. That is *conatus*.

However, a problem arises when considering immunity based on *conatus* because conatus is considered to apply to all beings, including inanimate objects, not just living organisms.

What did Spinoza think of the *conatus* in living beings? In this regard, Part III, Proposition IX contains the following statement that relates *conatus* to mental faculties in humans:

> The mind, both in so far as it has clear and distinct ideas, and also in so far as it has confused ideas, endeavours to persist in its being for an indefinite period, and of this endeavour it is conscious.

Thus, *conatus* includes both the organism's ability to strive to maintain its existence and its ability to be aware of that effort. Furthermore, in the Note to Part III, Proposition IX, he brings up psychological concepts to explain the nature of *conatus* in living organisms.

> This endeavour, when referred solely to the mind, is called will, when referred to the mind and body in conjunction it is called appetite; it is, in fact, nothing else but man's essence, from the nature of which necessarily follow all those results which tend to its preservation; and which man has thus been determined to perform.
> Further, between appetite and desire there is no difference, except that the term desire is generally applied to men, in so far as they are conscious of their appetite and may accordingly be thus defined: Desire is appetite with consciousness thereof.

Spinoza here refers to "will" (*voluntas*) when *conatus* concerns only the mind and "appetite" (*appetitus*) when it concerns both mind and body and says that this is the essence of human nature. He further defines "desire" (*cupiditas*) as being fundamentally the same as appetite, but "desire" is the state of being aware of "appetite" and is limited to human beings. The definitions of "appetite" and "desire" are not further detailed in Spinoza's philosophy. It may have been inescapable to limit "appetite" to human beings during Spinoza's time, but given recent developments in cognitive science, the faculty of "appetite" can be expanded to other species and interpreted as fundamental activities broadly distributed across living organisms. If we accept this interpretation, "appetite" is the primordial state of consciousness, or consciousness involved in the reception of information from the external world, and "desire" is the state of being aware of "appetite" and can be seen as referring to a higher level of consciousness.

In other words, the mental faculties in Spinoza's "appetite" and "desire" appear to correspond to two levels of consciousness as currently defined: one that is receptive to the information it receives from the environment surrounding itself and from its own body and another that is aware of what it is receptive to. These two levels appear to correspond to Ned Block's phenomenal and access consciousness (Block, 1995) or Gerald Edelman's primary and secondary consciousness (Edelman, 2003), introduced in Section 4.4, Chapter 4. Some people refer to the former simply as "consciousness" and the latter as "self-awareness" or "cognition." Recent neuroimaging analyses suggest that the brain regions responsible for these two types of consciousness differ (Denton et al., 1999; Laureys, 2005). Thus, it would be consistent to think that the consciousness involved in perception and sensation corresponds to "appetite," while the higher level of consciousness involved in interpreting or reflecting on such appetite corresponds to "desire."

Now what did Spinoza think about memory, an essential element for immunity? What is the relationship between *conatus*, which is concerned with the persistence of existence, and memory? Generally, memory is interpreted as the persistence of images or physical traces of things perceived in the past but not present. In Part II of *The Ethics*, "On the Nature and Origin of the Mind," Spinoza defines memory as follows: Memory "is simply a certain association of ideas involving the nature of things outside the human body, which association arises in the mind according to the order and association of the modifications (*affectiones*) of the human body" (Proposition XVIII, Note).

The human mind tries to represent as much as possible that which increases or promotes the active capacity of the body (*The Ethics*, Part III, Proposition XII). Conversely, if there is something that decreases or inhibits the active capacity of the body, it tries to recall as much as possible that which excludes its presence (Part III, Proposition XIII). Pain diminishes or constrains a person's power of activity (i.e., the endeavor to persist in one's own being [*conatus*]; Part III, Proposition XXXVII, Proof). Humans in pain turn away from it and try to recreate passed joys in the present.

Pain opposes the *conatus*, and the stronger the pain, the stronger the *conatus* trying to eliminate the pain. Therefore, memory is incorporated into the *conatus*, the essence of existence, as an important element, and its status overlaps with memory as an essential element in immunity.

The analysis of immunity in the biological world has led to the common understanding that it has the same extensity as life and is indispensable for the maintenance of life and that it has neural-like functions such as recognition and memory and can control mental and psychological states through the "psycho-neuro-endocrino-immune" networks. If we reinterpret the *conatus* proposed by Spinoza from a present-day perspective, there are "appetite," which is involved in the reception of information from the outside world and is inferred to be present in organisms other than humans, and "desire," which indicates a higher level of consciousness and is restricted to humans. If that is the case, "appetite" appears to be consistent as corresponding to immunity, and immunity constitutes the essence of the organismal beings in light of Spinoza's metaphysics.

Antonio Damasio (1944–) also used the concept of *conatus* to study the regulatory mechanisms of humans and unicellular organisms. Damasio's *conatus* is specific and includes the various chemicals transmitted by the brain, or the signaling involved in electrophysiology that generates general emotions and self-preservation drives. In other words, Damasio believes that the *conatus* is rooted in brain and neurobiological control activity. At the same time, he sees the essence of emotional reactions and feelings in unicellular organisms that do not have brains, such as *Paramecium* (Damasio, 2003a). In a sense, this conclusion represents a logical contradiction because he is applying the *conatus*, which he assumes to be rooted in the brain and nerves, to organisms without brains or nerves. Furthermore, it does not conform to Spinoza's concept of *conatus*, which he considered present in all beings, including inanimate objects. Damasio also presents a model of the tree for emotions that places immunity at the lowest level, the same level as reflexes and metabolic regulation, and sensation and emotion at the highest level (Damasio, 2003b). This model is based on the anthropocentric view and must be modified when looking at the broader biological world. As discussed in detail in Chapter 4 and elsewhere (Yakura, 2019b, 2019c), the position of immunity in bacteria, for example, is not so low; instead, it must be reconsidered as playing a central role in that organism.

Another aspect of *conatus* is also important for a deeper understanding of the phenomenon of immunity. Spinoza noted the close connection between *conatus* and moral considerations. In the Note to Proposition IX of Part III of *The Ethics*, he writes the following:

> It is thus plain from what has been said, that in no case do we strive for, wish for, long for, or desire anything, because we deem it to be good, but on the other hand we deem a thing to be good, because we strive for it, wish for it, long for it, or desire it.

In this observation, Spinoza reverses the logic that we do not seek because it is good; it is good because we seek. We do not repress our inner desires. Furthermore, in the Proposition XXXIX of Part IV, "Of Human Bondage, or the Strength of the Emotions," we find the following words:

> Whatsoever brings about the preservation of the proportion of motion and rest, which the parts of the human body mutually possess, is good; contrariwise, whatsoever causes a change in such proportion is bad.

The idea that the existence of humans, and more broadly, each living organism, is ensured by a balance between two polarities (i.e., motion and rest) is consistent with the holistic view that a balance of relative factors controls the pathophysiology of all living organisms. More importantly, Spinoza notes that efforts to maintain balance are good, and those that disturb the balance are bad. In other words, the Note to Proposition IX of Part III and Proposition XXXIX of Part IV of *The Ethics* show that Spinoza sees a moral element in the control function of the organism (i.e., in the *conatus*). If we accept the conclusion that the essence of immunity corresponds to Spinoza's *conatus*, or, more strictly speaking, to the "appetite," we would also have to rethink the phenomenon of immunity from the perspective of normativity.

5.3   IMMUNITY IN LIGHT OF CANGUILHEM'S "NORMATIVITY OF LIFE"

As we have discussed, immunity and life are inseparable since immunity is tightly integrated into life and is essential for maintaining life. In his magnum opus *The Normal and The Pathological*, Georges Canguilhem discusses human normality and pathology, emphasizing normativity (Canguilhem, 1991h). In this section, I will proceed to reflect on immunity from the perspective of the normativity of the organism in light of Canguilhem's philosophy.

First, let us briefly examine how the question of normality and pathology was considered in French medicine before Canguilhem. In the late 18th century, Xavier Bichat (1771–1802) attempted to define physiological functions based on a large number of autopsies performed in a very short period. At only 30 years of age, he wrote the four-volume *General Anatomy* (Bichat, 1801). Remarkably, he established the concept of "tissue" through anatomical studies without using a microscope and is called the founder of histology. According to Bichat, there are two states in the phenomenon of life (health and disease), which are the nature of all living individuals. He asserted that all disease is merely a symptom derived from the destruction or dysfunction of tissues. There is nothing pathological in homogeneous physical phenomena, but the biological world is essentially dynamic when we look at it from there. The so-called "life force" is unstable, oscillating between health and disease. For Bichat, normality was not determined by medical science or statistical concepts but by life itself. In this sense, he saw the normal as personal and subjective, and life as a polarity with a biological norm.

François Brousset (1772–1838), who was taught by Bichat, Philippe Pinel (1745–1826), Georges Cabanis (1757–1808), and others, believed that the essential difference between disease and health was only in degree and that all disease could be seen as an excess or deficiency in the normal function of various tissues. In other words, there was only a quantitative difference between pathology and physiology; otherwise, they were identical. Auguste Comte, who was strongly influenced by the ideas of Bichat, Pinel, and especially Brousset, believed that there was continuity and homogeneity between normality and pathology. Like Bichat, Comte opposed the "mathematization of biology," which introduced physical and statistical methods into the analysis of biological phenomena, but believed disease was a quantitative deviation from the healthy or normal state. However, unlike Brousset, Comte's ambition was to establish a theory to explain biological, psychological, and sociological phenomena and, in some cases, to modify them.

Claude Bernard also held that health and disease are not two different states but that there is only a difference in degree between them. He believed that physiology existed to explain all pathology. For example, almost all of the symptoms of diabetes he modeled were not new but already present in the normal state, meaning that the difference in symptoms between those with and without diabetes was only a difference in intensity and quantity and that there was continuity between the two states. From there, he expands on this idea to say there is no antagonism between life and death, plants and animals, and inorganic and organic matters. Bernard introduced the quantification of physiological concepts into experimental analysis, which shows a difference in approach from Comte's.

Canguilhem emerged in this historical context to criticize empirical and materialist interpretations of health and disease. In his doctoral dissertation, "Essay on Some Problems Concerning the Normal and the Pathological" submitted to the University of Strasbourg in 1943 (Canguilhem, 1991a), Canguilhem focused his analysis on the concepts of normal and pathological as they relate to medicine and reflected on humans more specifically. What was his conception of medicine? He stated, "Medicine seemed to us and still seems to us like a technique or art at the crossroads of several sciences, rather than, strictly speaking, like one science" (Canguilhem, 1991g).

In order to reflect on the seemingly opposite issues of health and disease, it is necessary to understand the concept of normativity as defined by Canguilhem. The word "normativity" was defined as "the state of conformity to a norm or rule," but to this, he added the opposing meaning of "the ability to change the norm and sometimes create new norms." In other words, being normative is not only a passive state of conforming to rules made by someone else but also includes behavior that is left to the active nature of the individual to create new norms. As discussed in Canguilhem's *The Normal and The Pathological*, normativity is imbued with a new meaning in which creativity is implied (Debru, 2015).

Canguilhem argued that normality is the value of life determined by each individual, and that statistical numbers do not determine it. Life is a normative activity, and one must be a direct actor in establishing norms, not a third-party subordinate to those who establish norms from the outside. The normal is highly personal, active, and equipped to change its relationship to its environment (i.e., to create its own norms). This concept is also helpful in considering how we should respond when dramatic changes occur, such as the COVID-19 pandemic. Normativity is a biological activity that actively adapts itself to the environment rather than being subordinated to something else, which is considered a characteristic of life itself. Furthermore, Canguilhem newly proposes the concept of the dynamic polarity of life and normativity as a regulator of this polarity.

As Kurt Goldstein (1878–1965) noted, Canguilhem also believed that being ill did not mean a lack of norms but rather a great opportunity to create new norms. Viewed in this way, actively creating norms may create a sense of control over one's body, freeing one from the psychological stress of passively relying on numbers calculated from an unspecified group. In reality, however, normativity is often used in a passive sense, and the statistical view still prevails in the scientific approach. Understandably, scientists would like to define the normal state objectively in numbers, but is it really possible to know normality in numbers?

Oddly enough, when it comes to the immune system, there is no immunological definition of normal or healthy in humans. In light of this situation, a group of immunologists proposed establishing a database of parameters such as cytokines, cell types, CD antigens, signaling pathways, and genome and regulatory factors from thousands of human materials (Davis, 2008; Hayday and Peakman, 2008). By statistically analyzing such data, they believed that they could infer the state of health in humans. Common sense suggests that the more parameters available, the clearer the definition of health becomes, but this may make the definition of normality more difficult. Furthermore, as noted in Chapter 3, immune phenomena involve elements throughout the body. In that case, is it possible to establish a definition of normal based solely on parameters within the classical immune system?

It can be inferred that there is something of the same nature as Adolphe Quetelet's (1796–1874) thought behind such an approach. The statistical methods and the concept of the "average man" (l'homme moyen) developed by the Belgian astronomer and mathematician Quetelet profoundly influenced thought in the biomedical field. This influence can be seen in the Quetelet or body mass index, which is still used to assess obesity worldwide. However, because it is difficult to define the boundary between the normal and the pathological for even a single parameter, one can imagine that it would be even more difficult to determine the criteria for normality for all parameters studied. While unexpected spin-offs may emerge while analyzing a large number of parameters, one is tempted to question how meaningful it is to talk about normality based on detailed figures obtained in this way. Instead, discussion of health and disease may have more meaningful effects on life if subjective and personal concepts are incorporated, as Canguilhem argues. In other words, we must not forget that the patient's condition, reduced to a number, is not the sole criterion for judgment but also that which is produced by objective observation at the organismic level and subjective reflection.

Life is in constant dynamism. Pathological conditions confer on the organism the ability to adapt to changes in the environment and to establish norms adapted to the new environment. Pathology is not confined to one part of the body or one function but affects the entire body and remodels the individual. If we recognize disease as a human "effort" to reach a new equilibrium, Canguilhem explains that we can also see the continuity between the pathological and the normal and the interdependence of all elements and functions in the body. This recognition leads to a holistic view of life, which, as discussed in Chapter 3, is supported by the vast amount of experimental data accumulated since Canguilhem. He also believed that disease was not merely a matter of increase or decrease but an innovative and creative experience of the organism. What happens with disease, he held, is not a change in the dimension of health but the acquisition of a new dimension of life. For Canguilhem, disease was both a deprivation and a remodeling (Canguilhem, 1991e). Comte or Bernard did not share this creative thinking.

In his discussion of the biological polarity of the normal and the pathological, or natural selection and the healing power of nature (*vis medicatrix naturae*), Canguilhem quotes the following words of Émile Guyénot (1885–1963):

> It is a fact that the organism has an aggregate of properties which[sic] belong to it alone, thanks to which it withstands multiple destructive forces. Without these defensive reactions, life would be rapidly extinguished. [...] The living being is able to find instantaneously the reaction which is useful vis-à-vis substances with which neither it nor its kind has ever had contact. The organism is an incomparable chemist. It is the first among physicians. The fluctuations of the environment are almost always a menace to its existence. The living being could not survive if it did not possess certain essential properties. Every injury would be fatal if tissues were incapable of forming scars and blood incapable of clotting.
>
> **Canguilhem (1991f)**

Canguilhem uses the term "immunity" in *The Normal and The Pathological* only when contrasting normal immune reactions with abnormal immune reactions such as allergy and anaphylaxis (Canguilhem, 1991d). The year 1943, when Canguilhem's dissertation "Essay on Some Problems Concerning the Normal and the Pathological" was written, was before Burnet's clonal selection theory (Burnet, 1957) but long after von Behring (von Behring and Kitasato, 1890), Ehrlich (Ehrlich, 1900), and Metchnikoff (Metchnikoff, 1883). Canguilhem saw the essence of disease as "an alteration (modification) of the total organism" (Canguilhem, 1991c), which can be seen as a manifestation of the immune response. Guyénot's assertion that what keeps an organism alive is its intrinsic and essential properties is also very much consistent with our analysis of immunity. It is very likely that by citing Guyénot, Canguilhem saw the phenomenon of immunity as the decisive factor controlling biological polarity.

As already mentioned, Canguilhem uses the term "effort" to describe the nature of the disease. For example:

> But disease is not simply disequilibrium or discordance; it is, and perhaps most important, an effort on the part of nature to effect a new equilibrium in man. Disease is a generalized reaction designed to bring about a cure; the organism develops a disease in order to get well.
>
> **Canguilhem (1991b)**

Canguilhem does not use the term "immunity" or "immune response" for this situation either. However, what he calls nature's "effort" can be seen as another name for "immunity." It appears to be a kind of indescribable force inherent in life or what Spinoza calls *conatus*. Canguilhem's view of disease as a response toward recovery echoes Metchnikoff's view that disease in the form of inflammation is not a passive state of being at the mercy of microorganisms but is an expression of an active response by the host. It is evident that Canguilhem viewed disease as something that dynamically affects the whole organism, which is a representation of immune responses.

Nature, including humans, is in harmony and equilibrium, and disease was interpreted as a disturbance of this harmony and equilibrium. Based on Canguilhem's view of the normal and the pathological, we can see that the immune function supports the normality of life and controls biological polarity. From this perspective, Kourilsky's view of the immune system mentioned in Section 1.7.6, Chapter 1 may be highly Canguilhemian in its view that maintaining the integrity of the organism is a fundamental function of the immune or biological defense mechanism.

I have always thought that "to be ill is like living in a foreign country" (Yakura, 2019a). If humans generally think elsewhere, then travel invites us to contemplate. However, unlike ordinary travel, illness is more likely to lead to serious contemplation of one's existence. We are forced to confront existential questions, which may be somewhat like living in a foreign country. When we fall ill, we all hope medical treatment will restore us to our original state. However, the problem with this idea is that our lives are in a constant state of change and cannot be reversed. When we truly understand the truth of our life, we realize that we must modify our previous norms and create new norms that are different from those we had before, which requires a certain kind of creativity. The attempt becomes an expression of the person's humanity. Becoming ill is a test of one's creativity. Becoming ill and living in a foreign country are connected in the sense that we have to remake the norms of life. The reality of life emerges where immunity, pathology, environment, and normativity are intricately intertwined.

Recently, a paper was published analyzing the issue of normativity in the human immune system based on Canguilhem's definition of biological normativity (Turki, 2011). The question was whether normativity is an actual capacity of organisms or whether normative capacities are differentially expressed at different levels of organization, such as genes, molecules, organs, and systems. The conclusion was that normative competence is observed at the level of organisms and organismal systems but not necessarily at the level of molecules and genes. Because the immune system is so well studied in vertebrates, it is easy to assume that the vertebrate system is typical. However, as we saw in Chapter 4, a broader examination of the biological world reveals that the vertebrate system is somewhat unique. If we were to focus our discussion of normativity solely on the vertebrate immune system, we might lose sight of its essential aspects. That was the lesson learned from the phylogenetic analysis.

The bacterial immune system CRISPR–Cas uses gene- and enzyme-mediated mechanisms. Bacteria also have a phenomenon called autoimmunity. Because of the potential for self-destruction, autoimmunity must be avoided for survival. When a self-destructive situation arises in bacteria, a mechanism is in place to avoid it. That is not to say that the genes comprising the immune system are in a passive state, but instead that they adapt to changes in the environment and create new norms, meaning that normativity can be seen not only at the organism or system level but also at the gene level. Considering the previous discussion on the normal and the pathological, it would be consistent to assume that immunity supports the normativity of life and regulates biological polarity.

5.4 THE MENTAL ELEMENTS WITH NORMATIVITY IN THE ESSENCE OF IMMUNITY

In this section, I summarize the fundamental characteristics (or essence) of immunity that can be deduced from the preceding analyses. The studies in Chapter 4 indicate that immunity's smallest functional units shared by the immune system of almost all species are recognition, information integration, appropriate response, and memory formation. However, marked differences exist in the mechanisms and supporting structures constituting the cognitive process. These functional units are well represented in the bacterial CRISPR–Cas system (Bolotin et al., 2005; Mojica et al., 2005; Pourcel et al., 2005; Lillestöl et al., 2006; Brouns et al., 2008; Marraffini and Sontheimer, 2008; Sorek et al., 2008; Karginov and Hannon, 2010; Marraffini and Sontheimer, 2010; Westra et al., 2012; Sorek et al., 2013), which recognizes invading DNA sequences, integrates that information, uses it to destroy the reinvading DNA, and stores the DNA information for future use. Since this process is essential for the existence and survival of organisms, it is one of the conditions for life. Furthermore, immunity was the earliest cognitive apparatus to support specific recognition and memory during evolution. Immunity also bears functional similarity or identity to the nervous system. These facts led me to answer the question about minimal cognition with the following proposal: CRISPR–Cas is a system with a minimal cognitive capacity (Yakura, 2019b, 2019c). When we ask what constitutes immunity or examine the presence of a particular system in other species, it is not the structure or mechanism that interests us but rather the functional identity or similarity; this is the lesson of the above analysis. Indeed, the structures that constitute the immune system vary so widely from species to species that anyone accustomed to the human immune system alone would find it difficult to recognize CRISPR–Cas as constituting an immune system. Overcoming that difficulty requires adopting a function-centered view.

Thus far, I have attempted to review these scientific results in an integrated manner, examining them from a philosophical perspective to identify immunity's universal properties. Spinoza defined *conatus* as the force or effort that sustains animate and inanimate beings, considering it the essence of existence. When applied to living organisms, the function that extends beyond the physical to the basic mental realm was defined as "appetite." Since immunity is concerned not only with the control of physical states through cognitive activity but also with the regulation of mental and psychological functions, I concluded that Spinoza's concept of "appetite" well describes the characteristics of immunity. In addition, Spinoza's *conatus* is accompanied by moral judgments of good or bad. For example, maintaining the balance between an organism's polarities, such as motion and rest, is deemed good, whereas failing to maintain the balance is deemed bad. This balance brings to mind what Canguilhem refers to as the normativity of life. Normativity controls the polarity of the normal and the pathological, and it is reasonable to suppose that the immune system determines this polarity. In other words, the essence of immunity is a physical and mental activity with a normative nature that controls the biological polarity. That appetite was considered the essence of biological existence gives rise to the possibility that immunity constitutes the essence of biological organisms.

The subjective mental world of any perceiving subject is unknowable by third parties, which is an inherent obstacle to determining whether other organisms are conscious. The term "consciousness" was originally introduced to describe our human state of awareness of both ourselves and the world around us. For a long time, consciousness was thought to exist only in highly evolved organisms with complex brains. Therefore, our anthropocentric imaginations and reflexive assumptions lead us to disregard the possibility of consciousness in other organisms. In his 1974 article "What it is like to be a bat," Thomas Nagel (1937–) shows that even if we can objectively characterize the structure and function of the bat's brain, it is difficult to imagine what it is like to perceive external objects through echolocation (Nagel, 1974). In other words, he concludes that a physicochemical understanding of biological phenomena cannot explain how an organism feels or experiences. This problem is known as the "explanatory gap" (Levine, 1983), and despite many attempts, no one has managed to bridge it (Chalmers, 1995; Searle, 2007; Feinberg and Mallatt, 2016; Godfrey-Smith, 2019).

However, even while acknowledging that the relationship between the nervous system's physical properties and the subjective experience of consciousness cannot be fully explained, research from neurobiology, animal behavior, and philosophy has suggested that many organisms may have phenomenal or primary consciousness (Low et al., 2012; Allen and Trestman, 2016; Feinberg and Mallatt, 2019). Phylogenetic studies of the immune system have taught us that the structures supporting a single function can vary dramatically across different species, and we may expect the same cross-species structural variation for the function of consciousness.

Human beings may have the highest level of consciousness and cognitive ability of any living organisms. However, if we could recognize and eliminate the anthropocentric perspective that affects our perceptions, how we see nature would change dramatically. When will science be able to unravel the subjective inner world? That question presumes that our current science can address the problem; perhaps it cannot. Therefore, it would make sense to humbly consider whether other organisms possess consciousness while reserving judgment and maintaining an attitude of *epoché*. Furthermore, to approach the question about consciousness with a broad perspective—as opposed to one limited to human consciousness—it may be important to apply an inclusive, "biologized" definition. This approach to the question of consciousness seems inevitable, given the conclusion drawn from the analysis in this book: namely, that cognitive capacity is the essence of immunity, which is inherent in all living organisms. This view also seems to be reflected in the ideas of Alain Prochiantz (1948–), who proposes a definition of the mental activity of thinking (*la pensée*) in purely biological terms as "an adaptative relationship of an individual and the species to their milieu" (Prochiantz, 2001). When thrown into a hostile environment, organisms are forced to adapt to survive, partly by exercising their cognitive capacities. The immune system senses information from the internal and external environment, integrates it, reacts appropriately to the original information, and stores the experience in memory for the future. If we accept the reasoning presented so far, we may say that, in some sense, the organism thinks through its immune system.

As mentioned in Section 4.4, Chapter 4, Anne-Marie Moulin has identified three paradigms in immunology: defense, selection, and recognition (Moulin, 1995). The first paradigm centers on defense against external microorganisms. The second paradigm is based on the clonal selection theory, in which our bodies are equipped with cells bearing receptors with one type of antigenic specificity, and antigens select cells with corresponding receptors. This paradigm implies that the immune system itself is natural selection's target. The third cognitive paradigm implies that the receptors on T and B cells specifically recognize antigens, and the immune system has functions similar to those of the nervous system.

According to Irun Cohen's cognitive paradigm mentioned in Section 1.7.3, Chapter 1, the immune system should be viewed as an inherently self-recognizing sensory or homeostatic system because the clonal selection theory does not successfully explain physiological autoimmunity (Cohen and Young, 1991; Cohen, 1992a, 1992b, 2000). In this book, the metaphysical analysis of immunity found that normative mental properties belong to immunity's essence. They may be considered a candidate for what Heidegger calls internal possibility. As Metchnikoff had sensed more than a century ago, these points suggest the possibility that cognition, including memory, is the primary function of immunity, whereas the defense function is secondary (Tauber, 1992). I hope that reappraising immunity from the perspective of cognition, as has been widely discussed (Tauber, 1997, 2011, 2013), will provide clues that lead to a deeper understanding of immunity, which constitutes the basis of life.

One additional issue to consider is autoimmunity or self-recognition, which appears to be embedded in the immune system. An interesting possibility emerges if we examine embedded self-recognition from a perspective that emphasizes that immunity is a necessary condition for life and is partially characterized by the mental property of normativity. Perhaps self-reflection is an essential activity of life. As discussed in Section 2.1.8, Chapter 2, Socrates' maxim reminds us that examining life is critical to a fully human life, and this activity has been the backbone of philosophy throughout its history. The metaphysicalization of immunity supports these ideas, and at the same time, the question arises as to how well we humans are examining ourselves compared to the immune system.

5.5 FROM A METAPHYSICS OF IMMUNITY TO PANPSYCHISM

The attempt to consider immunity from the perspective of metaphysics has raised the possibility that the essence of immunity encompasses neural-like cognitive functions and mental properties. This possibility, which at first glance seems to go beyond the physicalism or materialism espoused by modern science, seems to have an affinity with the panpsychist world, in which all beings are endowed with mental properties. To examine this point, we must know more about the panpsychist view. In this section, I review the historical background of the panpsychist worldview, looking at representative philosophers who hold this view (Skrbina, 2017; Yakura, 2020b, 2020d, 2020a; Goff et al., 2022).

A literal definition of panpsychism would be that the mind (consciousness) is everywhere or that all beings have a mental component. However, there is no consensus on the definition that is circulating, showing the difficulty of its definition. Furthermore, what do we mean by "mental component" or "all beings" here? According to modern scientific convention, the mind is limited to humans or animals with highly evolved brains and is the product of physicochemical processes in the brain. From this understanding, panpsychism appears to be entirely foreign. Conversely, we cannot see what panpsychism would look like unless we free ourselves from its common sense. A review of >2,500 years of human history reveals that the panpsychist view has shown an amazing vitality, surviving from ancient Greece to the present day. However, the name panpsychism was given to this view during the Renaissance by Francesco Patrizi (1529–1597), a Croatian-born philosopher active in Italy said to have defended Plato and harshly criticized Aristotle.

I begin our examination with pre-Socratic philosophers. Considered by Aristotle to be the first philosopher, Thales of Miletus (c. 626/623–c. 548/545 BC) held that the *arche* (first principle) of all things is water. His attempt to explain the entire world in terms of a single principle, away from mythology, led to Aristotle's reputation as the first philosopher. Thales, who believed that beings with minds could move themselves, not only held that magnets had *psyche* (souls) but also saw the universe as alive and full of spirit. Anaximenes (c. 585–c. 525 BC) considered the *pneuma* (air), which is associated with the soul, to be the *arche* of all things, and he believed that all things are endowed with soul-like qualities since air permeates all things. Empedocles (c. 494–434 BC) believed that the four elements (water, air, fire, and earth) constitute all things and that various phenomena are caused by the two forces of "love" (attraction) and "strife" (repulsion) acting on them. He held that each element is endowed with a soul and the power to think.

Plato also posited that the human body and the universe are composed of Empedocles' four elements (water, air, fire, and earth) and that the universe has a soul just as our bodies have a soul (Plato, 1871). Furthermore, he holds that the demiurge created the universe as a truly living being with a soul and intellect in its own image (Plato, 1888). It should be noted here that the idea that the universe has a soul does not immediately imply panpsychism. As we will see later, modern panpsychism requires, as a condition, the existence of a mental nature in the smallest component of the world. As a result, the universe has a mental nature, but not vice versa.

Aristotle believed that living beings have souls but that nonliving things do not (Aristotle, 1907). Judged by modern standards, he would not be considered a panpsychist. However, because he was aware that the boundary between the inanimate and the animate is impossible to determine (Aristotle, 1910), he seems to have been open to the idea that all beings are inherently endowed with something like a soul. He also uses Anaximenes' *pneuma* to advance his argument. According to him, *pneuma* is not the soul itself (which is said to exist only in living beings) but soul-like, and he writes that all beings in nature are full of soul-like *pneuma* (Aristotle, 1943).

Later, as Christianity prevailed, panpsychism was no longer discussed, but the situation changed during the Renaissance when it was labeled "panpsychism" by Francesco Patrizi, as mentioned above. Giordano Bruno (1548–1600) preached a panpsychist worldview that life and consciousness were born at the level of the universe and that everything is alive and has a soul within it, no matter how small (Knox, 2019). In the 17th century, unlike Descartes, who developed a mind-body dualism (Section 5.2, Chapter 5), Spinoza posited that the entity underlying reality is both eternal and infinite, both God and nature (*Deus sive natura*), and described a monistic world in which everything that exists contains both extended entities and thought entities corresponding to Descartes' conception. Leibniz developed an interesting metaphysics in his *Monadology*, published in 1714 (Section 1.7.1, Chapter 1). He arrived at the monad, as the constituent elements of the universe, which is an entity with no parts that cannot be ultimately divided. Because monads have no extensions (physical properties), the basic building blocks of nature are assumed to be mental properties. Each monad was considered a living mirror reflecting the universe and possessing its complete information. This ontology is interesting because it holds that the universe is composed of mental elements, but it also encourages us to invite the grandeur of the universe into our consciousness.

In the 19th century, the German psychologist and philosopher Gustav Fechner (1801–1887), considered the founder of experimental psychology and psychophysics, advanced panpsychist thought. His experience of seeing the spirit of a flower (Seele) rising around it one day after he had recovered his sight following a serious eye disease led him to believe that consciousness pervades the universe and that the soul never dies. However, if seeing the psychic element in the basic units that make up the world is a requirement for panpsychism, Fechner may not be a true panpsychist. He also distinguishes between the "night view," which sees nature as composed of dead matter and analyzes it through mathematics and physics, and the "daylight view," which holds that the world is alive and has consciousness and stresses the latter's importance.

Ernst Haeckel (1834–1919), a strong proponent of evolutionary theory, developed a monistic view that there are no clear boundaries between animals and plants, humans and other animals, inorganic and organic matters, and matter and spirit and that all matter has a soul. Interestingly, he divided the existence of the mind into three categories: panpsychism as a universal principle of the world; biopsychism, which holds that only living beings have a mind; and zoopsychism, which holds that only highly evolved animals have a mind (Haeckel, 1892). Johann Wolfgang von Goethe (1749–1832), whom Haeckel respected, also believed that matter could not exist or operate without a mind.

In the 20th century, William James (1842–1910), an American philosopher, psychologist, and advocate of pragmatism, presented an idea based on neutral monism (the view that the substance of the world is composed of a single neutral element that is neither mental nor physical). In a strict sense, it appears to differ from panpsychism, which holds that the world's essence is both matter and spirit. However, according to James, if evolution is continuous, consciousness must exist at the origin of everything, and each atom must be related to the primordial atom via consciousness, which has an affinity with modern panpsychism (James, 1890). James' argument appears in the case of a thoroughgoing physicalism and avoids or overcomes the question of how the mental is generated from the physical.

The English philosopher and social activist Bertrand Russell (1872–1970; Nobel Prize in Literature 1950) wrote with his teacher Whitehead, *Principia Mathematica* (Whitehead and Russell, 1910–1913). This book is considered one of the leading mathematical works of the 20th century. He proposed a neutral monism, also known as "Russellian monism," which went unnoticed for a long time (Russell, 1927). In other words, there is no clear boundary between mind and matter, but only a difference of degree. The essential element of the mind is memory, but inorganic matter also has something like memory. Russell's logic is that if memory is taken broadly to be all the effects of past experiences on present reactions, then the river bottom remembers experiencing violent currents, and if "thinking" means transforming one's behavior by past events, the river bottom must also be said to be thinking. Russell's monism also allows us to avoid the past problems that dualism and physicalism have had. For example, the problem of the physical causal closure, which is faced when explaining how the physical and mental worlds influence each other, cannot be explained if dualism is adopted. However, if consciousness were an intrinsic property of matter, Russellian monism would seem to be one option in that these problems would seem to be eliminated.

In the subsequent discussion of panpsychism from the late 20th century to the present, we can find materials for examining the problems and possibilities of panpsychism. In his 1979 book, *What It Is Like to Be a Bat* (originally titled *Mortal Questions*), Thomas Nagel discussed panpsychism, which had been forgotten for about half a century, and called attention to this issue (Nagel, 1979). Nagel's panpsychism is the view that the basic physical components of the universe have psychic properties. Because of his concise and powerful formulation of the problem, he is sometimes considered the father of contemporary panpsychism (Coleman, 2018). He develops his argument based on the following four premises:

1. Material composition: Any living organism is wholly composed of a vast number of physical particles.
2. Non-reductionism: An organism's conscious experiences are not explained by any physical properties alone.
3. Realism about consciousness: Consciousness belongs to the organism; it is a feature of its material constitution.
4. Non-emergence: All global properties of a complex system intelligibly derive from the properties of its constituents, and their arrangement.

The argument from this point forward is this. The fact that an organism is composed entirely of matter and yet has consciousness means that consciousness is derived from matter. However, because consciousness cannot be explained by the physical properties of its constituents, it must be explained by non-physical properties. If this is the case, then the constituent elements of a conscious organism must have some mental elements of their own. Moreover, the physical components with a mental component must be the most basic ones at the bottom of the hierarchy of structures, such as elementary particles, because if we assume that the mental component is first seen at a slightly higher level (e.g., in proteins and cells), the question arises of how to go from the absence of consciousness to a conscious state, as we have seen in previous discussions. Nagel believed that consciousness cannot arise from the absence of consciousness.

Almost 20 years after Nagel's panpsychism, Australian philosopher David Chalmers (1966–) published *The Conscious Mind*, in which he addressed fundamental issues in the philosophy of mind (Chalmers, 1996). Among his arguments were that materialism is false because physical things cannot explain all of reality, that consciousness is a fundamental fact of nature, and that science and philosophy must cooperate to find the fundamental laws of consciousness. He also noted that there are two different problems of consciousness: the easy problem and the hard problem. Easy problems can be solved in principle within the framework of current science, although they may be technically complex. In contrast, hard problems are subjective, phenomenal experience problems that are difficult to solve through physicalism or reductionism.

In the 21st century, he has argued favorably for panpsychism, including its problems, after stating that he is not confident whether it is true or false. Chalmers' panpsychism is the view that consciousness exists in the basic physical categories that make up the world (e.g., quarks and leptons), and in the Nagel fashion, the subjective aspect of "what it feels like to be..." is there. This view would be what is called panexperientialism, in the sense that consciousness and experience are all that is real (Griffin, 1997). His argument uses a dialectic of thesis, antithesis, and synthesis; the thesis is materialism, the antithesis is dualism, and the synthesis that emerges from there is panpsychism. Consciousness is fundamentally physical, according to materialism, but not physical, according to dualism. Moreover, panpsychism synthesized from there asserts that everything is fundamentally physical and mental simultaneously (Chalmers, 2013).

To advance the discussion, Chalmers introduces the concepts of macroexperience and microexperience. The former is the conscious experience of humans and human-equivalent organisms, while the latter is the conscious experience of minuscule physical elements, which are imagined to be much simpler than human experience. He then brings up constitutive and non-constitutive panpsychism (a typical example is emergent panpsychism). Constitutive panpsychism holds that macroexperience is constituted or realized by microexperience. In contrast, non-constitutive panpsychism holds that there are macroexperience and microexperience, but the microexperience does not ground the macroexperience, creating a gap between them. In this case, an explanation of how we get from the microexperience to the macroexperience is needed, as in dualism (Chalmers, 2013).

Chalmers also comes up with versions of Russellian panpsychism and constitutive Russellian panpsychism. Physics can provide answers about the structure of matter and what it does, but it remains mute about the properties inherent in that matter. Russellian panpsychism believes that the fundamental properties that physics does not teach are microlevel phenomenal properties. The constitutive Russellian panpsychism believes that microphenomenal properties are fundamental and constitute macrophenomenal properties, meaning that laws connect microphenomena and macrophenomena. Chalmers himself believes that constitutive Russellian panpsychism is the most likely panpsychism because we do not have to bother with the mental causation problem of how the mind affects the body that dualism poses (Chalmers, 2013). However, as William James noted at the end of the 19th century, the "combination problem" of how the simple experience of microscopic particles can ultimately produce the complex experience we feel will follow (Chalmers, 2016).

One philosopher who has recently been active in the discussion of panpsychism is Galen Strawson (1952–), originally from England but now at the University of Texas at Austin. In 2006, he published an influential paper entitled "Realistic monism? Why physicalism entails panpsychism?" (Strawson, 2006). The title suggests that the relationship between panpsychism and physicalism differs from what common sense would suggest. In 2020, as a prolegomenon to panpsychism, he published a paper entitled "What does 'physical' mean?" (Strawson, 2020d). In it, he develops a "pure panpsychist materialism." Materialists and physicalists believe that everything that concretely exists is physical. Pure panpsychist materialists are also materialists, and they are not at odds with physics in that they hold that the universe exists regardless of the nature of our minds. If the fundamental inner nature of reality is not a phenomenal experience, we would have to consider the emergence of the experiential from the nonexperiential. Strawson takes the terms "mental" and "mind" in the sense that they are commonly used as encompassing emotions, simple phenomenal experiences, and complex thoughts. According to Gerald Edelman's classification, this would include both primary and secondary consciousness. However, some philosophers use the term "mental" in a very exclusive manner and exclude primary consciousness from the mental. For example, Russell considered higher cognitive functions or the capacity for memory to be a necessary condition for the mind. In that case, some mental activities are not included in the mental, but my personal position is closer to Strawson, who takes an inclusive view.

Strawson went on to define "physical" or "physicalism" (materialism) as follows: "If x is physical, it is concrete," "If x is physical, it is a subject matter of physics," "If x exists in the universe, it is physical," and "If x is physical, it is a spatio-temporal entity" (Strawson, 2020c). Then, as a pure panpsychist materialist, he added "If experience exists in the universe, it is physical" (Strawson, 2020b), maintaining that any clear-headed materialist cannot think there is a fundamental distinction between the physical and the experiential or mental. In other words, the ultimate inner nature of our universe is experience. However, some philosophers have criticized this theory, because the definition of "physical" does not conform to the traditional discussion of the mind-body problem. Strawson simply responds that a major reason why the mind-body problem is at a standstill is that the traditional definition of what is physical is problematic (Strawson, 2020a).

Panpsychism may seem strange to many people, but it does not seem to me that it would take much effort to understand it if we leave our intuitive judgments behind and rely only on logic to think about the mental component. Once we overcome this hurdle, we find that how we see the world has changed dramatically compared to when we were unaware of it. Panpsychism can expand our consciousness by recognizing the mental nature of the world around us, both microlevel and macrolevel, and animate and inanimate. It also can potentially create consciousness as an inhabitant of this planet and this universe. Therefore, it is expected to change our attitude toward the environment and ecosystems that we had previously considered to exist outside of us and for our benefit because sensing a mind or sentient being there may give rise to a moral sense. From there, we may be able to offer a new perspective to counter the scientism (including objectivity, moral neutrality, and the elimination of value judgments), globalism, or single thought and value that underlie the problems of our time.

The immune system constitutes an ecosystem (Tauber, 2008; Swiatczak and Tauber, 2020). However, from now on, it seems to me that it will be important to take a viewpoint that includes immunity in the workings of the ecosystem or the world beyond the individual. If immunity is interpreted as synonymous with life, it is an inevitable consequence. The COVID-19 pandemic that swept the world has also highlighted the need for such a perspective. I have come to this shift in viewpoint not because I have tried to confront contemporary problems based on abstract speculation and conjecture from the beginning but rather because I have advanced my thinking based on ideas derived from scientific facts concerning a natural phenomenon called immunity. The path from metaphysical consideration of immunity to panpsychism was not in my initial vision, and it turned out to be a surprising journey. If it leads us to a foothold for confronting problems deeply rooted in the present age, it will show the potential of the MOS that I advocate. I will continue to reflect on this issue, and I hope that unexpected developments await us in the future.

NOTE

1 Whitehead, A. N. (1920). *The Concept of Nature. Tarner Lectures Delivered in Trinity College, November 1919.* Cambridge University Press. 163.

REFERENCES

Allen, C., & Trestman, M. (2016). Animal consciousness. (E. N. Zalta Ed.). *The Stanford Encyclopedia of Philosophy.* https://plato.stanford.edu/cgi-bin/encyclopedia/archinfo.cgi?entry=consciousness-animal.

Aristotle. (1907). *De Anima.* (R. D. Hicks, Trans.). Cambridge University Press.

Aristotle. (1943). Book III. (A. L. Peck, Trans.). *Generation of Animals.* William Heinemann.

Aristotle. (1910). Book VIII. (D. W. Thompson, Trans.). *Historia Animalium.* Clarendon Press.

Bichat, X. (1801). *Anatomie générale, appliquée à la physiologie et à la médecine.* Brosson, Gabon.

Block, N. (1995). On a confusion about a function of consciousness. *Behavioral and Brain Sciences, 18,* 227–247. doi: 10.1017/S0140525X00038188.

Bolotin, A., Quinquis, B., Sorokin, A., & Ehrlich, S. D. (2005). Clustered regularly interspaced short palindrome repeats (CRISPRs) have spacers of extrachromosomal origin. *Microbiology, 151,* 2551–2561. doi: 10.1099/mic.0.28048-0.

Brouns, S. J., Jore, M. M., Lundgren, M., Westra, E. R., Slijkhuis, R. J. H., Snijders, A. P. L., Dickman, M. J., Makarova, L. S., Koonin, E. V., & van der Oost, J. (2008). Small CRISPR RNAs guide antiviral defense in prokaryotes. *Science, 321,* 960–964. doi: 10.1126/science.1159689.

Burnet, F. M. (1957). A modification of Jerne's theory of antibody production using the concept of clonal selection. *Australian Journal of Science, 20,* 67–69. doi: 10.3322/canjclin.26.2.119.

Canguilhem, G. (1991a). *The Normal and the Pathological.* (C. R. Fawcett & R. S. Cohen, Trans.). Zone Books. (Originally published 1966). 27–229.

Canguilhem, G. (1991b). *The Normal and the Pathological.* (C. R. Fawcett & R. S. Cohen, Trans.). Zone Books. (Originally published 1966). 40–41.

Canguilhem, G. (1991c). *The Normal and the Pathological.* (C. R. Fawcett & R. S. Cohen, Trans.). Zone Books. (Originally published 1966). 41.

Canguilhem, G. (1991d). *The Normal and the Pathological.* (C. R. Fawcett & R. S. Cohen, Trans.). Zone Books. (Originally published 1966). 206–207, 211–212.

Canguilhem, G. (1991e). *The Normal and the Pathological.* (C. R. Fawcett & R. S. Cohen, Trans.). Zone Books. (Originally published 1966). 186.

Canguilhem, G. (1991f). *The Normal and the Pathological.* (C. R. Fawcett & R. S. Cohen, Trans.). Zone Books. (Originally published 1966). 130–131.

Canguilhem, G. (1991g). *The Normal and the Pathological.* (C. R. Fawcett & R. S. Cohen, Trans.). Zone Books. (Originally published 1966). 34.

Canguilhem, G. (1991h). *The Normal and the Pathological.* (C. R. Fawcett & R. S. Cohen, Trans.). Zone Books. (Originally published 1966). 1–327.

Chalmers, D. J. (1995). Facing up to the problem of consciousness. *Journal of Consciousness Studies, 2,* 200–219. doi: 10.1093/acprof:oso/9780195311105.003.0001.

Chalmers, D. J. (1996). *The Conscious Mind.* Oxford University Press.

Chalmers, D. J. (2013). Panpsychism and panprotopsychism. *Amherst Lecture in Philosophy, 8,* 1–35.

Chalmers, D. J. (2016). The combination problem for panpsychism. (G. Brüntrup, & L. Jaskolla, Eds.). *Panpsychism: Contemporary Perspectives.* Oxford University Press. 179–214.

Cohen, I. R. (1992a). The cognitive paradigm and the immunological homunculus. *Immunology Today, 13,* 490–494. doi: 10.1016/0167-5699(92)90024-2.

Cohen, I. R. (1992b). The cognitive principal challenges clonal selection. *Immunology Today, 13,* 441–444. doi: 10.1016/0167-5699(92)90071-E.

Cohen, I. R. (2000). *Tending Adam's Garden: Evolving the Cognitive Immune Self.* Academic Press.

Cohen, I. R., & Young, D. B. (1991). Autoimmunity, microbial immunity and the immunological homunculus. *Immunology Today, 12,* 105–110. doi: 10.1016/0167-5699(91)90093-9.

Coleman, S. (2018). The evolution of Nagel's panpsychism. *Klēsis, 41,* 180–202.

Comte, A. (1893). *The Positive Philosophy of Auguste Comte.* Vol. 1. (H. Martineau, Trans.). Kegan Paul, Trench, Trübner. (Originally published 1830). 1–4.

Damasio, A. (2003a). *Looking for Spinoza: Joy, Sorrow, and the Feeling Brain.* Harcourt. 40–41.

Damasio, A. (2003b). *Looking for Spinoza: Joy, Sorrow, and the Feeling Brain.* Harcourt. 37.

Davis, M. M. (2008). A prescription for human immunology. *Immunity, 29*, 835–838. doi: 10.1016/j.immuni.2008.12.003.

Debru, C. (2015). *Au-delà des normes: la normativité (Beyond Norms: The Normativity)*. Hermann. 11–15.

Denton, D., Shade, R., Zamarippa, F., Egan, G., Blair-West, J., McKinley, M., Lancaster, J., & Fox, P. (1999). Neuroimaging of genesis and satiation of thirst and an interoceptor-driven theory of origins of primary consciousness. *Proceedings of the National Academy of Sciences of the United States of America, 96*, 5304–5309. doi: 10.1073/pnas.96.9.5304.

du Bois-Reymond, E. H. (1874). The limits of our knowledge of nature. *Popular Science Monthly, 5*, 32.

Edelman, G. M. (2003). Naturalizing consciousness: A theoretical framework. *Proceedings of the National Academy of Sciences of the United States of America, 100*, 5520–5524. doi: 10.1073/pnas.0931349100.

Ehrlich, P. (1900). Croonian lecture. On immunity with special reference to cell life. *Proceedings of the Royal Society of London, 66*, 424–448. doi: 10.1098/rspl.1899.0121.

Feinberg, T. E., & Mallatt, J. (2019). Subjectivity "demystified": Neurobiology, evolution, and the explanatory gap. *Frontiers in Psychology, 10*, 1686. doi: 10.3389/fpsyg.2019.01686.

Feinberg, T. E., & Mallatt, J. M. (2016). *The Ancient Origins of Consciousness: How the Brain Created Experience*. MIT Press.

Godfrey-Smith, P. (2019). Evolving across the explanatory gap. *Philosophy, Theory, and Practice in Biology, 11*, 1. doi: 10.3998/ptpbio.16039257.0011.001.

Goff, P., Seager, W., & Allen-Hermanson, S. (2022). Panpsychism. (E. N. Zalta, Ed.). *The Stanford Encyclopedia of Philosophy*. https://plato.stanford.edu/archives/sum2022/entries/panpsychism/.

Griffin, D. R. (1997). Panexperientialist physicalism and the mind-body problem. *Journal of Consciousness Studies, 4*, 248–268.

Haeckel, E. (1892). Our monism: The principles of a consistent, unitary world-view. *Monist, 2*, 481–486. doi: 10.5840/monist18922444.

Hayday, A. C., & Peakman, M. (2008). The habitual, diverse and surmountable obstacles to human immunology research. *Nature Immunology, 9*, 575–580. doi: 10.1038/ni0608-575.

Heidegger, M. (1987). *De l'essence de la liberté humaine: Introduction à la philosophie (The Essence of Human Freedom: An Introduction to Philosophy)*. Gallimard. (Originally lectured 1930). 173–176.

James, W. (1890). *Principles of Psychology*. Henry Holt and Company.

Karginov, F. V., & Hannon, G. J. (2010). The CRISPR system: Small RNA-guided defense in bacteria and archaea. *Molecular Cell, 37*, 7–19. doi: 10.1016/j.molcel.2009.12.033.

Knox, D. (2019). Giordano Bruno. (E. N. Zalta Ed.). *Stanford Encyclopedia of Philosophy*. https://plato.stanford.edu/entries/bruno/.

Laureys, S. (2005). The neural correlate of (un)awareness: Lessons from the vegetative state. *Trends in Cognitive Sciences, 9*, 556–559. doi: 10.1016/j.tics.2005.10.010.

Levine, J. (1983). Materialism and qualia: The explanatory gap. *Pacific Philosophical Quarterly, 64*, 354–361. doi: 10.1111/j.1468-0114.1983.tb00207.x.

Lillestöl, R. K., Redder, P., Garrett, R. A., & Brugger, K. A. (2006). A putative viral defence mechanism in archaeal cells. *Archaea, 2*, 59–72. doi: 10.1155/2006/542818.

Low, P., Panksepp, J., Reiss, D., Edelman, D., van Swinderen, B., & Koch, C. (2012). The Cambridge Declaration on Consciousness. https://fcmconference.org/img/CambridgeDeclarationOnConsciousness.pdf.

Marraffini, L. A., & Sontheimer, E. J. (2008). CRISPR interference limits horizontal gene transfer in straphylococci by targeting DNA. *Science, 322*, 1843–1845. doi: 10.1126/science.1165771.

Marraffini, L. A., & Sontheimer, E. J. (2010). CRISPR interference: RNA-directed adaptive immunity in bacteria and archaea. *Nature Reviews Genetics, 11*, 181–190. doi: 10.1038/nrg2749.

Metchnikoff, E. (1883). Untersuchungen über die intracelluläre Verdauung bei wirbellosen Thieren (Research on the intracellular digestion of invertebrates). *Arbeiten aus den Zoologischen Instituten der Universität Wien und der Zoologischen Station in Triest, 5*, 141–168.

Mojica, F. J., Diez-Villasenor, C., Garcia-Martinez, J., & Soria, E. (2005). Intervening sequences of regularly spaced prokaryotic repeats derive from foreign genetic elements. *Journal of Molecular Evolution, 60*, 174–182. doi: 10.1007/s00239-004-0046-3.

Moulin, A. M. (1995). Clés pour l'histoire de l'immunologie (Keys for the history of immunology). *Le Système immunitaire ou l'immunité cent ans après Pasteur (The Immune System or Immunity a 100 years after Pasteur)*. Nathan. 122–131.

Nagel, T. (1974). What is it like to be a bat? *Philosophical Review, 83*, 435–450. doi: 10.2307/2183914.

Nagel, T. (1979). *Mortal Questions*. Cambridge University Press.

Plato. (1871). *Philebus*. (B. Jowett, Trans.). Scribner's Sons.

Plato. (1888). *The Timaeus*. (R. D. Archer-Hind, Trans.). Macmillan.

Pourcel, C., Salvignol, G., & Vergnaud, G. (2005). CRISPR elements in *Yersinia pestis* acquire new repeats by preferential uptake of bacteriophage DNA and provide additional tools for evolutionary studies. *Microbiology, 151,* 653–663. doi: 10.1099/mic.0.27437-0.

Prochiantz, A. (2001). *Machine-Esprit (Machine-Mind)*. Odile Jacob. 153–169.

Russell, B. (1927). *An Outline of Philosophy*. Allen and Unwin.

Searle, J. R. (2007). Dualism revisited. *Journal of Physiology-Paris, 101,* 169–178. doi: 10.1016/j.jphysparis. 2007.11.003.

Skrbina, D. (2017). *Panpsychism in the West*. MIT Press.

Smith, J. T. (2014). David Hilbert's Radio Address. https://www.maa.org/press/periodicals/convergence/david-hilberts-radio-address-german-and-english.

Sorek, R., Koonin, V., & Hugenholtz, P. (2008). CRISPR--a widespread system that provides acquired resistance against phages in bacteria and archaea. *Nature Reviews Microbiology, 6,* 181–186. doi: 10.1038/nrmicro1793.

Sorek, R., Lawrence, C. M., & Wiedenheft, B. (2013). CRISPR-mediated adaptive immune systems in bacteria and archaea. *Annual Review of Biochemistry, 82,* 237–266. doi: 10.1146/annurev-biochem-072911-172315.

Spinoza, B. (2009). *The Ethics*. (R. H. M. Elwes, Trans.). Project Gutenberg, May 28, 2009. https://www.gutenberg.org/files/3800/3800-h/3800-h.htm.

Strawson, G. (2006). Realistic monism: Why physicalism entails panpsychism? *Journal of Consciousness Studies, 13,* 3–31. doi: 10.1093/acprof:oso/9780199267422.003.0003.

Strawson, G. (2020a). What does "physical" mean? A prolegomenon to panpsychism. (W. Seager, Ed.). *The Routledge Handbook of Panpsychism*. Routledge. 331.

Strawson, G. (2020b). What does "physical" mean? A prolegomenon to panpsychism. (W. Seager, Ed.). *The Routledge Handbook of Panpsychism*. Routledge. 325.

Strawson, G. (2020c). What does "physical" mean? A prolegomenon to panpsychism. (W. Seager, Ed.). *The Routledge Handbook of Panpsychism*. Routledge. 324–325.

Strawson, G. (2020d). What does "physical" mean? A prolegomenon to panpsychism. (W. Seager, Ed.). *The Routledge Handbook of Panpsychism*. Routledge. 317–339.

Swiatczak, B., & Tauber, A. I. (2020). Philosophy of immunology. (E. N. Zalta, Ed.). *The Stanford Encyclopedia of Philosophy*. https://plato.stanford.edu/archives/sum2020/entries/immunology/.

Tauber, A. I. (1992). The birth of immunology. III. The fate of the phagocytosis theory. *Cellular Immunology, 139,* 505–530. doi: 10.1016/0008-8749(92)90089-8.

Tauber, A. I. (1997). Historical and philosophical perspectives concerning immune cognition. *Journal of the History of Biology, 30,* 419–440. doi: 10.1023/a:1004247922979.

Tauber, A. I. (2008). The immune system and its ecology. *Philosophy of Science, 75,* 224–245. doi: 10.1086/590200.

Tauber, A. I. (2011). The cognitive paradigm 20 years later. Commentary on Nelson Vaz. *Constructivist Foundations, 6,* 342–344.

Tauber, A. I. (2013). Immunology's theories of cognition. *History and Philosophy of the Life Sciences, 35,* 239–264.

Turki, A. T. (2011). On the normativity of the immune system. *Medicine Studies, 3,* 29–39. doi: 10.1007/s12376-011-0061-9.

Umehara, T. (2013). *An Introduction to the Philosophy of Humankind*. Iwanami Shoten. 161–174.

von Behring, E., & Kitasato, S. (1890). Über das Zustandekommen der Diphtherie-Immunität und der Tetanus-Immunität bei Thieren (On the establishment of Diphtheria immunity and Tetanus immunity in animals). *Deutsche Medizinische Wöchenschrift, 16,* 1113–1114. doi: 10.17192/eb2013.0164.

Westra, E. R., Swarts, D. C., Staals, R. H., Jore, M. M., Brouns, S. J., & van der Oost, J. (2012). The CRISPRs, they are a-changin': How prokaryotes generate adaptive immunity. *Annual Review of Genetics, 46,* 311–339. doi: 10.1146/annurev-genet-110711-155447.

Whitehead, A. N. (1929). *Process and Reality: An Essay in Cosmology*. The Free Press.

Whitehead, A. N. (2006). *The Concept of Nature. The Tarner Lectures Delivered in Trinity College, November 1919*. Cambridge University Press. 163.

Whitehead, A. N., & Russell, B. (1910–1913). *Principia Mathematica*. Cambridge University Press.

Yakura, H. (2015). Epistemological and metaphysical problems posed by immunology. (Ph.D. thesis), Université Sorbonne Paris Cité, Paris, France. 194.

Yakura, H. (2019a). Disease and cosmopolitanism, or the remaking of the norms of life. *Igaku no Ayumi (Journal of Clinical and Experimental Medicine), 268*, 884–887.

Yakura, H. (2019b). A hypothesis: CRISPR-Cas as a minimal cognitive system. *Adaptive Behavior, 27*, 167–173. doi: 10.1177/1059712318821102.

Yakura, H. (2019c). Response to Fred Keijzer's comments. *Adaptive Behavior, 27*, 179–180. doi: 10.1177/1059712319834503.

Yakura, H. (2020a). Contemporary panpsychism, or its problems and possibilities. *Igaku no Ayumi (Journal of Clinical and Experimental Medicine), 275*, 311–314.

Yakura, H. (2020b). CRISPR-Cas, or what opens us to panpsychism. *Igaku no Ayumi (Journal of Clinical and Experimental Medicine), 274*, 623–626.

Yakura, H. (2020c). Immunity in light of Spinoza and Canguilhem. *Philosophies, 5*, 38. doi: 10.3390/philosophies5040038.

Yakura, H. (2020d). Panpsychism, can it overcome physicalism? *Igaku no Ayumi (Journal of Clinical and Experimental Medicine), 274*, 1149–1152.

Yakura, H. (2022). *Meditative Life of an Immunologist in Paris*. Ishiyaku Publishers. 241–287.

Yakura, H. (2023). *From Immunity to Science as Philosophy*. Misuzu Shobo. 246–252.

6 Toward a New Philosophy of Life

It's time to change our paths to protect the planet and humanize society.[1]

Edgar Morin

There is a school of philosophy that holds that the most important thing is to search for the essence of things, and it has a long history. On the other hand, there are philosophers who deny this. In this book, we first examined the results of research in the scientific world to eventually ask the question: what is the essence of immunity? As a result, it was revealed that immunity is a function that exists ubiquitously in the biological world and is inseparably linked to life. Immunity may also be the oldest and most universal cognitive apparatus supporting recognition and memory, the functions that form the basis of life, meaning that we cannot discuss life without considering immunity. To discuss immunity, we must also deepen our thought on the cognitive functions of recognition and memory, which are thought to be monopolized by the nervous system. Or, conversely, we may be unable to ignore the results of research on immunity when considering the function of the nervous system.

Furthermore, in conducting metaphysical reflection on the essential elements of immunity based on the scientific results, we see a similarity with *conatus*, which Spinoza defined as the primordial "effort" to maintain existence. When this concept, which covers all beings, animate and inanimate, is applied to living beings, it includes a mental element in addition to the physical element: "appetite" (*appetitus*), consciousness related to sensation and perception, and "desire" (*cupiditas*), the capacity to be conscious or aware of "appetite," which is said to be limited to humans. Given that immune functions are involved in perception and reaction, the "appetite" overlaps with the essence of immunity. According to Spinoza, the *conatus* contains a moral element; it is good to move toward maintaining existence and bad to disturb it. This view, together with Canguilhem's reflection on the normativity of life, led us to conclude that the essence of immunity includes mental elements with normativity that balances biological polarity. This is the present state of the metaphysical reflection on immunity.

The German sociologist and philosopher Georg Simmel (1858–1918) wrote a work entitled *The View of Life* (Simmel, 2010), originally published as *Lebensanschauung*, meaning an intuition of life, in 1918. Reading this book, one can see that the object of contemplation is limited to human life. One imagines that this was due to the constraints and limitations of the times or the fact that we are most concerned with human life. However, Hans Jonas (1903–1993), a disciple of Heidegger, wrote in his *The Phenomenon of Life* (Jonas, 2001b), originally published in 1966, that to talk about life, one must not only philosophize about humans but also about other living beings, and at the same time not only about their physicochemical aspects but also about their mental nature (Jonas, 2001a). Indeed, the subtitle of this book is *Toward a Philosophical Biology*. Jonas could be viewed as our contemporary and was witnessing the development of science, including biology, which may have led him to broaden his vision. This broadening is an important transformation, considering that many did not necessarily extend their thinking beyond humans. If we accept Jonas' view—and I also agree with it—then the phenomenon of immunity, which has the same scope as life and encompasses both physicochemical and mental natures, could be the inexhaustible source of the philosophy of life.

Among the themes that emerge from the discussions in this book, we see some that require further deepening toward a new philosophy of life. First is the problem of recognition, memory, and consciousness. The phenomenon of immunological memory has been observed since ancient

DOI: 10.1201/9781003486800-6

Greece, but even now, more than 2,000 years later, its details remain a mystery. According to the classical view, consciousness and memory are cognitive functions assigned to the nervous system, but new findings on immunity have prompted us to question the validity of this view.

Second, there is the issue of symbiosis with other organisms, including bacteria, which is essential for the existence of most plants and animals. Symbiosis is a condition of existence for living organisms and influences how we view organisms. Further reflection will be required in the future.

Third, a close observation of the actual state of immunity based on philosophical considerations of normality and pathology reveals that the boundary between normal and pathological states is ambiguous. For example, even in a state considered normal, inflammation is induced by symbiotic bacteria in the intestines. While this is considered a physiological change because it does not produce obvious pathology, it is also physiological in that the changes are involved in processes essential to the organism such as the maturation of the immune system. The question of how to interpret these baseline maintenance functions becomes increasingly important.

Fourth, it has also become apparent that pathological conditions must not be viewed as local reactions but must be reconsidered as reactions of the whole body, including the mind. Historically, this understanding can be traced back to the holistic view of the human body by Hippocrates in ancient Greece and Galen in ancient Rome, and in modern times to the ideas of Claude Bernard's milieu intérieur, Walter Cannon's homeostasis, and Hans Selye's stress theory, among others.

Furthermore, a panpsychist view of the world has emerged from analyzing immunity from a metaphysical perspective. For example, in Whitehead's metaphysics, there is no separation between subject and object or organism and nonorganism; everything is considered an organism. Matter and spirit are identical. In addition, perception implies a fusion of the perceiving organism with the object or world. This view recalls Bergson who stated that there are two ways of knowing: one is to look at things from the outside, and the other is to enter into them with intellectual sympathy. The former is the science of inert things in time and space, whereas the latter is the metaphysical method of entering into and harmonizing with things through imagination. He called the type of sympathy that works there "intuition," while everything else is "analysis" (Bergson, 2007). The subject's becoming one with the world requires us to extend our contemplation not only in the direction of the tiniest atoms or subatomic particles but also to the Earth and even to the universe. It has the potential to lead to the contemplation of "nature," or all that exists, which the ancient Greeks named *physis*. This makes our relationship to the world stronger and denser, and as discussed in Chapter 5, the world of panpsychism might also create the empathy involved therein.

In this book, I have analyzed immunity, sometimes relative to the environment, but basically, I have developed philosophical reflections based on the results of science at the cell, tissue, and organism levels. However, the COVID-19 pandemic that emerged in Wuhan, China, in the fall of 2019 continues to teach us that immunological and virological analysis at the individual level is indispensable but that there are problems that cannot be solved while we remain there. First, the obvious reality became apparent that we cannot save the ailing unless we can build effective logistics to reach people with the results of science. In addition, as COVID-19 spread, we came to realize that there is no purely personal property or space in the face of a virus that spreads across boundaries and that we cannot overcome this crisis without cooperating with others. For example, we were reminded once again that getting vaccinated is not only for our protection but also an obligation to protect our fellow humans who make up the collectivity. Therefore, there is a need to rethink immunity from a broader perspective that extends beyond the individual in the natural environment to immunity in society and community or even on a global scale.

This situation corresponds well to what the German philosopher Peter Sloterdijk (1947–) described with the term "co-immunism" (Sloterdijk, 2011). The co-immune system he refers to concerns feelings of solidarity that transcend the individual and their family. The basis of "co-immunism" is serving the multiracial, institutional, or intergenerational level of the extended self rather than defining what is inherent to the self according to the egoism of organism. He sees herd immunity as a form of symbiosis, although it does not seem to be easily established in the case of COVID-19.

A study analyzing his philosophy describes our existence, which begins with symbiosis in the womb, as "coexistence precedes and conditions existence" (Wambacq and van Tuinen, 2017), which reminds us of Jean-Paul Sartre's (1905–1980) description of the essence of existentialism as "existence precedes essence" (Sartre, 1946). However, Sloterdijk seems to be looking beyond that and believes that what he calls "universal immunology," which requires transcending the opposition of self and foreign body or friend and foe, will be the successor to the metaphysics and religion of the past. After a long period of ecological reflection and the unexpected event of the COVID-19 pandemic, one can sense a new philosophy in gestation.

In Chapter 1, I mentioned that the word "immunity" derives from the ancient Roman word *immunitas*, which denoted exemption from political obligation or burden (*munus*). It was not until the 19th century that the medical meaning of "immunity from disease" was added to the originally political word, and the word "immunity" has been considered a metaphor. However, the COVID-19 pandemic reminded us once again that it is not enough for related disciplines such as virology and immunology to produce results to save lives; there must be politics accompanied by integrated thinking to translate the results to the field effectively. And the integrated thinking must necessarily incorporate the moral and normative nature encompassed in the essence of immunity, as revealed in this book. The political meaning of the word "immunity," which was the word's origin but buried in history, was alive and well. At the same time, this suggests that a new metaphysics of immunity from a perspective beyond the individual is required. We must continue to watch developments in the science world, seek our own direction without being bound by past methods, and move forward to weave a new philosophy of life.

Also, in Chapter 1, I discussed the opposing views on immunity presented by Élie Metchnikoff and Paul Ehrlich, who laid the foundation for immunology. While Metchnikoff believed that cells are the principal actors of immunity, Ehrlich and Emil von Behring argued that humoral antibodies are the main actors of immunity. In addition, the two appear to have differed in their approach to doing science and, more importantly, in their philosophy of life. Looking back at the course of research in the 20th century, the problems of antibody specificity and diversity became a central theme from the beginning of the 20th century, and physicochemical approaches were used to analyze them. These approaches are consistent with the reductionist way of advancing science, which is limited in scope and seeks technical rigor. This trend continued unabated into the latter half of the 20th century, with the addition of analyses at the genetic level, which are convincing and persuasive. It may be seen as the biology of "things."

However, phagocytes, which Metchnikoff considered the primary immunocompetent cells, lacked specificity and were difficult to handle in experiments, so they did not take center stage in immunological research in the first half of the 20th century. Nonetheless, in the latter half of the 20th century, the cells responsible for immunity were clearly defined, many new cell types were discovered and classified, and their isolation became possible. In 1996, Jules Hoffmann's group discovered that the Toll protein, whose role in fly development had already been clarified, was also important in the defense against infection in the fly and that similar mechanisms were conserved from sponges to humans. Since then, the previously disparaged innate immunity has become one of the centers of immunological research and has produced many results that have forced a revision of our understanding of the phenomenon of immunity itself. The explanation of immune phenomena at the cellular level has also become more rigorous, and the combination of philosophy and practice represented by Ehrlich and Metchnikoff can be seen as advancing modern immunology.

Indeed, Ehrlich's imagination and foresight were remarkable. The general framework of the basic structure and mechanism of immunity he imagined 120 years ago, via Burnet, has not faded even today. Not only did he achieve this theoretical result, but also a practical one, as he and Sahachiro Hata (1873–1938) discovered Salvarsan as a therapeutic agent for syphilis. Ehrlich gave the term "magic bullet" (Zauberkugel) to these chemotherapeutic agents and developed a very modern research approach involving both the basic theory and its practical application. In the 1970s, monoclonal antibody technology was developed and used for diagnosis and treatment as initially expected, and it can be said that modern medicine is full of "magic bullets."

In contrast, what is unique about Metchnikoff, who placed phagocytes at the center of immunity? From his youth, he was strongly influenced by the idea of civilization's progress through the development of science. Starting from histology and embryology, and strongly influenced by Darwin's theory of evolution, he had an eye to see things on a large time scale, such as phylogeny and ontogeny, and beyond the field. He could also think about phagocytosis beyond the framework of biological defense. For example, he imagined the involvement of phagocytes in the resorption of the tadpole tail during metamorphosis and in eliminating unnecessary items in the organism. In them, I see a rich and dynamic imagination at work that approaches the essence behind the phenomena. As Metchnikoff himself wrote in his dedication to Émile Duclaux (1840–1904) and Émile Roux (1853–1933) in *Immunity in Infective Diseases*, his theories "seemed to you too vitalistic, and not sufficiently physico-chemical" (Metchnikoff, 1905); his science was initially perceived as lacking in rigor and empirical power.

Indeed, the research approach of establishing a rigorous scientific theory and proceeding from there to practice is expected to continue unabated. However, to reach a deeper understanding of nature, we must approach local phenomena in pursuit of rigor and analytical precision and imagine invisible structures and hidden functions. From there, we must think philosophically to approach the essential things that connect to the whole. Metchnikoff traveled and studied throughout Europe for about 25 years until Pasteur invited him to the newly established institute in Paris in his early 40s. While there were indeed circumstances that compelled him to do so, there is an air of aloofness about his itinerary. In addition, perhaps because of the impression one gets from his appearance and the philosophical atmosphere of his writings, especially in his later years (Metchnikoff, 1903; Metchnikov, 1910), it seems to me that there is a grand world inside Metchnikoff that is created by slow but persistent thinking. The advice Japanese novelist Natsume Sōseki (1867–1916) sent to his students and novelists Ryūnosuke Akutagawa (1892–1927) and Masao Kume (1891–1952) in the summer of 1916, "You must keep pushing like a cow, not a horse" (Natsume, 1997) seems to encourage us in our future steps.

Twenty years have already passed since the beginning of the 21st century. Even if we only review the history of science, focusing on the 20th century, we cannot help but acknowledge the achievements and destructive influence that science has brought about. The thought based on physicalism and reductionism that underpins modern science has an exclusive aspect that recognizes no other, and its influence seems to extend beyond science to ordinary people's way of thinking. Indeed, while a logical and empirical attitude is essential, history has taught us that we must not discard anything else. Modern science does not include the autocritical activity of reflecting on science. The task of looking critically at science is left to those outside science or the very few scientists inclined to think in this way. Reflection within science is left to chance. As an antithesis to this trend, this book has advocated a method called metaphysicalization of science (MOS), in which scientific results are reconsidered from a philosophical perspective. This method can be seen not only as a new attempt to internalize philosophy into science but also as an attempt that, once its importance is recognized, is expected to influence ordinary people's thinking (Yakura, 2020, 2022). This book's attempt to be the first step in that direction is, of course, destined to be revised.

NOTE

1 Brenot, P. (2020). Edgar Morin: 15 leçons du coronavirus (H. Yakura, Trans.). *Le Monde* (June 19, 2020).

REFERENCES

Bergson, H. (2007). *The Creative Mind: Introduction to Metaphysics*. (M. L. Andison, Trans.). Dover Publications. (Originally published 1934). 133–136.

Jonas, H. (2001a). *The Phenomenon of Life: Toward a Philosophical Biology*. Northwestern University Press. (Originally published 1966). 1–6.

Jonas, H. (2001b). *The Phenomenon of Life: Toward a Philosophical Biology*. Northwestern University Press. (Originally published 1966).

Metchnikoff, E. (1903). *The Nature of Man: Studies in Optimistic Philosophy*. (P. C. Mitchel, Trans.). Putnam.

Metchnikoff, E. (1905). To Messieurs É. Duclaux et É. Roux. *Immunity in Infective Diseases*. (F. G. Binnie, Trans.). Cambridge University Press. vii.

Metchnikov, I. (1910). Médecine et philosophie. *La Revue de Paris, 17*, 475–494.

Natsume, K. (1997). *The Complete Works of Soseki. Vol. 24*. Iwanami Shoten. 558–562.

Sartre, J. P. (1946). *L'existentialisme est un humanisme (Existentialism Is a Humanism)*. Nagel.

Simmel, G. (2010). *The View of Life: Four Metaphysical Essays with Journal Aphorisms*. (J. A. Y. Andrews & D. N. Levine, Trans.). University of Chicago Press. (Originally published 1918).

Sloterdijk, P. (2011). Co-immunité globale. Penser le commun qui protège (Global co-immunity. On the need to elaborate a protective common). *Multitudes, 45*, 42–45. doi: 10.3917/mult.045.0042.

Wambacq, J., & van Tuinen, S. (2017). Interiority in Sloterdijk and Deleuze. *Palgrave Communications, 3*, 1–7. doi: 10.1057/palcomms.2017.72.

Yakura, H. (2020). Immunity in light of Spinoza and Canguilhem. *Philosophies, 5*, 38. doi: 10.3390/philosophies5040038.

Yakura, H. (2022). *Meditative Life of an Immunologist in Paris*. Ishiyaku Publishers. 241–287.

Epilogue

Immunology has always seemed to me more a problem of philosophy than a practical science.[1]

Frank Macfarlane Burnet

Immunology is for me becoming a mostly philosophical subject.[2]

Niels Jerne

This book is a collection and reconstruction of the traces of reflection spun out during more than a decade of philosophical contemplation in France after more than 30 years of experience as a scientist. The process of writing this book has been an invaluable journey of discovering what I have learned and what I have not learned while in the realm of science and what and how I must contemplate in the future. It was also a journey into the metaphysical dimension, where scientific thought and philosophical speculation resonated and sometimes merged in the sense that neither science nor philosophy could have created such a mass of thought without the other.

As the two predecessors of immunology similarly noted in the epigraph, the results produced by immunology are full of philosophical problems. These problems inherent in the phenomenon of immunity should be reflected not only in what has already been discussed but also in the newly discovered facts. My approach was to begin with a scientific analysis of the phenomenon of immunity, search for philosophical themes latent in the findings, and reflect on the natural phenomenon of immunity as a whole. In the sense of using scientific knowledge as material to extract the most fundamental things contained therein, it was somewhat like looking into the mind of an alchemist. At the same time, it was like an attempt to breathe new life into the now-forgotten natural philosophy.

In Chapter 4, I pointed out that when looking at the immune system from the perspective of phylogeny, it is not the aspect of its structure or mechanism that is important but the function of what it is doing. By that criterion, it is evident that almost every species has an immune system acting in a completely different structure and mechanism. This conclusion means that while we analyze structure and mechanism in the physical world, we cannot determine what immunity is by that criterion. The question of what immunity is in the first place belonged to the metaphysical world before there were philosophical questions in the immune phenomena as pointed out by Burnet and Jerne.

Since Heraclitus (c. 540–c. 480 BC), nature has been considered to love to hide and is often represented as a woman who covers herself with a veil. Pierre Hadot (1922–2010), a scholar of ancient philosophy, analyzed how the concept of nature emerged historically and found two ways to lift nature's veil (Hadot, 2006). One is the "Promethean" attitude, which holds that technology reveals the secrets of nature, that man has been given the right to dominate nature, and that he is allowed to do violent things for his own ends. This attitude has been carried over into modern science and remains a strong belief today. In contrast, the basis of what Hadot describes as the "Orphic" attitude is the recognition that nature behaves in a hide-and-seek manner because it is dangerous to humans. Since confronting nature with technology can have dangerous consequences, humans seek to uncover nature's secrets through philosophical and aesthetic methods, rational discourse, poetry, and art.

However, it would be unwise to reject the Promethean attitude simply because it is dangerous. Even if it is dangerous, this method has not only revealed nature's remarkable and exquisite workings but has actually produced things that are beneficial to us. These results also have the potential to enrich our inner world. For example, by analyzing the nature revealed by the Promethean method with an Orphic attitude, we will deepen our understanding of nature and bring science into our culture. Furthermore, we will also be able to observe the workings of science itself critically. The mobilization of these two methods to understand nature is the substance of what I have described as the MOS (Yakura, 2020, 2022). According to Friedrich Schelling (1775–1854), "primordial knowledge" is in the identity of the real with the ideal, and the merest claim to knowledge implies a search for this identity to resolve the real in the ideal and vice versa (Schelling, 1966). If we interpret the real as what science studies and the ideal as what philosophy produces, then the MOS is an attempt to seek what Schelling calls "primordial knowledge." Richard Dawkins considers the original contribution to science as follows:

> Rather than propose a new theory or unearth a new fact, often the most important contribution a scientist can make is to discover a new way of seeing old theories or facts. [...] But a change of vision can, at its best, achieve something loftier than a theory. It can usher in a whole climate of thinking, in which many exciting and testable theories are born, and unimagined facts laid bare. [...] I prefer not to make a clear separation between science and its "popularization." Expounding ideas that have hitherto appeared only in the technical literature is a difficult art. It requires insightful new twists of language and revealing metaphors. If you push [the] novelty of language and metaphor far enough, you can end up with a new way of seeing. And a new way of seeing, as I have just argued, can in its own right make an original contribution to science.

Dawkins (2009)

The MOS is expected to contribute to science in the sense that Dawkins meant.

For a long time, the function of the immune system was assumed to be biological defense, often spoken of in metaphors of war, and this tendency is still evident today. However, due to the first attempts to "metaphysicalize immunity," the "appetite," which Spinoza identified as the mental and physical component of the essence of life, and the normative nature of life associated with it, emerged as an internal possibility latent in immunity. Concepts related to cognitive functions such as recognition and memory, which are involved in mental activity, are susceptible to an anthropocentric view, and their relationship to entities can change dramatically depending on their definition.

In this book, I have developed speculations by adopting an inclusive view that redefines the functions of living organisms more broadly rather than the exclusive view that emerges from an anthropocentric perspective. When I look around the natural world in which we exist from this perspective, I feel that the immune systems of all organisms, including invisible ones like bacteria, arise with neural cognitive functions, and a completely different world emerges from the previous one. That world seems connected to the world of panpsychism, which has survived persistently from ancient Greece to the present. There is a view that metaphysics includes both the universal (*metaphysica generalis*) and the particular (*metaphysica specialis*) and that there is a divergence between them. From this perspective, while beginning with a speculation on the specialized field of immunity, this book is moving toward a more universal philosophy of life, which includes the philosophy of the mind and organism. Therefore, this may have been an attempt to bridge the gap between the two metaphysics.

NOTES

1 Burnet, F. M. (1965). The Darwinian approach to immunity. *Molecular and Cellular Basis of Antibody Formation* (J. Sterzl, Ed.). Academic Press. 17.
2 Söderqvist, T. (2003). *Science as Autobiography: The Troubled Life of Niels Jerne.* Yale University Press. 278.

REFERENCES

Dawkins, R. (2009). *The Selfish Gene.* Oxford University Press. xvi.
Hadot, P. (2006). *The Veil of Isis: An Essay on the History of the Idea of Nature.* (M. Chase, Trans.). Harvard University Press.
Schelling, F. W. J. (1966). *On University Studies.* (E. S. Morgan, Trans.) Ohio State University Press. (Originally published 1803). 9–11.
Yakura, H. (2020). Immunity in light of Spinoza and Canguilhem. *Philosophies, 5*, 38. doi: 10.3390/philosophies5040038.
Yakura, H. (2022). *Meditative Life of an Immunologist in Paris.* Ishiyaku Publishers. 241–287.

Index

Note: *Italic* page numbers refer to figures.